When a publisher requests a third edition of a text you know it must be good! This edition highlights the many new developments in spiritually integrated psychotherapy. As always, Len Sperry writes in an engaging and practical manner, weaving research and clinical best practices in a way that is easy to follow, understand, and implement. Mental health and spiritual health professionals should have this book and will find this new edition of tremendous value. I know I will!

Thomas G. Plante, *Ph.D., professor, Santa Clara University & Stanford University School of Medicine; editor,* Spirituality in Clinical Practice

This outstanding book provides valuable updates and new theoretical research and clinical insights about spiritually integrated psychotherapy. Dr. Sperry, a renowned expert on this topic, has again demonstrated his scholarly and clinical expertise and wisdom in this updated edition. I enthusiastically recommend it to all researchers, practitioners, educators, and students.

P. Scott Richards, *PhD., president, Bridges Institute for Spiritually Integrated Psychotherapies; editor,* Handbook of Spiritually Integrated Psychotherapies

This thoroughly updated version of Sperry's classic text is well-grounded in current research on both spirituality and psychotherapy and provides clinically valuable guidance in not just incorporating but actually *integrating* spirituality into the treatment process. Special attention is given to critical topics including spiritual assessment, case conceptualization, the cutting-edge interventions, outcomes monitoring, and cultural and ethical issues. This book will be a valued resource for students and experienced therapists seeking to deepen their integration of spiritual concerns in everyday clinical practice.

Harold G. Koenig, *M.D., professor of Psychiatry and Behavioral Sciences, Duke University Medical Center*

Spiritually Integrated Psychotherapy

As integrating spiritual concerns becomes commonplace in psychotherapy, this new edition of *Spiritually Integrated Psychotherapy* leads the way in describing and illustrating its effective clinical practice from the first through to the last session.

Effective clinical practice is emphasized with individual chapters on assessment and case conceptualization, intervention, outcome assessment and termination, and cultural and ethical considerations. The text highlights new developments in spirituality, neuroscience, and moral injury, while continuing to provide a concise, theory-based framework for understanding the spiritual dimension. Readers can use this framework as the basis for competently integrating spirituality in effective, evidence-based psychotherapy practice.

This practical book is essential for clinicians who wish to incorporate spirituality into their practice, as well as students and trainees preparing to practice spiritually integrated therapies.

Len Sperry, MD, PhD, is Emeritus Professor at Florida Atlantic University and Clinical Professor of Psychiatry and Behavioral Medicine at the Medical College of Wisconsin. He has over 1200 publications and was a founding editor of *Spirituality in Clinical Practice*.

Spiritually Integrated Psychotherapy

Infusing Spirituality in Clinical Practice

Third Edition

Len Sperry

Routledge
Taylor & Francis Group
NEW YORK AND LONDON

Designed cover image: © Getty Images

Third edition published 2025
by Routledge
605 Third Avenue, New York, NY 10158

and by Routledge
4 Park Square, Milton Park, Abingdon, Oxon, OX14 4RN

Routledge is an imprint of the Taylor & Francis Group, an informa business

First edition published by Routledge 2001
Second edition published by Routledge 2011

ISBN: 978-1-032-54653-7 (hbk)
ISBN: 978-1-032-54654-4 (pbk)
ISBN: 978-1-003-42599-1 (ebk)

DOI: 10.4324/9781003425991

Typeset in Sabon
by SPi Technologies India Pvt Ltd (Straive)

Contents

Introduction

Today, more individuals are seeking added meaning and fulfillment in their lives and believe that spirituality is essential for dealing with their problems and concerns. Many are pursuing a spiritual journey and are practicing spiritual disciplines like mindfulness, but find themselves trapped in old feelings, attitudes, and habits that seem to undo their progress. Even those who have made progress can encounter spiritual struggles and roadblocks to such growth. Psychotherapy may be sought with the expectation that therapists will address both their psychological and spiritual issues. However, finding a therapist who is willing and able to address both sets of issues can be quite challenging as the number of sufficiently trained therapists is small compared to the need.

Since publication of the first and second editions of this book, psychotherapists have become somewhat more receptive to focusing on spiritual issues in therapy yet are faced with limited formal training opportunities. The publication of this third edition of *Spiritually Integrated Psychotherapy* comes at a time when more faculty, supervisors, and therapists are expanding their teaching, supervision, and practice to include the spiritual dimension. It also comes at a time when more courses, graduate programs, research articles, book chapters, and books are available.

It appears that a shift is beginning to occur from an awareness of the need to change clinical practice patterns to actually changing these practice patterns by integrating the spiritual dimension in clinical practice. In time, spiritual and religious competencies can be expected to likely inform the training of all therapists and be reflected in accreditation standards. Overall, the shift has been from being sensitive to the spiritual needs of clients, to gaining specialized training, and eventually to exhibiting spiritual sensitive competency in everyday clinical practice.

Another necessary and critical shift will be from "incorporating" to "integrating." Here the word incorporate means to "to add" a spiritual intervention or practice. The challenge in the coming years will be to "integrate" or "infuse" spirituality into clinical practice. Integrating and

DOI: 10.4324/9781003425991-1

infusing mean introducing an element that transforms a given process. Spiritually integrated psychotherapy requires infusing the spiritual dimension within the essential psychotherapy processes of therapeutic alliance, assessment, case conceptualization, interventions, and outcomes monitoring into a seamless, integral whole. Simply "adding" spiritual interventions or practices to a therapist's usual clinical practice pattern might qualify as spiritually "incorporated" therapy but would not technically qualify as spiritually "integrated" psychotherapy.

This new edition emphasizes the therapeutic processes in spiritually integrated psychotherapy with individual chapters on the therapeutic relationship, assessment and case conceptualization, intervention, and clinical outcomes and termination. It also recognizes the importance of cultural and ethical factors in psychotherapy practice, including scope of practice and related legal considerations in the practice of spiritually integrated psychotherapy. New developments in clinical approaches, evidence-based and practice-based treatment, neuroscience, and innovative training are highlighted in the various chapters.

Overview of Chapters

Chapter 1 begins by describing the evolution of psychotherapy sensitive to the spiritual dimension in terms of four eras and time frames. It provides a context for understanding why this psychotherapy specialty has developed so slowly over the past several decades and why it has only recently begun to flourish. Next, it describes the components of spiritually integrated psychotherapy—psychology and spirituality—and their relationship. Then, it discusses and compares forms of psychotherapy with two related disciplines: pastoral counseling, and spiritual direction.

Chapter 2 describes five basic dimensions of human experience: psychological, social, moral, somatic, and the spiritual. A basic premise of this book is that the spiritual dimension is central to and integrally related to the other four dimensions. The moral dimension is then described as the "neglected" dimension not only in the psychological and behavioral sciences but also in spiritual theology. The recent increase in moral injury appears to be fostering a recovery of the moral dimension. Then, six perspectives or frames of reference for understanding the spiritual dimension and the process of spiritual development are described.

Chapter 3 describes seven developmental stage models that directly or indirectly address the spiritual dimension. These include Psychosocial Development, Moral Development, Faith Development, Self-Development, Spiritual Development, Spiritual Growth, and the Full Spectrum models. Some of these models have generated considerable research support while others are theoretical models which therapists have found clinically useful. Clinical implications are discussed.

Chapter 4 focuses on differentiating healthy from pathological spiritual and religious experiences. The differential diagnosis of psychosis, depression, and other psychiatric disorders from "mystical voices and visions," "dark night of the soul," and other "spiritual emergencies" is described. Then seven personality styles and their characteristic God representations, prayer styles, and other spiritual behaviors are detailed. Finally, it discusses the unique religious and spiritual dynamics and issues operative in individuals seeking psychotherapy.

Chapter 5 begins with an overview of basic elements that reflect the current theory, research, and practice, and their evolution in the practice of psychotherapy. They are: clinical outcomes, empirically supported treatments, practice-based evidence, the therapeutic alliance, client factors, and therapist factors. Similar changes are occurring in spiritually integrated psychotherapy. It then discusses current terminology in spiritually integrated psychotherapy. Finally, it describes developments in psychotherapy competencies as well as spiritual and religious competencies. This discussion serves as an introduction to Chapters 6–10.

Chapter 6 focuses on the development and maintenance of an effective therapeutic alliance. Because such an alliance is essential in achieving positive treatment outcomes, incorporating spiritual issues in the treatment process may complicate the alliance for various reasons. This chapter focuses on the development and maintenance of an effective relationship. It begins with a discussion of establishing an effective therapeutic relationship and the importance of maintaining that relationship in the face of resistance and countertransference, and provides strategies for dealing with these processes. Finally, it illustrates key points in the case of Maria.

Chapter 7 describes a comprehensive and integrative assessment strategy that includes assessment of personality dynamics, spiritual dynamics, cultural dynamics, and family dynamics. As in conventional psychotherapy, case conceptualization is the link between assessment and treatment planning. Also discussed and illustrated are how spiritual issues can be incorporated in the case conceptualization and how treatment interventions can be tailored to client need, personality style, and expectation. The continuing case of Maria illustrates these points.

Chapter 8 describes psychotherapeutic interventions useful in spiritually integrated psychotherapy. These include cognitive restructuring, cognitive and behavioral replacement, interpretation, and experiential methods, particularly as they relate to spiritual issues. Spiritual interventions are then described. These include focusing, mindfulness, acceptance, and self-awareness. Then spiritual practices such as centering meditation, forgiveness, recognizing the sacred in all, living ethically, fasting, and prayer therapy are discussed. The continuing case of Maria illustrates these points.

Chapter 9 describes termination issues that arise when spiritual concerns have been a focus of therapy. These include a discussion of referral, collaboration with ministers and spiritual guides, medication evaluation, and relapse prevention. Then the importance of assessing clinical outcomes, particularly session-by-session monitoring of therapeutic progress, is discussed and illustrated. The continuing case of Maria illustrates these points.

Chapter 10 begins by discussing cultural considerations that are present in spiritually integrated psychotherapy. Then, the unique ethical considerations, particularly with regard to informed consent, boundaries, and praying with a client, are addressed. These ethical considerations are described and illustrated. Of particular concern for licensed clinicians is the matter of scope of practice, which refers to the type and extent of practice that a licensure board considers acceptable professional practice. These considerations are discussed as well as guidelines for expanding scope of practice. The continuing case of Maria illustrates these points.

Chapter 11 begins with a recap of the four eras and the current status of this psychotherapy specialty. It suggests how new and cutting-edge developments can foster further development in spiritually integrative psychotherapy practice. It begins with two new clinical approaches or strategies: spiritually integrated cognitive processing therapy for moral injury, and spiritually integrated psychotherapy for sacred moral injury. Then it describes some cutting-edge research developments. Next, it reviews some of the clinical implications for spirituality from the neuroscience research. Finally, it discusses important developments for training spiritually integrated psychotherapists.

Spiritually Integrated Psychotherapy: Infusing Spirituality in Clinical Practice, Third Edition, will be of interests to students and trainees from all the mental health professions. It will also be of value to practicing psychotherapists as well as spiritual directors and pastoral counselors who want to become more familiar with the clinical aspects of the spiritual dimension. My hope is that by engaging with the contents of this book readers will more fully appreciate the psychological and spiritual concerns of their clients, as well as the value and impact that effective spiritually integrated psychotherapy can have for those clients.

Chapter 1

Spiritually Integrated Psychotherapy

From the Past to the Present

Spirituality continues to be important in the lives of many today. As noted in the Introduction, clients seeking psychotherapy increasingly expect that their spiritual concerns will be addressed in psychotherapy. While finding an adequately trained psychotherapist to meet that expectation is more likely today than it was a decade ago, the number of such trained therapists is still insufficient. As a result, some clients have either not formally addressed these concerns or have sought out practitioners of two related professions for help with their spiritual and religious concerns: spiritual direction and pastoral counseling.

This chapter begins with a discussion of the evolution of psychotherapy sensitive to the spiritual dimension in terms of four eras and time frames. Hopefully it provides a context for understanding how and why this psychotherapy specialty developed rather slowly. Next, it describes the components of spiritually integrated psychotherapy—psychology and spirituality—and their relationship. Then, it compares spiritually integrated psychotherapy with two related disciplines: pastoral counseling, and spiritual direction.

Evolution of Spirituality in Psychotherapy: Four Eras

Based on my observation and knowledge of the literature on spirituality and psychotherapy, the following four eras can be identified and described. As with most human endeavors that evolve, "growing pains" are inevitably part of the growth process. The same appears to be the case as the spiritually integrated psychotherapy emerges and evolves and seemingly resolves issues and "pains."

Era I: Prior to 1975

Some of the early leaders in the field of psychology like William James and G. Stanley Hall were fascinated by religious experiences and its influence

DOI: 10.4324/9781003425991-2

on human behavior. However, other leaders who endeavored to make psychology a scientific discipline were outspoken about their anti-religious views. For instance, Freud (1927/1961), the founder of psychoanalysis, insisted that religion was an illusion, a form of neurosis, and an attempt to fulfill childhood wishes or feelings of emptiness. Likewise, B. F. Skinner (1971), one of the founders of behaviorism, believed that God was an "explanatory fiction."

As a result of this anti-religious sentiment, by the mid-twentieth century the moral and spiritual dimensions began to disappear from the field of psychology and the practice of psychotherapy. As psychology sought to become a scientific discipline, some leaders endeavored to disengage it from its roots in moral philosophy. The result was that psychology established a scientific and value-free foundation for understanding human behavior and actions distinct from moral philosophy and other elements of the moral dimension.

Psychology was not the only discipline that sought to distance itself from moral philosophy. Economics was another. Adam Smith, one of the founders of economics and best known for his book the *Wealth of Nations*, actually called himself a moral philosopher. His earlier book, *The Theory of Moral Sentiments*, explains the role of moral philosophy and the common good in economic considerations. However, as economics shifted its focus to capitalism it is not surprising that it distanced itself from moral philosophy.

It should also be noted that as a group, psychologists are much less religious than the clients to whom they provide therapy (Shafranske & Cummings, 2013). Some 48% of psychologists consider religion to be unimportant in their lives, while only 15% of the general public share that belief (Delaney et al., 2007). While 89% of the public believes in God, only 50% of psychology professors share that belief, which makes them the least religious of the top 20 academic disciplines (Gross & Simmons, 2009). Based on such anti-religious sentiment and low levels of religiousness among psychologists as a group, it should not be too surprising that the American Psychological Association (APA) has been much slower than the other mental health professional organizations in responding to client needs and the expectations of its members for the type of training and accreditation standards required.

This may explain why many of my generation had little or no access to coursework dealing with the psychology of spiritual and religious issues during their undergraduate and doctoral training in the 1960s. It was only later in a master's degree program in Contemporary Spirituality in a religious studies department that I had access to coursework on spirituality, albeit from a theological rather than a psychological perspective. This was a common experience at the time, and I knew of no one who was integrating spirituality in psychotherapy practice. Needless to say, there was very little to read in this area.

Professional support plays an important role in the development of a psychotherapist. Typically, a trainee learns not only the knowledge and skills but also attitudes regarding a given profession from teachers, supervisors, and mentors. I can recall being an undergraduate with the dream of specializing in the psychology of religion and spirituality. One day I approached one of my esteemed psychology professors and asked his advice on how I might plan such a career trajectory. His response was gracious and cautious. He suggested that I complete training as a clinical psychologist, take an academic position, go through the ranks, and specialize in something other than the psychology of religion and spirituality. He seemed to imply that if I were research to and publish in this area before then I could jeopardize my career. Needless to say, I was taken aback by his caution.

This occurred in the mid-1960s during this first era. Yet he was correct, and it was not until the beginning of the second era that I, along with some other likeminded colleagues, shifted to my original career focus. While I had become a member of APA in 1971, it was not until 1976 when Division 36 was launched that I felt a sense of kinship and some validation of my dream.

Research in this area in Era I can be easily summed up: there was little or no research on spirituality related to psychotherapy. Yes, there was the occasional study on religious experience and correlations of religious practice and health that would continue into Era II, but not on spiritual issues in psychotherapy.

Era II: 1975–2004

At the beginning of Era II, I became more hopeful that my interest in integrating spirituality in clinical practice would someday be acknowledged by my profession and psychology colleagues. When asked to sign a petition requesting APA to establish a new division on Psychology and Religion I gladly agreed. Then at the annual APA conference in 1976 members of the new division called *Psychologists Interested in Religious Issues* met for the first time. It was there that Eugene Kennedy, PhD, the newly elected President of Division 36, proudly proclaimed "mission accomplished," in recognition of the long journey and challenges undertaken to accomplish this goal. Years later, Ralph Piedmont summarized this journey:

> Originally established in 1949 as the *American Catholic Psychological Association*, it was renamed in 1970 as *Psychologists Interested in Religious Issues*, becoming an official division in the APA in 1976. In 1993

> the name was changed to *Psychology of Religion*, and finally in 2012 we became *The Society for the Psychology of Religion and Spirituality*.
>
> (Piedmont, 2013, p. 1)

He indicated that these name changes reflected the evolving professional identity of this division and its members. Furthermore, these changes would serve to define the emerging specialty of spiritually oriented psychotherapy in broader and more scientific terms and "to keep pace with the increasing sophistication of the emerging models, methods, and measures of the field" (Piedmont, 2013, p. 1).

During this era, client expectation for therapy that incorporates the spiritual dimension continued to increase. But while more coursework and workshops became available, formal therapist training was insufficient, and certification non-existent, to meet this expectation. Limited theory development and spiritual interventions also characterized this era. Fortunately, the beginning of this era saw a steady increase in the numbers of new books and first edition textbooks.

Despite this recognition by APA, there were relatively few faculty members and colleagues to serve as role models for students and clinicians interested in the spiritual domain. It was for this reason that I decided to devote a full chapter in the first edition of this book to profiles of the lived experience of therapists who were known for incorporating spirituality in their professional and personal lives (Sperry, 2001). This chapter consisted of firsthand accounts of how six psychotherapists incorporated spirituality in their clinical practice, teaching, or supervision, as well as in their personal lives. They were from differing faith traditions—Jewish, Catholic, Mormon, Buddhist, and Evangelical Christian—and all incorporated spiritual assessment and spiritual interventions in clinical practice, and some in their teaching or supervision. All incorporated spiritual practices in their personal lives. Not surprisingly, all served as role models for those aspiring to practice therapy that integrated the spiritual domain.

Research during much of this era focused largely on the relationship of religion with various dimensions of health and well-being. For instance, researchers commonly reported that attendance at religious services was related to positive health indices. Unfortunately, much research of this era was largely correlational, relied on global measures of religiousness, and failed to identify how religious practices affected health and other behaviors (Pargament, 2023).

Era III: 2005–2019

Early during this era, several national surveys identified an increasing interest in spirituality in the general public. This led to the observation that a "twenty-first century spirituality" was evolving in America (Lesser, 2000). Among those surveyed were not just potential clients, but also psychotherapists, academics, and researchers. It seems that many of the developments of this era were influenced by this growing sentiment.

Presumably this lead to more books, articles, coursework, and workshops on religion and spirituality. Clinical competencies for spiritual and religious practice were likewise developed. So too were more sophisticated research projects funded and undertaken. Not surprisingly, the religious and spiritual concerns of clients were more likely and adequately addressed as more therapists became sufficiently trained and experienced in dealing with these concerns and issues.

In 2008 APA began publishing *Psychology of Religion and Spirituality* through Division 36 with the goal of publishing religion and spirituality research from a psychological perspective. Under the leadership of Ralph Piedmont, PhD, it began publishing cutting-edge research. Five years later the APA Publications Committee approved another journal, *Spirituality in Clinical Practice*, that would publish clinically focused articles on spirituality. Lisa Miller, PhD, and I proposed the journal, and we became founding editors. The first issue appeared in 2014 and clinicians now had a place to publish clinical applications and commentaries.

During this era evidence-based practice, empirically supported treatments, and practice-based treatments were promoted for clinical practice and research. Whereas evidence-based treatment focuses on controlling the treatment process in research settings, practice-based treatment focuses on measuring and tracking treatment in routine practice settings. Beginning in 2016 the Bridges Research-Practice Network was funded to study practice-based treatments at 20 clinical sites (Richards et al., 2015). Chapter 5 discusses both evidence-based and practice-based treatments and research in more detail. While not all training programs required students to learn and master specific empirically supported treatments, many did.

During this era two psychotherapeutic interventions were commonly and increasingly incorporated in therapy that was spiritually integrated. These included forgiveness (Worthington, 2013) and mindfulness (Lykins, 2014). Both of these have an extensive research base and are taught in graduate courses and workshops. They are described in greater detail in Chapter 8.

In 2017 APA formally recognized the multicultural domain in clinical practice (American Psychological Association, 2017). Unfortunately, while religion and spirituality were considered to be in the multicultural domain, relatively little appeared to have changed in training and in clinical practice. Some suggest that part of the reason for this lies in the distinction between visible and invisible forms of diversity. Visible diversity refers to what can be seen and not readily changed like age, physical appearance, or intellectual disability, while invisible diversity refers to traits that are not readily observed or seen. Based on that distinction, it was suggested that "(l)ike sexual orientation, socioeconomic status (SES), or disability, R/S [religion/spirituality] is often an invisible form of diversity, and without inquiry by the psychologist, may not be surfaced by the client" (Vieten & Lukoff, 2022, p. 30). When therapists do not inquire, research shows that many clients do not raise or discuss their R/S beliefs and concerns in therapy, even when these beliefs and concerns may interact with their behavioral and relational problems (Hodge, 2013).

During this era, more researchers focused on integrating the findings of spiritual and religious research into mainstream psychological theories. They examined the richness and complexity of religious life and the impact of religious and spiritual practices. It is not all that surprising that there has been a dramatic increase in this research given the increased interest in "twenty-first century spirituality." This produced findings that were applicable to clinical practice more so than in previous eras (Pargament, 2023). The second edition of this book attempted to capture these and other developments (Sperry, 2012).

Era IV: 2020–Present

The current Era IV is already notable for a number of key achievements that have moved the field forward. One of the first of these is an increasing consensus on the designation: "spiritually integrated psychotherapy." While Kenneth Pargament (2007) was one of the first to use the term in the previous era, based on a review of the titles of recent articles, books, workshops, and certification programs, most professionals now prefer "spiritually integrated psychotherapy" over other terms.

While evidence-based and practice-based treatments and research came into being in the previous era, both are firmly a part of the current era. Unexpectedly, practice-based treatments have become increasingly known largely because of Practice Based Research Networks. These networks engage groups of primary care clinicians—health care providers and psychotherapists—and practices who work together to address community-based health care questions and translate research findings into practice (Richards et al., 2015; Richards, Allen et al., 2023a). One of the largest is Bridges Research-Practice Network which involved 19 research teams who collected data from 400+ therapists and 40,000+ therapy sessions. Beginning at the end of Era III, the Bridges project was completed at the beginning of Era IV. As a member of the scientific advisory committee for Bridges, I was involved in planning parts of the project, choosing research teams, and reviewing data. The main finding was that clients' psychological and spiritual distress were significantly reduced (Richards, Allen et al.,

2023a). Chapter 11 provides an extended discussion of this network and the implications of its findings for spiritually integrated psychotherapies.

There was an increasing awareness of the moral dimension during this era, in the guise of moral injury (MI) as a diagnosable and treatable condition. An unexpected event, the COVID pandemic, unfolded during the early days of Era IV and left many therapists unprepared to offer effective treatment for the symptoms of depression, anxiety, and particularly MI, called the "invisible epidemic," that COVID has triggered. Briefly, MI is the trauma faced by individuals in situations that deeply violate their conscience or threaten their core values. While originally a concern of military personnel, estimates are that millions of health care workers, teachers, emergency workers, and other first line workers were and continue to be affected by COVID. The reason is that because of challenging circumstances, many of these individuals could only offer sub-par services. This led to guilt, anger, suicidality, and PTSD among many of them (Sperry, 2024b). Chapters 2 and 11 continue this discussion.

Training therapists to integrate spirituality in therapy continues to be a major focus of the current era. While it has been argued for some time that every therapist should develop competency in doing a basic spiritual assessment and then providing appropriate basic interventions in spiritual integration, there now exist empirically based competencies (Vieten & Lukoff, 2022) and an empirically based protocol for such training. Called the "Spiritual and Religious Competencies Project" and funded by a $5.1 million Templeton Foundation grant, this project aims to improve mental health care by ensuring that all mental health professionals are trained in the basic competencies to attend to their clients' religious and spiritual concerns (Currier et al., 2023).

This means that coursework, research, supervision, and publications must focus on integrating spiritual interventions and practices within the essential psychotherapy processes. In the current climate of accountability, therapists are increasingly required to utilize evidence-based practices and to demonstrate the effectiveness of their practice. The practice of spiritually integrated psychotherapy is not, and will not be, exempted from this requirement. Increasingly texts and professional books on spiritually integrated psychotherapy will be more focused on integrating the spiritual dimension with the therapeutic process and, of necessity, will focus on assisting trainees and clinicians to master strategies for enhancing the therapeutic alliance, assessment, case conceptualization, intervention, outcomes monitoring, and termination. In other words, therapists who are competent to practice the specialty of spiritually integrated therapy practice will likewise be competent to practice conventional psychotherapy.

Research in this fourth era is somewhat unique from research in previous eras. In addition to standard research protocols, some researchers and practitioners are collaborating to design and evaluate ways in which spiritual and religious resources, concerns, and struggles can be integrated into clinical practice (Pargament, 2023).

So, how might research efforts over the course of all four eras be characterized? A review of more than 1500 religious and spiritual studies published over the past 60 years is quite enlightening (Davis et al., 2024). Researchers examined published articles in three major R/S journals from the years 1962 through 2022. They found that 63% of the articles reviewed were empirical studies of which 90% used a quantitative-only methodology, while 6% used a qualitative-only methodology, and the remaining 4% utilized mixed-methods design. Their conclusion was that the: "psychology of R/S field is poised to make significant scientific and societal contributions, especially as it embraces open science practices; increased geographical, cultural, and methodological diversity; and enhanced scientific quality and rigor" (Davis et al., 2024, p. 7). Not only did the number of studies greatly increase as the decades went by but so did the sophistication of research and statistical methods used.

This current edition of *Spiritually Integrated Psychotherapy* attempts to chronicle the developments of this fourth era. Table 1.1 summaries the key points of the section and is followed by a brief commentary.

Commentary

Hopefully this description of the four eras has provided a context for understanding some of the reasons why spiritually integrated psychotherapy has developed slowly amid obstacles, and only recently has begun to flourish. The efforts and advocacy of a growing group of psychologists and other mental health professionals and researchers throughout these four eras has resulted in what is now called spiritually integrated psychotherapy. After being essentially orphaned during the first era and part of the second, religion and spirituality have largely returned to the mainstream of psychology in the current era. Quite an accomplishment!

Yet, the specialty of spiritually integrated psychotherapy still lags about a decade behind conventional psychotherapy research and practice. To "close the gap" is both reasonable and achievable, and it remains a major challenge for the remainder of Era IV. It will require attention in research, training, and clinical practice on routine outcome monitoring and the other essential psychotherapy competencies, particularly therapist effects and expertise. Because the mechanism of change in spiritually integrated psychotherapy has yet to be addressed, this too must begin in earnest. All of these factors are described in Chapter 5. Research on spiritual interventions and practices must be a priority. Besides mindfulness, yoga, and

Table 1.1 Evolution of Spirituality in Psychotherapy: Four Eras

Era I: Prior to 1975
- Attacks on S/R* from psychoanalysis and behaviorism
- Scientific psychology dissociates from moral philosophy → value-free stance
- Very limited S/R theory, clinical practice, training, and professional support
- Research: almost no research on spiritually related to psychotherapy

Era II: 1975–2004
- Client need for SIP** increases amid limited therapist training and support
- APA established Division 36 in 1976
- Limited S/R theory, clinical practice, training, and role models
- Research: some but mostly correlational with global measures of religiousness

Era III: 2005–2019
- APA recognizes multicultural domain but S/R "often an invisible form of diversity"
- More books, seminars, and clinical practice involving spirituality and psychotherapy
- Evidence-based interventions increase, e.g., mindfulness and forgiveness
- Practice-based funded initiatives, e.g., Bridges Research-Practice Network
- *Slightly more* training becomes available in S/R theory and clinical practice
- Research: dramatic upsurge largely due to the rise of interest in spirituality

Era IV: 2020–present
- Increasing agreement on the designation: SIP**
- Increasing focus on culture/religion/ethnicity research and practice
- Increasing awareness of moral dimension, especially moral injury
- Increasing number of evidence-based and practice-based treatments
- Increasing training in spirituality related to psychotherapy; Spiritual and Religious Competencies Project
- Research: increasing focus on integrating S/R resources into clinical practice

*S/R = Spirituality/Religious
**SIP = Spiritually Integrated Psychotherapy

forgiveness, there is also a need for robust research on other spiritual interventions and practices.

The increasing number of researchers, clinicians, and students as well as other resources such as training and research grants is heartening. Presumably Era V will build on these achievements and resources and further close the gap.

Spirituality, Religion, and Psychology

Spiritually integrated psychotherapy is a type of psychotherapy informed by spirituality and psychology. This section describes the similarities and differences between spirituality and religion, their relationship, and then the relationship between psychology and spirituality. While in the past the terms spirituality and religion were often interchangeable, that is not the situation today. In fact, many individuals go to great lengths to distinguish spirituality from religion in their lives. It is increasingly common for individuals to proclaim with conviction: "I am not a religious person, but spirituality is important to me." Exactly what they mean by religion and spirituality is not always clear. For mental health professionals, the meaning and definition of religion and spirituality—and the relationship between religion and spirituality—has not been very clear either.

Religion

In the past, defining religion seemed rather straightforward. Religion is a shared belief system, i.e., doctrine or dogma, which has some communal practices, i.e., ritual or liturgy (Ellswood, 1990). Usually, religion was understood in terms of an institutional dimension, i.e., an obligation to a particular faith tradition, or a means of codifying and capturing spiritual experiences within a system (Fontana, 2003). Even outside an institutional context, religion was considered the larger frame in which the spiritual dimension was embedded. This is exemplified in William James' description of religion in the *Varieties of Religious Experience* (1902/1985). He describes religion as the feelings, acts, and experiences of individuals in relation to the divine. For James, religion draws its significance from a spiritual world, and its true end is the attainment of union within the spiritual domain. Still, James viewed authentic religion as a dynamic experience that encompassed the spiritual dimension.

Relationship of Religion and Spirituality

Most agree that religion and spirituality are related but there is less agreement on the nature of their relationship. The Summit on Spirituality (Miller, 1999) defined spirituality as the innate, animating force in life which moves individuals toward love, knowledge, meaning, connectedness, and compassion. Notable is that spirituality is viewed as encompassing the religious dimension. This view contrasts sharply with James' view of the relationship of religion and spirituality.

Endeavoring to develop a more balanced relationship between the two, Pargament (1999) utilizes the concepts of search and sacred to describe the interrelationship of religion and spirituality. He defines religion as the search for significance through the sacred, and spirituality as the process through which individuals seek "to find, conserve, and if necessary, transform the sacred in their lives" (Pargament, 1999, p. 12). He insists that the search takes place in a larger religious context and that the sacred is what distinguishes religion and spirituality from other phenomena. Yet, the sacred, which includes concepts of God, the divine, or the transcendent, is understood to be the common denominator of religious and spiritual life.

Spirituality

Unlike religion, in which there is at least some agreement about its basic elements, there is no consensus on what constitutes spirituality. As a result, there are some 300 descriptions and definitions of spirituality in the professional literature (Zinnbauer et al., 1997). Here is a selective summary of these various definitions and descriptions. For some spirituality is basically a feeling state (Domasio, 2003), while others contend it is an instinct (Hamer, 2004). Some consider it a basic trait, such as of character (Cloninger, 2004), a striving (Emmons, 1999), or spiritual transcendence (Cloninger, 2004; Piedmont, 1999; Reed, 1991). Others consider it a peak or mystical experience (Maslow, 1968), a search (Pargament, 1999), a search for meaning (Frankl, 1985), an insatiable spiritual longing (Rolheiser, 1999), spiritual practices (Walsh, 1999), a form of intelligence (Emmons, 2000), quantum change (Miller & C'de Baca, 2001), integrating one's self toward ultimate value (Schneiders, 1986), or spiritual transformation (Stawski, 2003).

Since there is little agreement among either researchers or clinicians on what constitutes an adequate definition, clinicians have essentially two options when dealing with a client's spiritual issues or concerns. One is to choose an existing definition that has personal meaning for them and utilize it as the basis for conceptualizing client issues and concern in their practice. Another is to elicit and respect a client's unique view of spirituality and use it to conceptualize and respond to client concerns (McSherry & Cash, 2004).

In time, it is expected that a consensus definition will emerge. Such a consensus definition is likely to be systemically based which means that it can be characterized in terms of three systems theory variables: input, process, and output variables. More specifically, spirituality can be understood as an input or antecedent variable, a process or mediating variable, and an output or dependent variable. Most current definitions reflect only one or two of these variables. For example, spiritual longing (Rolheiser, 1999) is an antecedent variable while spiritual practices (Walsh, 1999) is a moderating variable, and spiritual transformation (Stawski, 2003) is an output or dependent variable. The assumption is that a systemic-based definition is more theoretically valuable and clinically useful than one that includes only one or two variables (Sperry, 2006).

There is theoretical value in framing spirituality in such a systemic context, particularly if it is centered on the concept of spiritual transformation. "Spiritual transformation can be defined as dramatic changes in world and self-view, purposes, religious beliefs, attitudes, and behavior. These changes are often linked to discrete experiences that can occur gradually or over relatively short periods of time" (Stawski, 2003, p. 425). Spiritual transformation involves much more than increasing one's level of physical health and/or psychological well-being. Parenthetically, this definition of spiritual transformation has been operationalized in more than two dozen research studies funded by the Templeton Foundation and sponsored by the Spiritual Transformation Scientific Research Program (Katz, 2004). Similarly, spiritual transformation has been described as an output or dependent variable, and spiritual longing (Rolheiser, 1999) represents an antecedent or independent variable (Sperry, 2006). Linking spiritual longings and spiritual transformation are various spiritual transcending practices (Walsh, 1999) which are mediating variables or dimensions. These practices include prayer, meditation, mindfulness, fasting, and service. Figure 1.1, based on Sperry (2006), portrays this multidimensional model which articulates the relationship of these three systemic variables. In this book, spirituality is framed in this multidimensional model as a process that is activated by spiritual longings, fostered by self-transcending spiritual practices, and results in spiritual transformation, which is an ongoing process.

Relationship of Spirituality and Psychology

Even though there is yet to be a consensus definition of spirituality (McSherry & Cash, 2004; Sperry, 2005), it is possible to describe the relationship of spirituality and psychology that has been discussed or implied in psychological and spiritual theories. It is possible to articulate the relationship between the domains of spirituality and psychology in terms of two sets of factors: whether the domains are the same or different, and which domain has primacy over the other. In terms of these two factors, it is possible to derive five different relationships between spirituality and psychology (Sperry & Mansager, 2007). It is a taxonomy or framework from which to generate theory building and empirical studies. These five relationships are briefly described here.

Spiritual Longing –> Self-Transcending Practices –> Spiritual Transformation

Figure 1.1 A Multidimensional Model of Spirituality.

1. Psychology and spirituality are viewed as essentially the same as psychology having primacy. There is little or no need for spiritual interventions or disciplines necessary to affect development. This is the epitome of psychological reductionism and is exemplified by the classical psychoanalytic approach (Freud, 1927/1961).
2. Psychology and spirituality are essentially the same as spirituality having primacy. This view is represented by classical Jungian psychotherapy (Jung, 1963) and a few traditional approaches to spiritual direction and pastoral counseling (May, 1992). This is the epitome of spiritual reductionism.
3. Psychology and spirituality are essentially different, with psychology having primacy. This view is representative of some spiritually oriented psychoanalytic approaches (Shafranske, 2005), as well as some existential-humanistic approaches (Elkins, 2005).
4. Psychology and spirituality are essentially different, with spirituality having primacy. In this view, growth in one domain such as the psychological can be reflected in the other but is not inevitable. Thus, one can be saintly but neurotic. This view is representative of a number of the transpersonal approaches to psychotherapy (Cortright, 1997), spiritually oriented interpersonal psychotherapy (Miller, 2005), as well as spiritually oriented cognitive behavior therapy (Tan & Johnson, 2005).y
5. Psychology and spirituality are essentially different, with neither having primacy nor being reducible to the other. When client concerns involve symptom or problem-resolution, psychotherapeutically oriented strategies are indicated, whereas when concerns involve ultimate questions and answers, spiritually oriented strategies are indicated. This view is representative of the holistic orientation (Sperry & Mansager, 2007).

This taxonomy identifies the first four orientations as being reductionist with the fifth as holistic, i.e., non-reductionist. Reductionist approaches are less likely to be developmentally oriented. On the other hand, holistic approaches are post-materialist in perspective, and more likely to be strengths-based and growth-oriented.

Growth-focused, spiritually oriented psychotherapies tend to emphasize constructing meaning and the transcendent over decreasing symptoms and impairment, i.e., an emphasis on meanings more than on observation of facts. Such therapy requires a focused listening to the client's experience to understand his or her meaning (Shafranske & Sperry, 2005).

Pastoral Counseling, Spiritual Direction, and Spiritually Integrated Psychotherapy

Before proceeding further, it will be useful to begin describing spiritually integrated psychotherapy as a professional entity. To accomplish this, it will be compared to two similar but different approaches that focus on spirituality and religious concerns: pastoral counseling and spiritual direction. While there are some similarities, spiritually integrated psychotherapy differs in a number of respects from pastoral counseling and spiritual direction with regard to: goals, clientele, process and interventions, and sponsoring professional organizations. This section specifies these differences and provides an introduction to the practice of spiritually integrated psychotherapy.

Pastoral Counseling

For centuries clergy have endeavored to help believers with personal problems and crises, as well to as to provide pastoral care for those with mental illness. Besides pastoral care provided by clergy, pastoral counseling is also rooted in clinical pastoral education and chaplaincy. Yet, it was recognized that specialized professional training was necessary to effectively treat some believers. The identity of pastoral counselors as professional counselors with specialized trained in theology, pastoral care, and psychology was crystalized with the founding of the American Association of Pastoral Counseling in 1963. Until recently, pastoral counseling was often viewed as an alternative to conventional psychotherapy. It had also been viewed as an alternative to spiritual direction for many Protestant and Jews, since in the past, spiritual direction was considered a Catholic "intervention."

Goals

The primary goal and functions of pastoral counseling is coping with physical, emotional, or moral stressors as well as coping with a crisis of meaning. Its secondary goal is psychological change which includes symptom reduction and problem resolution. A basic assumption of pastoral counseling is that addressing spiritual or religious needs is essential in effectively dealing with personal problems and crises, particularly for believers.

Currently, three forms of pastoral counseling are practiced: a brief situational form of counseling of a single session, a time-limited form that is problem-solving or solution-focused that typically lasts 2–5 sessions, and a long-term form, called pastoral psychotherapy, that is often psychoanalytically oriented that focuses on personality change and may continue for a year or more (Montgomery, 2010; Stone, 1999). Clergy and other ministry personnel who have some training in pastoral care and counseling provide the majority of short-term pastoral counseling. However, ministry personnel and others with formal supervised training in counseling and psychotherapy and are certified and/or licensed can practice what is called pastoral psychotherapy. Pastoral psychotherapy is variously defined (Wise, 1980) but tends to involve longer-term therapy, and in some instances is difficult to distinguish from psychotherapy.

Clientele

Clientele for pastoral counseling are typically troubled individuals presenting with life transitions, emotional or relational crises, or guilt, abuse, addictions, or low self-esteem (Benner, 2003; Stone, 1999). Pastoral counseling is well suited for such crises and concerns and is a unique form of counseling which uses religious and spiritual resources as well as psychological understanding for healing and growth. Its primary goal is problem resolution and restoration of psychological health; however, personality change may also be a goal in pastoral psychotherapy.

Process and Interventions

As in psychotherapy, the relationship between pastoral counselor and client is important and maintaining some measure of clinical distance is useful in diagnosis and therapeutic change. Nevertheless, many recently trained pastoral counselors advocate a mutually collaborative relationship with the client (Benner, 2003). Assessment may include a pastoral assessment or diagnosis. The dimensions of such an assessment include: awareness of God, acceptance of God's grace; repentance and responsibility, and involvement in one's faith community (Benner, 2003).

Treatment interventions usually include active listening and other problem-solving or solution-focused counseling methods. It may also include advice on religious or spiritual matters, e.g., forgiveness. Unlike spiritual direction, pastoral counseling typically does not bring to bear the resources of the client's faith community for healing, growth, or integration. Pastoral counseling usually involves just the client, but may include the client's spouse or even the family (Sperry, 2002). Sessions are usually scheduled weekly, more likely in a counseling clinic rather than in a church or synagogue community. Furthermore, pastoral counselors are likely to refer clients with certain presentations for spiritually integrated psychotherapy or even conventional psychotherapy.

Training

How are pastoral counselors trained and how do they practice? Pastoral counselors are often psychologically as well as theologically trained and it is not uncommon for the pastoral counselor or psychotherapist to possess graduate degrees in ministry and in pastoral counseling or another mental health discipline. An increasing number are licensed to practice, usually in a mental health specialty. Certification is available from the American Association of Pastoral Counselors, a professional organization representing 3000 pastoral counselors.

Professional Organization

Pastoral counseling is currently preoccupied with enhancing its identity as a recognized profession. As such training, licensure, and certification are central concerns (Sperry, 2002, 2013). An increasing number of pastoral counselors are licensed to practice, usually in one of the mental health specialties, e.g., licensed professional counselor, and certification is available from the American Association of Pastoral Counselors. This professional organization represents about 4000 pastoral counselors and is actively exploring ways of incorporating a focus on spiritual concerns and spiritual direction methods into the practice of pastoral counseling. It was founded in 1963 to certify pastoral counselors, accredit pastoral counseling centers, and approve training programs. It is an interfaith organization representing more than 80 faith groups including the Protestant, Catholic, and Jewish faiths. As a non-sectarian professional organization, it respects the spiritual and religious traditions of those who seek assistance without imposition of counselor beliefs.

While some are wary of extending the scope of pastoral counseling, citing major differences in epistemological perspectives and praxis stances between the two fields, others are supporting this extension (Galindo, 1997). Needless to say, the identity of pastoral counseling has been significantly impacted by such forces as managed behavioral health care and the increasing numbers of spiritual directors and mental health counselors who compete for many of the same clients as pastoral counselors (Stone, 1999).

Another organization, the Association for Clinical Pastoral Education (ACPE), has for years certified clinical pastoral education (CPE) training for chaplains, and distinguished chaplaincy from pastoral counseling. However, recently they have introduced a Spiritually Integrated Psychotherapy training and certification for licensed and pre-licensed counselors, social workers, marriage and family therapists, pastoral counselors, psychologists, psychiatrists, and addiction specialists, as well as graduate students in these disciplines.

Spiritual Direction

Spiritual direction is also known as spiritual guidance, spiritual friendship, and spiritual companionship (Lesser, 1999). While its roots extend from the third century where it was practiced primarily with monks, priests, and other religious, it has been rediscovered, evolved, and practiced in various forms in nearly all spiritual traditions, particularly in the past 40 years (Edwards, 1980, 2001). Today, spiritual direction in the US is still associated with the Catholic tradition, although it is also practiced in several Protestant denominations (Leech, 1977), as well as in Judaism and in Buddhism (Bhikku, 2003).

Spiritual direction can be described as the art of spiritual listening which focuses on movement of the divine within another's life story (Stairs, 2000). It involves a trained director who guides or companions another, called a directee. While spiritual direction can occur in a group setting, it most commonly is practiced in the context of a one-to-one trusting relationship. While there may be a candle, a bible, or some other non-verbal symbol representing the Holy, spiritual direction always occurs in the context of prayer.

Goal

Spiritual direction, also called spiritual companionship or spiritual guidance, is primarily concerned with spiritual growth and only secondarily with psychological growth and change. Its basic goal is to facilitate spiritual growth (Barry & Connolly, 2009; Gratton, 1992). It achieves this goal by emphasizing the relationship between the directee and God and utilizing spiritual resources, particularly prayer. The basic assumption of spiritual direction is that spiritual growth is fostered by a reflective process with another who guides and models this process (Ruffing & Ruffing, 2000). It can and does process crisis issues that impact spiritual growth.

Clientele

As already noted, clients are referred to as directees. Spiritual direction focuses on the maintenance and development of spiritual health and well-being, and it assumes that the person is already whole, but has not yet fully embraced this truth for themselves. Thus, spiritual direction is not for everyone, since it presumes a moderate degree of psychological health and well-being (Sperry, 2002).

Process and Interventions

Discernment is central to spiritual direction and usually involves recognizing the spiritual or ultimate meaning of events and circumstances in the directee's life (Barry & Connolly, 1982, 2009). The relationship between director and directee is one of mutual engagement based on the recognition that both are walking the same spiritual journey. The role of faith in the spiritual dimension and one's relationship to a faith community is central to Christian spiritual direction (Gratton, 1992). In addition, spiritual direction involves spiritual conversion, in that it is attentive to the "dynamics of change through conversion, the radical transformation... a relational, personal surrender to a personal, living God" (Galindo, 1997, p. 400).

Interventions in spiritual direction include instruction in prayer and the prescription of rituals and other spiritual practices. A focus on developing and monitoring the directee's prayer life, including meditation or contemplation, is central to spiritual direction. When indicated spiritual directors may refer directees with certain psychological problems for concurrent psychotherapy or will suspend spiritual direction until the course of therapy is completed (Culligan, 1983). Whether one professional can effectively and appropriately provide both spiritual direction and either psychotherapy or pastoral counseling is a matter of considerable debate (May, 1992). Spiritual direction is customarily provided in a one-to-one format and usually on a monthly basis, although spiritual direction can also occur in small group settings. Some spiritual directors and guides charge a fee or request a free will offering while others do not.

Training

How are spiritual directors trained and how is spiritual direction usually practiced? There are no set requirements to practice spiritual direction. Some contend that it is a vocation rather than a profession; a special calling for which formal coursework and supervision is not essential. Other contend that specialized training in selected areas of theology and psychology are helpful and essential (Lescher, 1997; Sperry, 2002). Currently, there are a number of formal graduate training institutes and programs in spiritual direction but no universally recognized certification or licensure for spiritual directors.

Professional Organization

As a profession, spiritual direction is represented by Spiritual Directors International, an organization with a worldwide membership. Compared to pastoral counseling and spiritually integrated psychotherapy, Spiritual Directors International has the least restrictive membership requirements. It appears that anyone interested in spiritual direction can join the Spiritual Directors International global learning community. This organization promulgates its own code of professional ethics for its members.

Spiritually Integrated Psychotherapy

Spiritually integrated psychotherapy is the most recent of the three approaches. Its development stems from theoretical developments, such as transpersonal psychology, but also from client considerations, the most important of which is the expectation that spiritual values and concerns will be respected and incorporated into the therapeutic process. Spiritually integrated psychotherapy is a broad characterization for a variety of psychotherapeutic approaches that are sensitive to the spiritual dimension. These approaches range from non-Christian approaches, to transpersonal psychotherapies (Cortright, 1997; Karasu, 1999), to theistic (Richards & Bergin, 2005) and various Christian approaches (Sperry, 2001, 2002, 2005, 2010; Steere, 1997).

Pargament (2007) described spirituality integrated psychotherapy as an "approach to treatment that acknowledges and addresses the spirituality of the client, the spirituality of the therapist, and the process of change" (Pargament, 2007, p. 176). He conceived it as drawing on a wide range of approaches and interventions and could be provided to clients from diverse spiritual or non-religious backgrounds by therapists from diverse spiritual or non-religious backgrounds. From his perspective, it differs from spiritually accommodative and spiritually oriented approaches that are not theory and research based. He believed that spirituality integrated psychotherapy "will not gain widespread use and acceptance until it has proved to be effective" (Pargament, 2007, p. 320).

Later, Sperry (2013) offered a more comprehensive definition of spiritually integrated psychotherapy as:

> a term that broadly characterizes a variety of psychotherapeutic approaches that are sensitive to the spiritual dimension... It draws on spiritual resources in addressing spiritual issues and struggles to resolve psychological and relational problems. Although it can also foster spiritual change and growth, spiritually integrated psychotherapy accomplishes this as a by-product that accompanies psychological change.
>
> (Sperry, 2013, p. 227)

As spiritually integrated psychotherapy has continued to evolve in terms of theory, research, essential psychotherapy competencies, and training, the following definition is offered.

> Spiritually integrated psychotherapy is a broad designation that refers to approaches provided by therapists that integrates the essential psychotherapy competencies as well as spiritual resources in addressing spiritual issues and struggles to resolve psychological and relational problems. Although it can also foster spiritual change and growth, spiritually integrated psychotherapy accomplishes this as a by-product that accompanies psychological change. It is distinct from pastoral counseling and spiritual direction in its treatment focus and training.
>
> (Sperry, 2024b, p. 11)

So why was "essential psychotherapy competencies" added to the definition? The reason is that spiritually integrated psychotherapy had significantly evolved and changed based on research and clinical experience. For me this change in understanding began with my ongoing consultation with groups of therapists in different clinics who were learning to use outcome measures to inform their treatment decisions. In working with them weekly for several months at a time, I observed that therapists who were open to integrating the client feedback received from outcomes monitoring had increased positive clinical outcomes. Not only was treatment more successful but the therapeutic alliance with the clients improved, and these therapists had a better understanding of their clients' basic patterns. Even if they had not formally developed a case conceptualization—for which maladaptive patterns is central—these therapists developed a firsthand understanding of these patterns based on their outcomes monitoring and were able to make changes in the treatment process. As they utilized this client feedback to better tailor treatment, there was a concomitant positive shift in the alliance with the clients as well as in treatment outcomes.

Later clinical trials and meta-analyses research would demonstrate the powerful therapeutic effect of routine outcomes monitoring (ROM). The use of client feedback to inform therapy—both conventional and spiritually integrated psychotherapy—began appearing in the latter part of the Era III, becoming a major force in the early days of Era IV (Barkham et al., 2023; Johnson et al., 2022). Not surprisingly, some suggested that "that ROM represents a major revolution in the practice of psychotherapy" (Miller et al., 2015, p. 449).

As part of the scientific advisory committee for Bridges, I witnessed again the powerful impact of outcomes monitoring as we planned and reviewed data from the various clinic sites throughout the treatment phase of this major Templeton Foundation funded study involving some 400+ therapists and 40,000+ therapy sessions. The results were unmistakable. It was not just the spiritual interventions that resulted in client changes; it was the intentional use of feedback from ROM along with these spiritual interventions that made the difference.

This definition of spiritually integrated psychotherapy informs the rest of this book. The essential psychotherapy competencies of therapeutic alliance, assessment, case conceptualization, intervention, and outcomes monitoring are described and illustrated throughout Chapters 5 and 10. Despite considerable variability among these spiritual psychotherapy approaches, some general observations about goals, clientele, the intervention process, and training, and professional considerations can be made.

Goals

The primary goal of spiritually integrated psychotherapy is the resolution of psychological and relational problems. Although it can also foster spiritual change and growth, spiritually integrated psychotherapy accomplishes this as a by-product that accompanies psychological change. Related to presenting psychological symptoms and concerns can be religious and spiritual issues such as struggles involving serious health problems, personal or professional loss, or interpersonal conflict; struggles involving betrayal, the death of a child, or other loss (Pargament & Exline, 2021; Sperry, 2013). These can reflect a crisis of faith or meaning in life (American Psychiatric Association, 2022).

Clientele

Individuals seeking spiritually integrated psychotherapy range from relatively healthy spiritual seekers to disordered clients presenting with symptomatic distress and/or impairment in one or more areas of life functioning (Sperry, 2012, 2013). The focus of treatment varies according to client presentation and need. This may include help with spiritual emergencies, the process of spiritual growth, increased psychological well-being, self-fulfillment or individuation, or the reduction of symptomatic distress and the restoration of baseline functioning (Sperry, 2002).

Process and Interventions

Unlike pastoral counselors and spiritual directors who offer spiritual resources or advice that is rooted in a particular religious or institutional framework, spiritually oriented psychotherapists are more likely to be non-committal about a particular religious solution. The therapeutic relationship typically involves mutual collaboration. Accordingly, spiritually integrated psychotherapists can be expected to show respect for the client's spiritual values and concerns.

Various psychotherapeutic and spiritual interventions are utilized depending on client need and indication (Pargament & Exline, 2021; Plante, 2024). If indicated, referral for a psychiatric evaluation for medication or hospitalization may occur. Spiritual interventions are also involved. These include spiritual practices, such as prayer and meditation, and when indicated, collaboration or referral to clergy or chaplain (Sperry, 2013).

Training

How are those who practice spiritually integrated psychotherapy trained? While some graduate programs offer coursework, such training has yet to be formalized in accreditation standards nor regulated by licensing bodies. However, despite the fact that several recommendations have been offered for training psychotherapists in spiritual and religious competencies to address spiritual concerns in the context of psychotherapy (Currier et al., 2023; Richards, Currier et al., 2023b), until recently very little training was available.

Organizations like the Association for Clinical Pastoral Education (ACPE) have begun to offer Spiritually Integrated Psychotherapy training and certification. Whether or not such programs will attract psychologists is yet to be seen. Presumably APA or APA sponsored programs will offer such training and certification programs.

Professional Organization

Two professional organizations represent a large number of spiritually integrated psychotherapists. These are APA and the American Counseling Association (ACA). Division 36 of APA, the Society for the Psychology of Religion and Spirituality, represents and advocates for psychologists practicing spiritually integrated psychotherapy and continues to develop ethical and practice guidelines for both trainees and practitioners (Piedmont, 2013). Similarly, ACA has a division called the Association for Spiritual, Ethical, and Religious Values in Counseling, which advocates for those practicing spiritually oriented counseling (Cashwell & Watts, 2010).

Table 1.2 summarizes much of the discussion of the goals, clientele, interventions, training, and professional organizations involving pastoral counseling, spiritual direction, and spiritually integrated psychotherapy.

Concluding Note

During the past several decades psychotherapy sensitive to the spiritual dimension has evolved over four eras. Today, psychotherapists are experimenting with different ways of integrating the spiritual dimension in their professional work, and also in their personal lives. The culture of accountability has already impacted the practice of conventional psychotherapy as clinicians are increasingly expected to utilize evidence-based treatments and demonstrate positive clinical outcomes. There is no question that these influences will also impact the practice of spiritually integrated psychotherapy. Accordingly, the practice of spiritually integrated psychotherapy will continue to evolve as it reflects these parameters.

Table 1.2 Comparison of Pastoral Counseling, Spiritual Direction, and Spiritually Integrated Psychotherapy

	Pastoral Counseling and Psychotherapy	*Spiritual Direction*	*Spiritually Integrated Psychotherapy*
Goals	Spiritual change and secondarily psychological change; may focus on symptom reduction and problem resolution	Primarily spiritual change, with focus on prayer; focus on crisis issues that impact spiritual life	Psychological change with spiritual growth and change as a by-product of psychological change
Clientele	Troubled individuals often concerned with religious issues and/or desire that their spiritual/religious values be respected	Usually relatively healthy spiritual seekers	Varies from relatively healthy to troubled or disordered individuals with spiritual or religious concerns
Process and Interventions	Listening, advice; other therapeutic interventions; may include religious or spiritual advice or practices; referral for psychotherapy	Listening, instruction in prayer and other spiritual practices; possibly referral for psychotherapy	Various counseling and psychotherapeutic interventions plus spiritual practices and interventions, including referral to clergy or chaplain
Training	Master's or doctorate in theology or pastoral counseling; supervised experience; endorsement by a religious body	Master's in spirituality or psychology; some formal training and supervised experience	Doctorate in psychology; may or may not have formal training and supervised experience
Professional Organizations	American Association of Pastoral Counseling	Spiritual Directors International	Society for the Psychology of Religion and Spirituality (APA); Association for Spiritual, Ethical, and Religious Values in Counseling (ACA)

References

American Psychiatric Association. (2022). *Diagnostic and statistical manual of mental disorders*, 5th ed., Text revision. American Psychiatric Association.

American Psychological Association. (2017). *Multicultural guidelines: An ecological approach to context, identity, and intersectionality*. www.apa.org/about/policy/multicultural-guidelines.pdf

Barkham, M., De Jong, K., Delgadillo, J., & Lutz, W. (2023). Routine outcome monitoring (ROM) and feedback: Research review and recommendations. *Psychotherapy Research*, *33*(7), 841–855. https://doi.org/10.1080/10503307.2023.2181114

Barry, W., & Connolly, W. (1982). *The practice of spiritual direction*. Seabury.

Barry, W., & Connolly, W. (2009). *The practice of spiritual direction* (2nd ed.). Seabury.

Benner, D. (2003). *Strategic pastoral counseling: A short-term structured model* (2nd ed.). Baker Academic.

Bhikku, T. (2003). Making a cup of tea: Some aspects of spiritual direction within a living Buddhist tradition. In N. Vest (Ed.), *Tending the holy: Spiritual direction across traditions* (pp. 3–18). Morehouse Publishing.

Cashwell, C., & Watts, R. (2010). The new ASERVIC competencies for addressing spiritual and religious issues in counseling. *Counseling and Values*, *55*, 2–5.

Cloninger, C. R. (2004). *Feeling good: The science of well-being*. Oxford University Press.

Cortright, R. (1997). *Psychotherapy and spirit: Theory and practice in transpersonal psychotherapy*. State University of New York Press.

Culligan, K. (1983). The counseling ministry and spiritual direction. In Estadt B. (Ed.), *Pastoral counseling* (pp. 37–49). Prentice-Hall.

Currier, J. M., Fox, J., Vieten, C., Pearce, M., & Oxhandler, H. K. (2023). Enhancing competencies for the ethical integration of religion and spirituality in psychological services. *Psychological Services*, *20*(1), 40–50. https://doi.org/10.1037/ser0000678

Davis, E. B., Lacey, E. K., Heydt, E. J., LaBouff, J. P., Barker, S. B., Van Elk, M., & Ladd, K. L. (2024). Sixty years of studying the sacred: Auditing and advancing the psychology of religion and spirituality. *Psychology of Religion and Spirituality*, *16*(1), 7–9. https://doi.org/10.1037/rel0000485

Delaney, H. D., Miller, W. R., & Bisonó, A. M. (2007). Religiosity and spirituality among psychologists: A survey of clinician members of the American Psychological Association. *Professional Psychology, Research and Practice*, *38*(5), 538–546. https://doi.org/10.1037/0735-7028.38.5.538

Domasio, A. (2003). *Looking for Spinoza: Joy, sorrow, and the feeling brain*. Harcourt.

Edwards, T. (1980). *Spiritual friend: Reclaiming the gift of spiritual direction*. Paulist.

Edwards, T. (2001). *Spiritual director, spiritual companion*. Paulist.

Elkins, D. N. (2005). A humanistic approach to spiritually oriented psychotherapy. In L. Sperry & E. P. Shafranske (Eds.), *Spiritually oriented psychotherapy* (pp. 131–151). American Psychological Association. https://doi.org/10.1037/10886-006

Ellswood, R. (1990). Religion. In R. Hunter (Ed.), *Dictionary of pastoral care and counseling* (p. 1054). Abingdon Press.
Emmons, R. (1999). *The psychology of ultimate concerns: Motivation and spirituality in personality.* Guilford.
Emmons, R. (2000). Is spirituality an intelligence? Motivation, cognition, and the psychology of ultimate concerns. *International Journal of Psychology of Religion*, *10*(1), 3–26.
Fontana, D. (2003). *Psychology, religion and spirituality.* BPS Blackwell.
Frankl, V. E. (1985). *Man's search for meaning.* Simon and Schuster.
Freud, S. (1927/1961). *The future of an illusion.* Norton.
Galindo, I. (1997). Spiritual direction and pastoral counseling. *Journal of Pastoral Care* 51(4), 395–402.
Gratton, C. (1992). *The art of spiritual guidance: A contemporary approach to growing in the spirit.* Crossroad.
Gross, N., & Simmons, S. (2009). The religiosity of American college and university professors. *Sociology of Religion*, *70*(2), 101–129. https://doi.org/10.1093/socrel/srp026
Hamer, D. (2004). *The God gene: How faith is hardwired into our genes.* Doubleday.
Hodge, D. R. (2013). Assessing spirituality and religion in the context of counseling and psychotherapy. In *APA handbook of psychology, religion, and spirituality (Vol 2): An applied psychology of religion and spirituality.* (pp. 93–123). American Psychological Association.
James, W. (1902/1985). *The varieties of religious experience: A study in human nature.* Harvard University Press.
Johnson, S. K., Galan-Cisneros, P., & Heaton, L. R. (2022). Outcomes of a practice-based evidence study of spiritually integrated psychotherapy in a mental health setting. *Journal of Religion & Spirituality in Social Work: Social Thought*, *41*(4), 437–453.
Jung, C. G. (1963). *Essays on a science of mythology (Vol. 22).* Princeton University Press.
Karasu, T. (1999). Spiritual psychotherapy. *American Journal of Psychotherapy*, *53*(2), 143–162.
Katz, S. (2004). *The Spiritual Transformation Scientific Research program.* Metanexus Institute on Religion and Science.
Leech, K. (1977). *Soul friend.* Harper & Row.
Lescher, B. (1997). The professionalization of spiritual direction: Promise and peril. *Listening*, *32*, 81–90.
Lesser, E. (1999). *The new American spirituality: A seeker's guide.* Random House.
Lesser, E. (2000). Insider's guide to 21st-century spirituality. *Spirituality and Health: The Soul/Body Connection*, Spring, 46–51.
Lykins, E. L. B. (2014). Mindfulness, consciousness, spirituality, and well-being. In C. Kim-Prieto (Ed.), *Religion and spirituality across cultures* (pp. 203–225). Springer Science. https://doi.org/10.1007/978-94-017-8950-9_11
Maslow, A. (1968). *Toward a psychology of being* (2nd ed.). Van Nostrand.
May, G. (1992). *Care of mind, care of soul: A psychiatrist explores spiritual direction.* HarperCollins.

McSherry, W., & Cash, K. (2004). The language of spirituality: An emerging taxonomy. *International Journal of Nursing Studies*, *41*, 151–161.

Miller, L. (2005). Interpersonal psychotherapy from a spiritual perspective. In L. Sperry & E. P. Shafranske (Eds.), *Spiritually oriented psychotherapy* (pp. 153–175). American Psychological Association. https://doi.org/10.1037/10886-007

Miller, S. D., Hubble, M. A., Chow, D., & Seidel, J. (2015). Beyond measures and monitoring: Realizing the potential of feedback-informed treatment. *Psychotherapy*, *52*(4), 449–457.

Miller, W. (Ed.). (1999). *Integrating spirituality into treatment: Resources for practitioners*. American Psychological Association.

Miller, W., & C'de Baca, J. (2001). *Quantum change: When epiphanies and sudden insights transform ordinary lives*. Guilford.

Montgomery, D. (2010). *Pastoral counseling and coaching*. Compass Works.

Pargament, K. (1999). The psychology of religion and spirituality? Yes and no. *International Journal of Psychology of Religion*, *9*, 3–16.

Pargament, K. I. (2007). *Spiritually integrated psychotherapy. Understanding and addressing the sacred*. Guilford.

Pargament, K. I. (2023). From research to practice: Three waves in the evolution of the psychology of religion and spirituality. *Spiritual Psychology and Counseling*, *8*(3), 207–225.

Pargament, K. I., & Exline, J. J. (2021). *Working with spiritual struggles in psychotherapy: From research to practice*. Guilford.

Piedmont, R. (1999). Does spiritual represent the sixth factor of personality? Spiritual transcendence and the five-factor model. *Journal of Personality*, *67*, 985–1013.

Piedmont, R. L. (2013). A short history of the *Psychology of Religion and Spirituality*: Providing growth and meaning for Division 36. *Psychology of Religion and Spirituality*, *5*(1), 1–4. https://doi.org/10.1037/a0030878

Plante, T. G. (2024). *Spiritually informed therapy (SIT): Wisdom and evidence-based strategies that work*. Cognella Academic Publishing.

Reed, P. (1991). Toward a nursing theory of self-transcendence: Deductive reformulation using developmental theories. *Advances in Nursing Science*, *13*(4), 64–77.

Richards, P. S., Allen, G. E., & Judd, D. K. (2023a). *Handbook of spiritually integrated psychotherapies*. American Psychological Association.

Richards, P. S., & Bergin, A. E. (2005). *A spiritual strategy for counseling and psychotherapy* (2nd ed.). American Psychological Association.

Richards, P. S., Currier, J. M., Jones, R. S., Pearce, M., & Stephens, D. (2023b). Training opportunities and resources for spiritually integrated psychotherapists and researchers. In P. S. Richards, G. E. K. Allen, & D. K. Judd (Eds.), *Handbook of spiritually integrated psychotherapies* (pp. 423–447). American Psychological Association. https://doi.org/10.1037/0000338-022

Richards, P. S., Sanders, P. W., Lea, T., McBride, J. A., & Allen, G. E. (2015). Bringing spiritually oriented psychotherapies into the health care mainstream: A call for worldwide collaboration. *Spirituality in Clinical Practice*, *2*(3), 169–179.

Rolheiser, R. (1999). *The holy longing: The search for a Christian spirituality.* Doubleday.
Ruffing, J. K., & Ruffing, J. (2000). *Spiritual direction: Beyond the beginnings.* Paulist Press.
Schneiders, S. (1986). Theology and spirituality: Strangers, rivals, or partners? *Horizons, 13*, 253–274.
Shafranske, E. P. (2005). A psychoanalytic approach to spiritually oriented psychotherapy. In L. Sperry & E. P. Shafranske (Eds.), *Spiritually oriented psychotherapy* (pp. 105–130). American Psychological Association. https://doi.org/10.1037/10886-005
Shafranske, E., & Sperry, L. (2005). Addressing the spiritual dimension in psychotherapy: Introduction and overview. In L. Sperry & E. Shafranske (Eds.), *Spiritually oriented psychotherapy* (pp. 11–29). American Psychological Association.
Shafranske, E. P., & Cummings, J. P. (2013). Religious and spiritual beliefs, affiliations, and practices of psychologists. In K. I. Pargament, A. Mahoney, & E. P. Shafranske (Eds.), *APA handbook of psychology, religion, and spirituality (Vol. 2): An applied psychology of religion and spirituality* (pp. 23–41). American Psychological Association. https://doi.org/10.1037/14046-002
Skinner, B. F. (1971). *Beyond freedom and dignity.* Knopf.
Sperry, L. (2001). *Spirituality in clinical practice: Incorporating the spiritual dimension in psychotherapy and counseling.* Brunner/Routledge.
Sperry, L. (2002). *Transforming self and community: Revisioning pastoral counseling and spiritual direction.* Liturgical Press.
Sperry, L. (2005). Integrative spiritually oriented psychotherapy. In L. Sperry & E. Shafranske (Eds.), *Spiritually oriented psychotherapy* (pp. 307–330). American Psychological Association.
Sperry, L. (2006). Is a consensus definition of spirituality possible? Theory construction in spiritually oriented psychotherapy. *Research in the Social Scientific Study of Religion, 17*, 10–22.
Sperry, L. (2010). Psychotherapy sensitive to spiritual issues: A post-materialist psychology perspective and developmental approach. *Psychology of Religion and Spirituality*, 2, 46–56.
Sperry, L. (2012). *Spirituality in clinical practice: Theory and practice of spiritually oriented psychotherapy* (2nd ed.). Routledge.
Sperry, L. (2013). Distinctive approaches to religion and spirituality: Pastoral counseling, spiritual direction, and spiritually integrated psychotherapy. In K. I. Pargament, A. Mahoney, & E. P. Shafranske (Eds.), *APA handbook of psychology, religion, and spirituality (Vol. 2): An applied psychology of religion and spirituality* (pp. 223–238). American Psychological Association. https://doi.org/10.1037/14046-011
Sperry, L. (2024a). Spiritually integrative psychotherapy: An impending paradigm shift in theory and practice. In L. Miller (Ed.), *The Oxford handbook of psychology and spirituality* (2nd ed., pp. 314–332). Oxford University Press.
Sperry, L. (2024b). The moral domain, moral injury, and the healing process. *Journal of Christian Healing, 40*(1), 5–14.

Sperry, L., & Mansager, E. (2007). The relationship between psychology and spirituality: An initial taxonomy for spiritually oriented counseling and psychotherapy. *Journal of Individual Psychology*, *63*(4), 360–370.

Stairs, J. (2000). *Listening for the soul: Pastoral care and spiritual direction*. Fortress.

Stawski, C. (2003). Definitions and hypotheses: William James, religion and spiritual transformation. *Cross Currents*, *53*(3), 424–437.

Steere, D. (1997). *Spiritual presence in psychotherapy: A guide for caregivers*. Brunner/Mazel.

Stone, H. (1999). Pastoral counseling and the changing times. *Journal of Pastoral Care*, *53*, 47–56.

Tan, S.-Y., & Johnson, W. B. (2005). Spiritually oriented cognitive-behavioral therapy. In L. Sperry & E. P. Shafranske (Eds.), *Spiritually oriented psychotherapy* (pp. 77–103). American Psychological Association. https://doi.org/10.1037/10886-004

Vieten, C., & Lukoff, D. (2022). Spiritual and religious competencies in psychology. *American Psychologist*, *77*(1), 26–38. https://doi.org/10.1037/amp0000821

Walsh, R. (1999). *Essential spirituality: The seven central practices to awaken heart and mind*. Wiley.

Wise, C. (1980). *Pastoral psychotherapy*. Jason Aronson.

Worthington, E. L. (2013). *Forgiveness and reconciliation: Theory and application*. Routledge.

Zinnbauer, B. J., Pargament, K. I., Cole, B., Rye, M. S., Butter, E. M., Belavich, T. G., Hipp, K. M., Scott, A. B., & Kadar, J. L., (1997). Religion and spirituality: Unfuzzying the fuzzy. *Journal for the Scientific Study of Religion*, *36*, 549–564.

Chapter 2

Dimensional Perspectives on Spiritual Development

This chapter introduces five basic dimensions of human experience and describes the spiritual dimension as the central dimension of human experience. Next it briefly reviews the results of research on the positive impact of the spiritual dimension and health and well-being. Then the decline and recovery of the moral dimension is described as a result of developments in moral psychology, positive psychology, and moral injury. Finally, six perspectives or frames of reference for understanding the spiritual dimension and the process of spiritual development are described.

The Dimensions of Human Experience

Historically, human experience has been described in terms of several dimensions. These have included the spiritual or religious, the moral, the social, the biological or somatic, and the psychological dimensions. While human experience has always been considered holistically from an Eastern perspective, it is only recently that it has begun to be viewed in this fashion from a Western perspective. Because of its allegiance to the scientific method and the law of parsimony (Ockham's Razor, i.e., the simplest explanation is preferable to a more elaborate one), Westerners have been content to explain all of human experience in terms of a single dimension. For example, in the early twentieth century scientists were content to conceptualize the theory and practice of medicine in terms of a single dimension of human experience, the biological or somatic dimension. Similar efforts were made to conceptualize individual human behavior or social and organizational processes in terms of either the psychological or the social dimension. Efforts to combine the dimensions of the psychological and the somatic were called "psychosomatic" medicine, while efforts to combine the psychological and social dimensions were called the "psychosocial."

Contemporary efforts in psychiatry and professional psychology to understand and change human behavior, and even organizational

DOI: 10.4324/9781003425991-3

behavior, have led to the adoption of the biopsychosocial model. First proposed by George Engel in 1977 (Engel, 1977), this model describes a way of conceptualizing human behavior in terms of three dimensions of human experience rather than previous models based on only one or two dimensions. Due to increasing scientific knowledge and clinical necessity over the past 20 years, the fields of psychiatry, family medicine, and internal medicine have come to adopt the biopsychosocial model as the theoretical and clinical basis for professional practice. Very recently, and based on scientific as well as political and economic considerations, the American Psychological Association officially adopted the biopsychosocial model as the basis for clinical practice.

The Centrality of the Spiritual Dimension

Five dimensions of human experience are commonly posited: psychological, social, moral, spiritual or religious, and somatic (Wilber, 1999). Figure 2.1 diagrams the interrelationship among the five basic dimensions of human experience. The spiritual dimension is placed at the core of the diagram to illustrate the belief that the spiritual dimension is foundational to all the other dimensions of human experience. This core may or may not involve any formal affiliation with a religious tradition, but it reflects the beliefs, affects, and behaviors associated with the basic spiritual hunger or desire for self-transcendence that all individuals experience.

Research on the Spiritual Dimension and Health and Well-Being

Currently, there is considerable interest in examining the impact of the spiritual dimension on the psychological, social, and somatic dimensions. Considerable research is underway or has already been reported on the so called "health effects" of religious and spiritual behaviors and physical health and psychological and relational well-being. Based on over 200

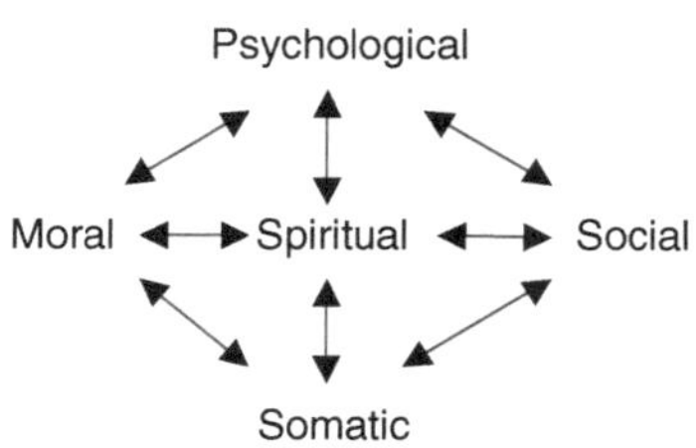

Figure 2.1 Centrality of the Spiritual Dimension Among the Dimensions of Human Experience.

published studies, it appears that higher levels of spirituality are related to lower risk for disease, fewer medical and psychiatric problems, and higher levels of psychosocial functioning. (Koenig, 1999; Levin, 1994; Levin & Chatters, 1998; Worthington et al., 1996). Interestingly, this finding seems to hold regardless of gender, ethnicity, the severity or type of the disease, how the concept of spirituality is measured or defined, or the type of research design used (Levin, 1994).

Looking more specifically at the somatic, psychological, and social dimensions, the following findings or results have been reported.

Somatic Dimension

Religious and spiritual commitment is related to a lower prevalence of illnesses, including heart disease, hypertension, stroke, and most cancers. Individuals with such commitment tend to live longer, have stronger immune systems, and respond better to treatment after being diagnosed with a disease. If they are undergoing surgery, they tend to have lower rates of postoperative mortality and faster recovery time from hip fractures and open-heart surgeries. Finally, they have a reduced likelihood of perceived disability.

Psychological Dimension

Individuals with higher levels of spirituality and religious commitment tend to report higher levels of subjective well-being and life satisfaction. They experience less anxiety, including less fear of death, and less worry and neurotic guilt. They have less depression and substance abuse and dependence, and report fewer suicidal impulses and less likelihood of committing suicide. Finally, they tend to show more empathy and altruism.

Social Dimension

Commitment and social involvement, which includes attendance at religious or spiritual services and activities, tend to have a prophylactic effect on health and well-being. Individuals who engage in spiritual practices such as prayer, meditation, reading sacred writings, and seeking spiritual counsel and support from religious leaders and community during stressful times tend to adjust better to crises and problems. Religious commitment is not usually associated with depression. Attendance at religious services is related to marital satisfaction and adjustment, less divorce, less use or abuse of alcohol or drugs, and lower rates of premarital sex, teenage pregnancy, and delinquency. Finally, there is less clinical depression among the elderly.

Parenthetically, this same line of research also studied the impact of the spiritual dimension on the moral dimension. Religious commitment is positively associated with moral behavior, in terms of adhering to higher moral standards and curbing personal desire or gain to promote the welfare of others. With regard to the other dimensions, these findings seem less surprising and newsworthy. Why is this? An examination of the tenuous relationship among the moral dimension with both the psychological and the spiritual dimensions suggests an explanation.

The Moral Dimension: Decline and Recovery

The moral dimension refers to moral thinking, decision making, and actions involving all the relationships in one's life: self, interpersonal, work, family, peers, and community. It includes conscience formation and the development of character and virtue, as well as moral codes and professional codes of ethical practice. It reflects the discipline of moral philosophy from which psychology emerged in the late nineteenth century.

Decline of the Moral Dimension

By the mid-twentieth century the moral dimension had all but disappeared from the study of human behavior and the practice of psychotherapy. As psychology evolved as a discipline and field of inquiry, it effectively disengaged from its roots in moral philosophy. While moral philosophy tended to emphasize the common good, character and virtue, rational judgment, and will, i.e., the volitional aspect of character, psychology increasingly focused on science, behavior, emotion, individuality, and the unconscious. Unfortunately, as a scientific discipline psychology became value neutral. As noted in Chapter 1, economics was another discipline that effectively distanced itself from its roots in moral philosophy.

The basic strategy psychology utilized to distance itself from moral philosophy was to disengage the study of personality from the study of character. Gordon Allport was one of the early academic psychologists to banish character from American psychology. His famous dictum: "Character is personality evaluated, and personality is character *devalued*" (Allport, 1937, p. 252, italics added) summarized psychology's disdain for the concept of character. Within a short time, psychology effectively succeeded in establishing a scientific and value-free foundation for understanding human behavior and actions distinct from moral philosophy. Essentially the concept of character, once a staple of everyday conversation, was nearly entirely replaced with the construct of personality (Taylor, 1997).

From the late 1950s through the early 1970s the profession of psychology endeavored to reformulate psychotherapy into the same scientific, value-free discipline framework as the rest of science. One of the results of these efforts has been that psychology students and mental health professionals have relatively limited acquaintance with the moral dimension except for a brief exposure to Kohlberg's stages of moral development usually in an Introduction to Psychology course.

Nevertheless, some psychotherapists became increasingly dissatisfied with this value-free, scientific view of psychotherapy as represented by the various editions of the *Diagnostic and Statistical Manual* (American Psychiatric Association, 2022), clinical practice guidelines, and treatment outcome measures. Many critiques of psychotherapy's value-free stance were forthcoming, including Rieff's provocative analysis in *Freud: the Mind of a Moralist* (1959) and in *Triumph of the Therapeutic* (Rieff, 1966), as well as Frank's *Psychotherapy and the Human Predicament* (1978).

Frank contended that nearly all psychotherapy approaches share a value system that accords primacy to self-fulfillment and views individuals as the center of their moral universe. He insists that this value system can easily become a source of misery because of its unrealistic expectations for personal happiness and because it downplays traditional values such as "the redemptive power of suffering, acceptance of one's lot in life, adherence to tradition, self-restraint and moderation" (Frank, 1978, pp. 6–7). Cushman (1990, 1995) argued that the goal of attaining and maintaining an "autonomous self" can be misguided and that preoccupation with an inner self which is self-soothing, self-loving, and self-sufficient eventually leads to an "empty self."

Others have observed that such a value-free psychotherapy fostered individual self-fulfillment over community well-being. Hillman and Ventura in *We've Had a Hundred Years of Psychotherapy and the World's Getting Worse* (1992) concluded that much of psychotherapy had effectively refocused our view of the problems of daily life into personal issues and reframed our view of the communal world in terms of psychopathology. They also noted that psychotherapy tends to draw sensitive, intelligent people away from the political arena and a focus on the common good into introspection and support groups. As a result, any motivation these individuals might have had to improve their local community by addressing issues such as hunger, illiteracy, and homelessness, were effectively displaced. Similarly, in their book, *Whatever Became of Sin?* (1973), Menninger and Tiedemann warn that if the concepts of sin and conscience are eliminated from open discourse, any hope of a moral society would vanish.

In *Re-envisioning Psychology: Moral Dimensions of Theory and Practice*, Richardson and his colleagues (1999) observed that most therapeutic approaches had little or nothing to say about character, conscience, or commitment. Nor did these approaches make a significant and positive contribution to human welfare and the struggle for a good society. They concluded that this value-free psychotherapy had effectively changed the moral calculus from a social ethic to an individual ethic (Richardson et al., 1999).

These and others have proposed that character, virtue, and conscience can and must be reintegrated into a scientific understanding of psychology and psychotherapy. Rather than being viewed as irrelevant to the science and practice of psychotherapy, key elements of the moral dimension—character, virtues, and conscience—must be recognized as integral to any science that systematically studies the human person. This reconceptualization acknowledges that psychology and psychotherapy are value-laden enterprises and require that psychotherapists intentionally integrate the moral dimension (character, virtue, and conscience) into their professional efforts. As a result, psychological science can better reflect the fullness of human life and fosters fulfillment and transformation for both clients and psychotherapists (Sperry, 2012, 2024a).

Recovery of the Moral Dimension

Three developments have been instrumental in the recovery of the moral dimension: character in moral psychology, virtue in positive psychotherapy, and conscience in moral injury. While their impact may not be immediately obvious, these moral factors influence the lives of individuals and the practice of psychotherapy. Unfortunately, specific implications and applications for psychotherapy practice are beyond the scope of this article.

Moral Psychology

Moral psychology is the field of study in psychology and philosophy of various topics at the intersection of psychology, ethics, and the philosophy of mind. It originated with Plato and Aristotle, notably in their philosophical works on moral education and later with Thomas Aquinas and faculty psychology on character and virtue (Aquinas, 1966). Today, moral psychology focuses on topics that include moral development, moral judgment, moral reasoning, moral sensitivity, moral responsibility, moral motivation, moral identity, moral action, moral diversity, moral forecasting, moral emotion, and moral character.

While relatively few mental health professionals know much about moral psychology, its research base is ever expanding. Recently, an extensive literature review yielded 1278 relevant research articles published between 1940 and 2017 (Ellemers et al., 2019). Five major research areas were identified: moral reasoning, moral judgments, moral behavior, moral emotions, and moral self-view. This last area, moral self-view, is essentially about moral character.

It is also noteworthy that a number of the studies on moral character and virtue have some serious research design issues. This is the case with some of the most well-known ones such as the Phone Booth Study, the Good Samaritan Study, the Obedience Experiments, and the Stanford Prison Study. Unfortunately, each of these studies of character show that situational factors impact behavior in seemingly arbitrary ways. In these and other studies, disappointing omissions and appalling actions have been induced by relatively minor situational features (Doris, 2015). It was not so much that individuals failed standards for good conduct and character, but that they were easily induced to do so. In response to these and similar studies, a group of so called "character skeptics" have insisted that since these studies found that moral conduct varied widely depending on minor situational circumstances, then "good" character does not seem to predict "good" conduct. It has become obvious that design flaws in these studies account for these unexpected findings.

Positive Psychology

Although Abraham Maslow first coined the term "positive psychology" (1954), it was not until Martin Seligman, as President of the American Psychological Association, challenged psychology and psychotherapy to adopt a positive perspective that the positive psychology movement gained traction (Seligman, 2018; Seligman & Csikszentmihalyi, 2000).

Positive psychology is rooted in moral philosophy, humanistic psychology, and psychotherapy. Its roots in moral philosophy are based in Aristotle's belief that happiness is constituted by rational activity in accordance with "virtue" and the "virtue tradition." This tradition was further developed by theologians and philosophers like Thomas Aquinas (Aquinas, 1966) who emphasized the four cardinal virtues—prudence, temperance, justice, fortitude—and the three theological virtues—faith, hope, charity—which served as a counterpoint to the seven deadly sins or vices centered on self-indulgence and narcissism.

Historically, before the advent of scientific psychology in 1879, virtue remained central to psychology. It was defined as the disposition that moves one to accomplish moral good, or more contemporaneously as a value in action (Peterson & Seligman, 2004). Then, virtue became increasingly "lost" for more than a century as scientific psychology developed. In large part the "recovery" of the virtue tradition occurred as the positive psychology movement emerged. The publication of *Character Strengths and Virtues: A Handbook and Classification* (Peterson & Seligman, 2004) represents a landmark research effort in identifying and classifying the positive psychological traits of persons. In addition, Seligman credits humanistic psychology's emphasis on fulfillment as another influence on the development of his version of positive psychology. Overall, the recovery of the virtue tradition has and will continue to positively influence the practice of psychotherapy.

Moral Injury

Despite these welcome developments, it was the COVID pandemic and the stunning increase in the incidence of moral injury that unexpectedly accelerated the recovery of the moral dimension. Unless psychotherapists, other healing professionals, and researchers had a personal or professional experience with moral injury before, during, or since the pandemic, they were unlikely to consider the moral dimension to be relevant to health and mental health care (Sperry, 2024b). Understandably, the importance and clinical implications of the moral dimension were seldom, if ever, a part of their academic and clinical training.

Moral injury has been defined as an injury to an individual's conscience or moral compass resulting from an act of perceived moral transgression on the part of themselves or others (Litz et al., 2009). The operative word here is conscience. Moral injury produces profound feelings of guilt, shame, moral disorientation, and societal alienation, and often anger and a sense of betrayal toward colleagues, leaders, organizations, or society (Molendijk, 2018). Moral injury is most accurately conceptualized as a moral, psychological, and spiritual trauma (Sperry, 2023).

In the past, moral injury was associated primarily with military personnel. Since the pandemic it is being called an "invisible epidemic affecting million" (Svoboda, 2022) as it affects health care professionals, psychotherapists, first responders, and others experiencing moral distress resulting from actions taken or observations made during traumatic events or circumstances (Koenig & Al Zaben, 2021). While surveys report that more than half of teachers and physicians have experienced it, these figures may be artificially low, since many do not yet have the vocabulary to describe what is happening to them (Svoboda, 2022). This holds true for many if not most mental health professionals who had not learned of it nor its treatment in their graduate training.

A common example of moral injury experienced by psychotherapists prior to, during, and since the pandemic was working in clinic settings with the explicit expectation for therapists to upcode diagnoses and billings with threats of reprisal, including termination, if not done (Griswold et al., 2022). Unexpectedly, during the pandemic there were a number of situations which fostered moral injury. Access to mental health treatment was difficult particularly in the public sector. Teletherapy was another. While teletherapy allowed clients remote access to therapists, issues of privacy and client safety became sources of moral injury. For instance, an adult client may feel unsafe and be hesitant to discuss domestic violence concerns when their partner is within earshot, or a hovering parent might walk into the room and cut off a child client's answer who is remotely conferring with their therapist. In both instances therapists might not be able to effectively protect their clients. Repeated instances could compound and reinforce feelings of guilt and shame that are characteristic of moral injury for therapists (Goldin et al., 2022) and possibly for clients.

Sacred Moral Injury

Sacred moral injury is a form of moral injury (Sperry, 2021b, 2023). It is a trauma syndrome in which the abused individual experiences a violation of conscience and loss of the sense of the sacred because of abuse in a religious context. Lasting spiritual, psychological, biological, social, and institutional effects may result from betrayal of a sacred trust perpetrated by an abuser whom the abused believes represents God (Sperry, 2021b). Because it is more than a psychological condition, it requires that the moral and spiritual dimensions be addressed. Furthermore, because it is both a failure of the individual perpetrator as well as institutional factors, recovery requires that institutional factors be addressed. This means that psychotherapists will likely need to collaborate with other specialized professionals (Sperry, 2021a, 2023).

Relationship of the Moral and Spiritual Dimensions

It seems self-evident that the moral dimension and the spiritual dimension should be closely linked. Just as the link between the psychological and moral dimensions has been strained in psychology and psychotherapy, the link between the moral and spiritual dimensions likewise has been considerably strained. Historically, in the Christian tradition, moral and spiritual theology were a single discipline until they began to separate in the late middle ages. While several factors influenced this split, the result was that morality became the province of the commoners, while spirituality became the province of a small elite. Morality became associated with goodness, moral codes, sin, and living in the real world with daily duties and responsibilities, while spirituality was associated with holiness, altered states, contemplative prayer, and living another worldly existence in a monastery or cloister. In short, the moral dimension is about goodness, while the spiritual dimension is about holiness. Everyone was expected to manifest goodness but only a few would achieve holiness. It should be noted that there was no such split between morality and spirituality in the Eastern religions.

Since the late 1960s there has been a gradual "reconciliation" not only among Western moral and spiritual theologies, but also among spiritual seekers. Now, anyone and everyone can aspire to both goodness and holiness whether they live in a monastery or cloister or not. Consumerism, materialism, and unbridled individualism seem to be fueling the pursuit for spiritual development. Many would say that the spiritual journey requires that the spiritual and moral dimensions be pursued simultaneously and integrated with the other three dimensions of human experience (Gelpi, 1998; Keating, 1998; Wilber, 1999). It appears that many so called "New Age" spiritualities place a premium on the pursuit of holiness while downplaying the pursuit of goodness. Whether spiritual seekers pursue the journey of both goodness and holiness or only the holiness journey is and should be a basic consideration in spiritually integrated psychotherapy and counseling.

Perspective on Spiritual Development

This section describes several perspectives involving the spiritual dimension and the process of spiritual development. Six perspectives can be described: character perspective, ethical perspective, transpersonal perspective, self-transcendence perspective, object relations perspective, and transformation perspective.

Character Perspective

Character can be thought of as that dimension of personality which describes how individuals conduct themselves in interpersonal and organizational situations and shaped through the simultaneous development of self-identity and self-regulation (Cloninger, 2004). When this learning or socialization process is reasonably adequate and without significant developmental arrests, adaptive, creative, and socially responsible or virtuous behavior—called "good character"—can be expected. Generally speaking, an individual with a good character or reputation is considered to be responsible, trustworthy, respectful, fair, caring, and a good citizen, which means they cooperate and play by the rules.

How is character different from personality? Currently, personality is described as the confluence of both character and temperament. Temperament refers to the more biologically or somatically determined aspect of personality, while character refers to the enduring component of personality based on learned, psychosocial influences (Sperry, 2003). Because character is essentially learned, it follows that it can be changed through such processes as psychotherapy. Largely due to the influence of Freud and the subsequent psychodynamic revolution, psychotherapy focused primarily on the dimension of character to the point at which personality essentially became synonymous with character. Before 1980 personality was often conceptualized in "character language," such as the oral character or obsessive character. Descriptions of personality disorders reflected this emphasis on character and psychodynamics (Sperry, 2016). Within the psychoanalytic community, character reflected specific defense mechanisms. Accordingly, the defense of isolation of affect, intellectualization, and rationalization were common in the obsessive character.

Another way of specifying the characterological component of personality is with the term "schema." Whether in the psychoanalytic tradition or the cognitive therapy tradition, schema refers to the basic beliefs individuals use to organize their view of self, the world, and the future. While the centrality of schema has historically been more central to the cognitive tradition and the cognitive-behavioral tradition than to the psychoanalytic tradition, this apparently is changing. While classical psychoanalysts focused on libidinal drives, some modern analysts have focused instead on relational themes, emphasizing the self, the object, and their interaction, while a number of ego psychology and object relations theorists have emphasized schema theory.

While the theoretical and clinical literature on character is quite extensive, the empirical literature is not. On the basis of extensive interview studies, C. Robert Cloninger and his colleagues concluded that individuals with mature personalities tend to be self-reliant, cooperative, and self-transcendent (Cloninger, 2008; Cloninger et al., 1993). In contrast, those with personality disorders were noted to have difficulty with self-acceptance, were intolerant and revengeful toward others, and felt self-conscious and unfulfilled. This suggested that the presence or absence of a personality disorder could be defined in terms of the character dimensions of self-directedness, cooperativeness, and self-transcendence. These three dimensions of character were subsequently incorporated into Cloninger's seven-factor model of temperament and character and can also be measured by the Temperament Character Inventory (Cloninger et al., 1993). Healthy personality reflects positive or elevated scores on these three character dimensions, while personality disorders reflect negative or low scores on them. Furthermore, individuals with a low score on one or more of the character dimensions and increased dysregulation of one or more of the temperament dimensions typically experience either considerable distress or impairment in life functioning or both. For example, the borderline personality disorder would likely rate high in two temperament dimensions but low in character dimensions of self-directedness and cooperation.

Self-Directedness

The basic concept of self-directedness refers to self-determination, which is an individual's ability to control, regulate, and adapt behavior in accordance with one's chosen goals and values. Individuals differ in their capacity for self-determination. Individuals with moderate to high levels of self-determination are considered to be mature, effective, and well-organized, who exhibit self-esteem, are able to admit faults and accept themselves as they are, feel their lives have meaning and purpose, can delay gratification in order to achieve their goals, and take initiative in overcoming challenges. On the other hand, individuals with lower levels of self-determination have low self-esteem, blame others for their problems, feel uncertain of their identity or purpose, and are often reactive, dependent, and resourceless (Cloninger, 2008).

Self-determination can be thought of as having various sub-components such as an internal locus of control, purposefulness, resourcefulness, and self-efficacy. Individuals with an internal locus of control tend to believe that their success is controlled by their own efforts, whereas individuals with an external locus of control tend to believe their success is controlled by factors outside themselves (Cloninger, 2008). Research on locus of control indicates that those with internal locus of control are more responsible and resourceful problem-solvers, whereas others are more alienated and apathetic, tending to blame other people and chance circumstances for problems.

Purposefulness and meaningful goal-direction is a motivating force in mature people. Such purposefulness varies widely between individuals. Initiative and resourceful problem solving, which define effective executives, is an important aspect of mature character. Self-efficacy is also related to resourcefulness and initiative in goal-directed behavior.

Self-esteem and the ability to accept one's limitations unapologetically without fantasies of unlimited ability and ageless youth are crucial aspects of the development of mature self-directed behavior. Individuals with poor adjustment and feelings of inferiority or inadequacy are often reactive and deny, repress, or ignore their faults, wishing to be best at everything always, whereas well-adjusted individuals are able to recognize and admit unflattering truths about themselves. Such positive self-esteem and ability to accept individual limitations is strongly correlated with responsibility and resourcefulness. The absence of self-directedness is the common characteristic of all categories of personality disorder. Regardless of other personality traits or circumstances, a personality disorder is likely to be present if self-directedness is low (Cloninger, 2008).

In short, self-directedness is a developmental process with several dimensions. These include: acceptance of responsibility for one's own choices vs. blaming other individuals and circumstances; identification of individually valued goals and purposes vs. lack of goal direction; development of problem-solving skills and resourcefulness vs. apathy; self-acceptance vs. self-striving; and, congruent second nature vs. personal distrust.

Cooperativeness

The character factor of cooperativeness was formulated to account for individual differences in identification with and acceptance of other people. This factor is a measure of character that is related to agreeability vs. self-centered aggression and hostility. Low cooperativeness scores contribute substantially to the likelihood of a concomitant personality disorder (Cloninger, 2008). In individuals who are high or only moderately low in self-directedness, the probability of a diagnosis of personality disorder was increased by low cooperativeness. All categories of personality disorder are associated with low cooperativeness. Cooperative individuals tend to be socially tolerant, empathic, helpful, and compassionate, while uncooperative individuals tend to be socially intolerant, disinterested in other people, unhelpful, and revengeful. Cooperative individuals are likely to show unconditional acceptance of others, empathy with other's feelings, and willingness to help others achieve their goals without selfish domination. It is not surprising that social acceptance, helpfulness, and concern for the rights of others are correlated with positive self-esteem. Empathy, which is a feeling of unity or identification with others, facilitates improved communication and compassion. Helpful generativity and compassion are frequently noted as signs of maturity in developmental psychology. For instance, such compassion involves the willingness to forgive and be kind to others regardless of their behavior, rather than to seek revenge or to enjoy their embarrassment or suffering; it involves feelings of brotherly love, and the absence of hostility. Mature persons are more likely to seek mutually satisfying, "win-win" solutions to problems than indulge personal gain. In addition, religious traditions also emphasize the notion of "pure-hearted" acceptance of principles that cannot be broken without the inevitability of grave consequences for individuals and society (Cloninger, 2008).

In short, cooperativeness is a developmental process with several dimensions. These include: social acceptance vs. intolerance; empathy vs. social disinterest; helpfulness vs. unhelpfulness; compassion vs. revengefulness; and pure-hearted principles vs. self-advantage (Cloninger et al., 1993).

Self-Transcendence

Self-transcendence and character traits associated with spirituality are typically neglected in systematic research and omitted from personality inventories (Cloninger, 2004). Nevertheless, observations about self-transcendence and self-actualization abound. Specifically, the subjective experiences and changes in behavior of people who attain the state of self-transcendence as a result of insight and meditation techniques have been well documented in the transpersonal psychology literature. The stable self-forgetfulness of self-transcendent individuals has been described as the same as experienced transiently when individuals are totally absorbed, intensely concentrated, and fascinated by one thing, such that they may forget where they are and lose all sense of the passage of time. Such absorption often leads to "transpersonal" identification with things outside of the individual self. The person may identify or feel a sense of spiritual union with anything or everything.

Self-transcendence is considerably lower in psychiatric inpatients than in adults in the general community (Cloninger, 2008). Except for individuals with schizoid and schizotypal personality disorder, self-transcendence was not a distinguishing factor between patients with and without personality disorders. Self-transcendence can be particularly useful in distinguishing schizoid from schizotypal patients because the latter tend to endorse questions about extrasensory perception and other aspects of self-transcendence. Also, individuals with schizoid personality disorder tended to exhibit low self-transcendence. In contrast, self-directedness and cooperativeness were low in all personality disorders (Svrakic et al., 1993).

Considered as a developmental process, self-transcendence has various dimensions. These dimensions can be simplified to some basic experiences and behaviors that have been described in a broad spectrum: self-forgetful vs. self-conscious experience; transpersonal identification vs. self-differentiation; and spiritual acceptance vs. rational materialism. Thus, it seems that psychologically healthy spiritual seekers would manifest appreciably more self-transcendence than less mature individuals (Cloninger, 2008).

Ethical Perspective

Psychotherapists and counselors are enjoined by the codes of ethics of their professional organizations and, in some cases by state licensing boards, to act ethically in their professional roles. Professional codes of ethics and state statutes are not intended to address all possible ethical and moral matters. Since research indicates that most clients expect helping professionals to assist them with moral issues and dilemmas (Richardson et al., 1999), it would not be unreasonable to anticipate that spiritual seekers and other clients with religious issues may need to or want to address ethical and moral matters in the course of therapy. Many questions arise. Is it ethical for therapists and counselors to discuss such matters? Should spiritual seekers and other clients be counseled to act ethically in their professional and personal lives? Is it or might it be unethical for psychotherapists and counselors to broach some ethical matters with spiritual seekers? Obviously, there are no easy answers to these questions. An ethical perspective is much broader than the provisions of a code of ethics.

Developing an ethical perspective involves not only learning ethical theories and principles but also incorporating such principles in one's own philosophy of life and then acting on these principles in one's daily personal and professional life. It means becoming a person of good character, i.e., someone who acts virtuously. In other words, developing an ethical perspective means becoming a "virtuous therapist."

The ethical theory that emphasizes character and virtue is *virtue ethics*. Virtue ethics defines certain traits of character which are understood to make one a morally good person. While rule and principle ethics focuses on morally good actions, virtue ethics focuses on morally good character. For virtue ethics the question is not: Is this action moral? but is rather: What kind of person am I becoming? According to virtue ethics, moral virtues are states of character concerned with controlling and directing not only one's thoughts and rational processes but also one's emotions and feelings. The repeated performance of virtuous actions leads to the acquisition of virtue. A morally virtuous person aims at morally good ends rather than being clever and goal oriented.

What, then, is a virtuous therapist? A virtuous therapist is a professional individual of good moral character whose actions reflect both the practice of virtue and their ability to incorporate professional standards in daily practice.

> A morally virtuous psychotherapist would seek to be honest with her clients not merely because this behavior is itself a way toward the goal of maximizing profit—supposing that "morality pays" by attracting clients—but because honesty itself is to be valued.
>
> (Cohen & Cohen, 1999, pp. 19–20)

These authors contend that a rule of principle ethics, i.e., the framework for professional codes of ethics, is a woefully inadequate basis for the ethical practice of counseling and psychotherapy. Instead, they propose a composite ethical theory that recognizes that moral action involves not only rules or professional standards but also emotions, human relatedness, virtue, and sensitivity to the nuances of a specific individual context.

Practicing psychotherapists and those in training often view ethics as a necessary evil. At a time when therapists are increasingly concerned about ethics complaints and malpractice suits, ethics is often taught as a defensive or risk-management strategy. This represent the negative perspective on ethics. On the other hand, positive ethics (Handlesman et al., 2002) counterbalances this view. It supplements negative ethics in acknowledging that risk-management is a necessary consideration, but it is not a sufficient condition for ethical decisions. Positive ethics views ethical values rather than laws and codes as the starting point for ethical practice. It emphasizes ethical sensitivity as essential for professional practice and considers ethical reasoning and decision-making to be contextual and not simply a linear process. In addition, positive ethics endorses ongoing self-care and personal and professional growth as essential to ethically sensitive, effective, professional practice (Sperry, 2007).

Transpersonal Perspective

Transpersonal psychology is broad term for approaches to therapy which focus on the spiritual dimension, i.e., consciousness, mystical experiences, altered states of consciousness and on questions relating to the value of life and the meaning of existence. Transpersonal psychology is considered by many to be the "fourth force" in psychology following psychoanalysis, behavior therapy, and humanistic psychology. Its precursors are to be found in Eastern religions and in the West. Both Augustine and Thomas Aquinas can be considered as early thinkers who combined a psychological awareness with a spiritual and philosophical focus. More recently, William James anticipated the claims of current transpersonal psychology that altered states of consciousness can be induced and can give access to special knowledge which cannot be gained through ordinary conscious processes.

In his articulation of analytic psychology, Carl Jung developed several ideas that are centrally relevant to transpersonal psychology. These include the Self, the collective unconscious, archetypes, and the process of individuation. Central to Jung's approach to psychotherapy is the value and importance of the spiritual dimension of human existence. Individuation, for example, includes the reintegration of the spiritual as well as the psychic.

Other approaches included under the umbrella of transpersonal psychology are Roberto Assagioli's Psychosynthesis, Stanislav Grof's Holotropic Model, existential transpersonal psychotherapy, transpersonal psychoanalytic psychotherapy, and body-centered transpersonal approaches (Cortright, 1997).

Perhaps the most known and influential theorist in transpersonal psychology in recent decades is Ken Wilber. He was the first to systematically demonstrate how the consciousness of mystical states related to the consciousness of neurosis and psychosis. Wilber has proposed and refined a Spectrum Model (1977, 1995, 1999; Wilber et al., 1986) which is an integrating structure in which all competing psychological systems and spiritual traditions are seen as containing partial and complementary truths about human consciousness. It is the foundation for his theories of development, psychopathology, and psychotherapeutic treatment. Reasoning that consciousness is composed of many different levels and that different psychotherapies are related to specific levels of his spectrum model, Wilber posited that traditional Western psychotherapy systems are directed to the lower end of this spectrum with psychoses representing the most limited level of consciousness, while the middle portions of the spectrum involve the neuroses and existential levels. Spiritual systems and transpersonally oriented approaches represent the upper levels of the spectrum where consciousness is the fullest. Based on this formulation, Wilber concludes, some would say erroneously that psychology and spirituality are integrally related into a single line or spectrum of consciousness.

Today, there is an emerging consensus in transpersonal psychology that "the psychological and spiritual dimensions of human experience are different, though at times overlapping, with the spiritual as foundational" (Cortright, 1997, p. 237). In its earliest formulation, transpersonal psychology assumed that the psychological and spiritual lines of development were identical or formed one continuous line or spectrum (Wilber, 1977). It was also assumed that an individual would first pursue psychological integration and then move on to spiritual integration. Usually that meant beginning in psychotherapy, and when successfully completed taking up spiritual practices and working with a spiritual guide. Basically, it was believed that only those who were sufficiently healed and psychologically integrated were capable of true spiritual development and realization.

Such beliefs do not match current clinical research and clinical practice. Some clients with highly advanced spiritual development may function at primitive levels psychologically and interpersonally, while psychological development far exceeds spiritual development in others. Then there are other clients where spiritual and psychological development are more balanced. Similarly, history records a number of disturbed, psychotic, and neurotic saints and spiritually advanced individuals. Furthermore, to presume that all saints, sages, and shamans throughout history have somehow spontaneously achieved a working through of childhood traumas and unconscious defenses leading to a high level of psychological integration prior to their spiritual development is extremely dubious (Cortright, 1997).

Transpersonally oriented clinicians have observed that psychological and spiritual development are composed of multiple and complex developmental pathways that mutually interact but are different. In other words, the spiritual emerges in and through psychological work rather than after it. Furthermore, clinicians espousing a transpersonal approach to psychotherapy tend to view their work within a context of spiritual unfolding since the basic assumption of transpersonal psychology is that individuals are spiritual beings rather than simply a self or psychological ego. Another basic tenet of transpersonal psychology is that achieving psychological integration is not essential for spiritual realization, nor does spiritual realization bring about psychological integration. Nevertheless, psychotherapy can be quite helpful for those on the spiritual journey in contending with avoidances and unconscious defenses, just as the inner deepening resulting from spiritual practices can be helpful in one's psychological work. In short, each can help the other but neither one is required for the other (Cortright, 1997).

Clinicians practicing transpersonal psychotherapy note that it is possible to pursue psychological wholeness and spiritual wholeness simultaneously, and that while "one or the other may predominate at times, it is a *both/and* process rather than *either/or* or even *first one/then the other*" (Cortright, 1997, p. 234). Psychotherapy may facilitate spiritual unfolding by breaking unconscious and defensive patterns and processes, and in passing through the self to find the spirit deeper within more skillfully than by spiritual practices alone. Finally, since it aims at expanding consciousness, psychotherapy can be thought of as a spiritual activity of sorts.

Consciousness is where spirituality and psychotherapy intersect. Both are methods for exploring, deepening, and expanding consciousness. Transpersonally oriented psychotherapy is primarily focused on consciousness. Such therapy is the exploration of consciousness and the contents of that consciousness. It has been said that the reason most individuals seek treatment is that they are stuck and underdeveloped, meaning they cannot function with full consciousness. Such individuals have blind spots or defenses which block awareness of essential aspects of themselves: feelings, bodily sensations, thoughts, etc. This blocked awareness results in symptoms, self-defeating patterns, and disease with life. Consciousness involves all the dimensions of human experience: cognitive, affective, moral, somatic, and spiritual. And the greater or more complete the level of consciousness, the greater the likelihood of psychological and spiritual change and development (Cortright, 1997).

It is a tenet of transpersonally oriented psychotherapy that engaging the consciousness of the client is considered the key to change and growth. Nevertheless, the clinician's own consciousness, presence, and inner clarity "provide the guiding light for the therapeutic journey" (Cortright, 1997, p. 238). It has been said that the consciousness of the clinician functions like a subtle energy field in inducing the client into a deeper experience of being.

Finally, transpersonal psychotherapies tend to be experiential. "It is only the experience of spirit that satisfies the soul's quest, and only by plunging into the depth of the inner heart and feeling can the realm of spiritual being be plumbed" (Cortright, 1997, p. 239). By viewing consciousness as multidimensional, the central focus on the client's consciousness implies an experiential process that involves the whole person.

Allowing for different dimensions of human experience in the therapeutic context, i.e., the affective, moral, intellectual, or the somatic dimension, means that an openness exists to alternate modes of experiencing beyond that of a traditional psychotherapy focused primarily or only on words.

Nevertheless, words are important, and the articulation of inner experience can be of inestimable value in "skillfully traversing inner worlds of feeling and meaning. Only when words become launching pads into deeper experiencing is their potential realized" (Cortright, 1997, p. 239).

According to Cortright (1997), the transpersonal paradigm has seriously challenged the distinction between psychology and spirituality, science, and spirit, and the sacred and the profane. By insisting that the roots of the psyche are spiritual, that the basis of consciousness is a spiritual reality, and by adopting a wider view of the self than traditional psychology, transpersonal psychology offers a more fully integrative and inclusive view of human experience than other psychological systems. As such it has considerable value to clinicians who choose to incorporate the spiritual dimension in counseling and psychotherapy.

Self-Transcendence Perspective

There is much in the Eastern and Western spiritual traditions and in the psychological and literature on the self. For the purpose of this chapter, only the concepts of true self, false self, and self-transcendence will be discussed. False self was the term Winnicott (1960) used to describe the defensive structure that develops during infancy when there is not a "good enough mother" to provide the nurturance and the facilitative conditions necessary for the development of the true self. As noted in Chapter 2, Keating describes the false self as the self that develops to cope with the emotional trauma of early childhood. It seeks happiness in satisfying the instinctual needs of survival, esteem, and control, and bases its self-worth on cultural or group identification. In contrast the true self is one's participation in the divine life manifested in one's uniqueness. Wilber (1999) makes a similar distinction between the false self and what he calls the real self. Interestingly, Thomas Merton's (1974) notion of the false self suggests that it is a failure in self-transcendence. For most spiritual writers, the movement from the false self to the real or true self involves the process of self-transcendence.

The concept of self-transcendence has much to offer for the clinician seeking to incorporate the spiritual dimension in psychotherapy. It is a term used widely in philosophy, theology, and psychology as a conceptual bridge between two seemingly contradictory constructs. For example, in theology, self-transcendence provides a way of understanding the apparent contradiction between love of self and love of others, while in philosophy it links autonomy and beneficence, and in psychology, it bridges the apparent contradiction of independence with intimacy.

Self-transcendence has been described as the most basic human desire and drive to move beyond or transcend the self (Cloninger, 2004; Conn,

1997; Lonergan, 1972). It is the most basic and encompassing of all human drives and is the source of everything that is uniquely human. Theologically, this drive represents divine life within a person and is fully realized in a personal relationship with God. Psychologically, self-transcendence differs from both self-sacrifice—when understood as a denial or other negation of the true self—and self-fulfillment—when understood as a collection of desires to be filled. "In contrast, the experience of self-transcendence supports the gospel's paradoxical view that authentic self-realization results not from a self-centered effort to fulfill one's every wish, but from a movement beyond oneself in an attempt to realize the good of others" (Conn, 1998, p. 324).

Self-transcendence is reflected in all the dimensions of human experience: affective, cognitive, moral, and spiritual or religious. Conn notes that the structure of the desire for self-transcendence,

> because it is conscious, also delineates the self by specifying distinct levels of consciousness... all interrelated as successive phases in the unfolding of the single desire of the human spirit for self-transcendence. From bodily nerves and psychic images, through sensitivity and intelligence to free choice and love, the radical desire for self-transcendence unifies the self in its heuristic dynamism and integrates it in its realization.
>
> (Conn, 1998, p. 325)

Thus, in addition to cognitive self-transcendence there is affective self-transcendence. It is present when individuals break out of their social isolation and act spontaneously for themselves as well as for others. "Affective self-transcendence thus grounds the real possibility of achieving moral self-transcendence in decisions to act for value. And, finally, beyond cognitive, affective, and moral self-transcendence, there is the possibility of religious self-transcendence" (Conn, 1998, p. 326).

What are the implications of self-transcendence for clinical practice? Self-transcendence is distinctly relational, and this relational understanding is reflected in the basic goal and strategy of spiritually integrated psychotherapy and counseling. The basic goal is: "empowering persons to realize even greater self-transcendence in their lives. To a great degree, this means helping people to liberate themselves from the countless defense mechanisms and other distortions of personality that constitute a drag on the desire for self-transcendence" (Conn, 1998, pp. 326–327). The strategy of therapy is to "deal with those limitations in order to increase the probability of self-transcendence in individual lives" (Conn, 1998, p. 327). In short, the goal of is to facilitate the development of self-transcendence.

Object Relations Perspective

Object relations theory is a relatively recent development in psychoanalytic thinking. It has made a major contribution to the understanding of an important component of the spiritual dimension: the formation of God representations (Guntrip, 1969). It has been observed that negative God representations can and do block progress on the spiritual journey.

> [The] spiritual journey may be blocked if we carry negative attitudes toward God from early childhood. If we are afraid of God or see God as an angry father-figure, a suspicious policeman, or a harsh judge, it will be hard to develop enthusiasm, or even an interest, in the journey.
>
> (Keating, 1998, p. 22)

Thus, it is important for those practicing spiritually oriented therapy and counseling to assess and to endeavor to modify negative God representations.

Object relations theory takes its name from "object relations" or "object representations." Object relations signifies the child's internalization of early significant individuals and the relational dynamics with such individuals, and the continuing psychic influence of these internalized object relations. It describes three phases of early childhood development: symbiosis, separation-individuation, and object constancy (Mahler et al., 1975). The basic development of one's God representation occurs during these phases, and specifically involves transitional objects.

Symbiosis

This is the stage of development wherein a child develops a sense of themselves in relation to other persons. The child needs caretakers, usually the parents who, from birth, will provide a self-regulating or "holding environment" for them. A holding environment is the parents' capacity to communicate to the child the message: "I'm strong enough to take care of you and protect you. I'm going to hold you. I'll take care of you. I'll comfort you. I'll soothe you." Things are perfect in the beginning, as the child's sense of self is merged with that the parents. The child most likely believes they are in control of everything, and they are as long as the parents are at their beck and call.

Separation-Individuation

A major change in the child's developmental needs are noted around the age of 10–14 months just as life begins expecting the child to gradually assume the holding and self-regulating function themselves. However, the child is not ready to direct assume this responsibility so they essentially "trick" themselves; it is as if they say to themselves, "Let me take that holding function that's not under my control, but transfer it to an object, that is going to be much more clearly under my control." Their blanket or teddy bear not only will be under their total control, but it soothes their anxiety of growing and becoming a separate person. There is a distortion of external reality because the child treats the object with the properties that previously were the properties of the parent, the one who really had the soothing capacity. Transitional objects allow all of us to progressively exercise this holding/soothing function by proxy. Transitional objects help one in exploring one's environment and learning how to master it. They represent an intermediate step in the process of internalizing this self-regulating capacity. By age three or four the child has developed enough capacity to understand and master the environment around them that they are now able reduce their distortion of reality (Mahler et al., 1975).

A transitional object is an intermediate experience between self and object which serves to soothe separation anxiety and facilitate individuality, the sense of one's own unique identity. A related term is "transitional phenomena" which includes both transitional objects and "transitional modes." Transitional modes refer to later life experiences in normal persons. A transitional mode is a resting place or temporary suspension of higher ego functions like logical thinking which can free the person to deeply experience other modes of reality, such as music, the performing arts, or creative expression (Mahler et al., 1975). In essence, the transitional mode has a soothing function, but for the purpose of further self-integration and self-transformation.

When speaking of God, the term transitional object is not used. This is because God is not an object, but rather a special type of object representation created by the child in that unique psychic space where transitional objects—whether toys, blankets or mental representations—are provided with their powerfully real illusory lives. He is a transitional phenomenon because he does not follow the usual course of other transitional objects. Generally, over the course of life the transitional object loses its meaning and value as the individual becomes their own self-regulating person. On the other hand, instead of losing meaning God becomes more meaningful over the years. When other transitional objects can be repressed or even forgotten, God cannot be fully repressed. God is always potentially available for further love, acceptance, anger, or even rejection. God is psychically useful for us. He remains a transitional phenomenon at the service of gaining leverage with oneself, with others and with life itself. According to Rizzuto (1979, 1991), God, like the teddy bear, has obtained half of his stuffing or holding function from his parents, and the other half comes from the child's capacity to "create" a God according to their own needs (1979, p. 179). This process of creating and finding God—this transitional phenomenon—never ceases in the course of life. It is further shaped and reinforced by culture. God has a special place in our culture such as in the dedication of our Constitution, our money system (coins and bills), holidays like Easter and Christmas, church buildings, tax credits, and the like.

Object Constancy

Assuming the child more or less successfully navigates through the first three to four years through to object constancy—the child's capacity to enter into stable and loving relationships with people perceived as fully separate and independent from themselves—the child's image of God becomes less concrete and more conceptual. This cognitive development is facilitated, in large part, through fantasy. The earliest stage of fantasy is the imaginary companion (Rizzuto, 1979). An imaginary friend or companion helps to solve daily problems in relating to others. The child's newly developing imagination serves as a buffer in the harsh world the child begins to experience. The imaginary companion plays a specific positive role in child development and once that role is fulfilled it tends to disappear. Specifically, it can serve as a scapegoat for badness or negative impulses, a playmate when no one else is available, a confirmer of the child's sense of omnipotent control, etc. The nature and structure of fantasy elaborates as the child grows and develops. For a male child, the sequence from three years onward is: monster—devil—hero—super hero (Rizzuto, 1979).

Imaginary companions and monsters help the child to tolerate his badness, rageful impulses, deceptions, and frustrations. They also represent the child's grandiose sense of power. It's been said that monsters help the child know, master, and forget the monster the child feels or fears himself to be. At the age of two the child learns that God is taken seriously by adults, that God will punish him, bless him, or love him. Though the child can't see God, be comes to sense that God is powerful, everywhere, and rules everything. Of necessity, the child's God image utilizes the representation of the most significant parent available at the moment.

At two and a half years of age the child discovers that things are made by people and then he questions how things like clouds or oceans are made and hears from another that God made them. The child needs to imagine that God is formidable to make big things like clouds. This kind of questioning and wonder continues through age 5 (Rizzuto, 1979).

At age six the child grasps the concept of God as creator of the world, of animals and beautiful things, and he begins to develop a feeling relationship with God. Prayer becomes important and he believes that prayer will be the answer. God's counterpart at this stage is the Devil. It probably reflects the child's hostile, sadistic parental representation. Later, as the child begins to experience disillusionment with his parents, he is likely to have elaborate fantasies about having a set of ideal, imaginary parents, and fantasies of having a twin or a guardian angel to play with and guide him. Actually, it may be that bible stories and pictures of heaven and a better life serve the same function as some of these fantasies.

Thus, by about the age of six a formal God representation is formed. Rizzuto (1979) notes that finally together with this colorful crowd of characters and amidst fantasies, wishes, fears, and sexual preoccupation, God formally arrives. God acquires a special and superior status because of multiple sociocultural religious, ritualistic, and family factors. This representation continues to be modified and reinforced throughout latency and adolescence particularly with images of heroes and super heroes: rock stars, sports figures, movie stars, and even politicians.

To summarize then, objects theory suggests this developmental sequence of the God representation: as the child grows and develops a transitional reality, an intermediate space in which he can momentarily shift from being centered and dependent on his mother to the larger outside world. When he is between the ages of approximately two and a half to five years old, he experiences this transitional reality as one which is "alive" with imagined people and monsters. These images provoke intense feelings of fright and vulnerability that heretofore had been buffered by mother's deeply reassuring words and very presence. Often in this period God arrives on the scene of the youngster's consciousness. Because of what he has been taught by others, God becomes supreme, God is the ultimate male. He is the strongest, the biggest, the best. As a result, monsters now lose their terrifying power and grip over the child's imagination. By the age of five or six, the young boy has internalized a simple cognitive notion of God which becomes part of how the child sees himself in the world. As the boy grows and begins the process of separating from his mother, he now can join the larger, male-oriented world of his particular culture. This process is facilitated because he has both his own father and a male God with whom to relate. It appears forming a God representation is somewhat different for a young girl (Heller, 1986), which this theory does not go into in detail.

If the developmental process proceeds normally, the child learns to differentiate the earthly father from the Heavenly Father who is all-knowing, all-powerful, and all-protective. In this process of differentiation, the earthly parent becomes less divine and more a fallible human being. In this critical time, the God image can become confused and distorted if differentiation is poorly accomplished. Distortions can also occur if the quality and consistency of his bonding to mother is compromised. The parent's own image of God also influences the formation of the young male's image of God. To the extent that the parental God image is relatively mature and that parent–adolescent relations are relatively harmonious, the adolescent is likely to have a realistic, balanced, and healthy God image. But to the extent that the parental God representation is distorted, and parent–adolescent relations are ambivalent and convicted, the young man is likely to develop a distorted representation and style of relating to God (Heinrichs, 1982). The quality of the relationship between parents cannot be overemphasized.

Clinical Implications

What is the clinical value of God representations? Rizzuto (1991) describes the potential therapeutic value of clinicians understanding their clients' God representation:

> Careful exploration of the subjective description of an individual's God may reveal precious information about the type of psychic and interpersonal events that led to the particular characteristics attributed to God... An understanding of an individual's God representation may provide, in turn, information about his or her psychic history and the types of obstacles that interfere with potential belief, or with the updating of the God representation. I am referring now to [intrapsychic] processes... that may obstruct the transformation of the God representation and of religious behavior to a level more compatible with the individual's developmental moment.
>
> (Rizzuto, 1991, pp. 56–57)

Transformation Perspective

Transformation, also known as conversion, is a central focus of spiritually integrated psychotherapy as well as spiritual guidance (Gratton, 1992, p. 122). Conversion can have several meanings and definitions (Rambo, 1993), from a change in religious affiliation to significant life transformation. The definition used here was first articulated by Bernard Lonergan (1972) and amplified and extended by Donald Gelpi (1998). Gelpi defines conversion as the decision to repudiate irresponsible behavior and to take responsibility for the subsequent development of some aspect of one's own experience. Two forms of conversions are initial and ongoing. Initial conversions involve moving from irresponsible to responsible behaviors in some dimension of experience, such as the affective, intellectual, or religious dimension. Ongoing conversion is the interaction between various dimensions of conversions and the continuous process of change throughout life. Gelpi presumes that ongoing conversion will be integral, meaning that there is a commitment to living out these fundamental changes in all areas of life: affective, moral, intellectual, religious, and sociopolitical. A somatic dimension of conversion has recently been added (Sperry, 1999). These six dimensions are described below.

Affective Conversion

Affective conversion involves taking responsibility for one's emotions and requires the willingness to acknowledge and forgive past hurts. Growing in emotional maturity is incompatible with racism, sexism, militarism, and other forms of social bigotry. Affective conversion requires moving from a self-oriented focus to the love of others. It presumes some measure of repentance, particularly the renouncement of the rage, fear, and guilt that separates the individual from God. As these negative affects are brought to healing in faith, individuals need to learn to own and express their positive affects, including love, friendship, compassion, sensitivity, and enthusiasm.

Ongoing affective conversion may require "sound spiritual direction and psychotherapy when necessary or helpful" (Gelpi, 1998, p. 197). Ongoing affective conversion demands a willingness to face one's own unconscious capacity for violence and destructive behaviors. Forgiveness is essential in this type of ongoing conversion as it inaugurates a new level of conscious integration. The measure of growth in this area of conversion is the increasing capacity to see God in all things, to respond with enthusiasm to the vision of the Kingdom, to translate that enthusiasm by working to bring about God's will on earth, and by sharing one's possessions and life with those in greatest need (Gelpi, 1998).

Moral Conversion

Moral conversions challenge the person to move from simple gratification of immediate personal needs to living by consistent principles of ethics and justice. It assumes a formed conscience, i.e., that individuals can distinguish right from wrong, and the capacity to deal with moral dilemmas and challenges faced in everyday life. It leads one to treat other persons as persons made in the image of God and to foster the common good. Ongoing moral conversions challenge and eliminate the likelihood and impulse to selfishness, acts of deceit, violation of laws and statutes, sins of omission, spitefulness, and destructive behavior. It requires that the individual grasps the practical consequences of dedication to the common good (Gelpi, 1998). It also requires an increasing capacity to criticize false value systems that corrupt one's conscience.

Intellectual Conversion

Intellectual conversion requires an individual to be able to understand and express their relationship to God in personally meaningful terms. It is not simply the capacity to recite passages from scripture or doctrinal statements, but rather to pursue the truth and confront any form of false ideology and personal prejudice that rationalizes immoral conduct. Ongoing intellectual conversion requires that individuals develop a balanced philosophy of life. In the process of ongoing intellectual conversion, they should have moved beyond mere knowledge of religious beliefs and tenets and have come to a personal appropriation of these beliefs. In terms of Fowler's stages of faith development, Gelpi contends that initial conversion requires at least at the synthetic-conventional level of faith, while ongoing conversion requires movement to or beyond the individuate-reflective level of faith (Gelpi, 1998). Accordingly, individuals would be able to sufficiently understand theological issues and controversies surrounding their faith tradition to formulate their own position or response to these issues.

Religious Conversion

This form of conversion challenges individuals to live for the true God rather than idols. While the dynamics of religious conversion are the same for all of the great religious traditions, Gelpi emphasizes Christian conversion where the goal is a commitment to unconditionally finding God's will revealed in the person of Jesus, and his vision of the Kingdom of God. True religious conversion transcends the concerns of narrow, denominational sectarianism, since the religiously converted individuals are committed to reaching out in compassion to anyone in need regardless of race, creed, or class (Gelpi, 1998). Repentance sensitizes the convert to natural beauty and Divine beauty. Strategies for ongoing religious conversion include a regular prayer and meditation, fasting, spiritual reading, and almsgiving. Finally, religious conversion mediates between affective and moral conversion.

Sociopolitical Conversion

While affective, intellectual, moral, and religious conversion are personally focused, sociopolitical conversion is socially focused, meaning it involves engaging social systems, such as corporations and government, to be accountable and responsible for their actions. Beyond personal moral principles, sociopolitical conversion generates its own moral principles. These include the right of all persons to share in the good things of life, and the principles of legal, distributive, and commutative justice. It challenges individuals to resist the social pressure to think and act with political correctness. Ongoing sociopolitical conversion involves a commitment to a reexamination of one's biases and prejudices against certain groups and subcultures and challenges a lifestyle of convenience and personal luxury that fosters insensitivity to the needs of the poor (Gelpi, 1998).

Somatic Conversion

Somatic refers to the human body, to body structure, and to bodily sensations, feelings—including sexual feelings—and memories. It involves the physical expression or manifestations of an individual's soul and spirit (Sperry, 1999). Subsequently, when the body is injured, as in a motor vehicle accident or by a stroke, this somatic expression becomes distorted and limited, and the individual may experience a reduced capacity in the expression of his or her full personhood. Likewise, if the individual's soul and spirit is pained, such as in mourning the loss of a loved one, a predictable somatic expression would be symptoms of grief and depression. Somatic conversion is primarily about wellness. Wellness is similar but not synonymous with health, because wellness can coexist with chronic illness, disease, and even terminal illness. Individuals with a high level of somatic conversion can be expected to experience a high level of wellness irrespective of their health status. To experience a high level of wellness, individuals need ongoing conversion in the somatic dimension. Preventive measures such as proper diet, exercise, and sleep can contribute effectively to one's degree of vitality, somatic wholeness, and conversion. However, preventive measures do not guarantee wellness since wellness is not dependent on health status. Finally, their individuals with a high level of somatic conversion are likely to have life-affirming attitudes toward their bodies—including sexuality—and will have integrated these attitudes into their philosophy of life (Sperry, 1999).

Concluding Note

Chapter 2 has described six perspectives on the spiritual dimension as they relate to the process of spiritual development. Presumably each of these perspectives can contribute something to one's understanding and appreciation of the process of spiritual development. What potential clinical value do these various perspectives offer for the practice of spiritually integrated psychotherapy and counseling? Table 2.1 indicates some key insights that are applicable in incorporating the spiritual dimension in a clinical setting.

Table 2.1 Key Insights for Incorporating Various Perspectives of the Spiritual Dimension

Perspectives	*Insights for Incorporating the Spiritual Dimension*
Object-Relations	Object relations are internalized relationships and God representations (images) reflect early parental object relations. Negative God images negatively impact the spiritual journey and can be modified in therapy.
Self-Transcendence	Spiritual hunger reflects one's basic drive for self-transcendence. Spiritual development means increasing self-transcendence which requires balancing autonomy and relationship. The goal of spiritual counseling and therapy is to facilitate the process of self-transcendence.
Transpersonal	Consciousness is the central concept. The spiritual and psychological dimensions differ but overlap; and the spiritual dimension is central to all human experience. Spiritual emergencies differ from psychopathology. *Self-transcendence* is a function of increased consciousness.
Character	Personality consists of character and temperament. Self-responsibility, cooperation, and *self-transcendence* are the basic components of character. Low levels of these components are associated with personality disorders.
Ethical	A virtuous therapist is a professional person of good moral character whose actions reflect both the practice of virtue and the ability to incorporate professional ethical standards in daily practice.
Conversion	Conversion means self-transformation. Self-transformation requires moving from irresponsible to responsible behavior in each of the dimensions of human experience; a continuous process of change.

References

Allport, G. (1937). *Personality: A psychological interpretation*. Holt.

American Psychiatric Association. (2022). *Diagnostic and statistical manual of mental disorders*, 5th ed., Text revision. American Psychiatric Association.

Aquinas, T. (1966). *Treatise on the virtues*. Prentice-Hall.

Cloninger, C. R. (2004). *Feeling good: The science of well-being*. Oxford University Press.

Cloninger, C. R. (2008). The science of well-being: An integrated approach to mental health and its disorders. *World Psychiatry*, *5*(2), 71–76.

Cloninger, R., Svrakic, D., & Przybeck, T. (1993). A psychobiological model of temperament and character. *Archives of General Psychiatry*, *50*, 975–990.

Cohen, E., & Cohen, G. (1999). *The virtuous therapist: Ethical practice of counseling and psychotherapy*. Brooks/Cole.

Conn, W. (1997). Understanding the self in self-transcendence. *Pastoral Psychology, 46*(1), 3–17.
Conn, W. (1998). Self-transcendence, the true self, and self-love. *Pastoral Psychology, 46*(5), 323–332.
Cortright, B. (1997). *Psychotherapy and spirit: Theory and practice in transpersonal psychotherapy*. State University of New York Press.
Cushman, P. (1990). Why the self is empty. *American Psychologist, 45*, 599–611.
Cushman, P. (1995). *Constructing the self, constructing America: A cultural history of psychotherapy*. Addison-Wesley.
Doris, J. M. (2015). *Talking to ourselves: Reflection, ignorance, and agency*. Oxford University Press.
Ellemers, N., Van Der Toorn, J., Paunov, Y., & Van Leeuwen, T. (2019). The psychology of morality: A review and analysis of empirical studies published from 1940 through 2017. *Personality and Social Psychology Review, 23*(4), 332–366.
Engel, G. L. (1977). The need for a new medical model: A challenge for biomedicine. *Science, 196*(4286), 129–136.
Frank, J. (1978). *Psychotherapy and the human predicament*. Shocken.
Gelpi, G. (1998). *The conversion experience*. Paulist Press.
Goldin, D., Cabán-Alemán, C., & von Harscher, H. (2022). Moral injury and telemental health services: An overview on clinician impact. *Journal of Psychosocial Nursing and Mental Health Services, 60*(11), 49–54.
Gratton, C. (1992). *The art of spiritual guidance: A contemporary approach to growing in the spirit*. Crossroad.
Griswold, S., Manzur, M. K., & Dean, W. (2022). What should clinicians do when health services are improperly billed in their names? *AMA Journal of Ethics, 24*(11), 1049–1055.
Guntrip, H. (1969). Religion in relation to personal integration. *British Journal of Medical Psychology, 42*, 323–333.
Handlesman, M., Knapp, S., & Gottlieb, M. (2002). In C. Snyder & S. Lopez (Eds.), *Handbook of positive psychology* (pp. 731–744). Oxford.
Heinrichs, D. (1982). Our father which art in heaven: Parataxic distortions in the image of God. *Journal of Psychology and Theology, 10*, 120–129.
Heller, D. (1986). *The children's God*. University of Chicago Press.
Hillman, J., & Ventura, M. (1992). *We've had a hundred years of psychotherapy and the world's getting worse*. Harper San Francisco.
Keating, T. (1998). *Invitation to love: The way of Christian contemplation*. Continuum.
Koenig, H. (1999). *The healing power of faith: Science explores medicine's last great frontier*. Simon & Shuster.
Koenig, H. G., & Al Zaben, F. (2021). Moral injury: An increasingly recognized and widespread syndrome. *Journal of Religion and Health, 60*(5), 2989–3011.
Levin, J. (1994). Religion and health: Is there an association, is it valid, and is it casual? *Social Science and Medicine, 38*, 1475–1484.
Levin, J., & Chatters, L. (1998). Research on religion and mental health: An overview and empirical findings and theoretical issues. In H. Koenig (Ed.), *Handbook of religion and mental health* (pp. 34–50). Academic Press.

Litz, B., Stein, N., Delaney, E., Lebowitz, L., Nash, W., Silva, C., & Maguen, S. (2009). Moral injury and moral repair in war veterans: A preliminary model and intervention strategy. *Clinical Psychology Review*, *29*(8), 695–706.

Lonergan, B. (1972). *Method in theology*. Herder & Herder.

Mahler, M., Pine, F., & Bergman, A. (1975). *The psychological birth of the human infant*. International Universities Press.

Maslow, A. (1954). *Motivation and personality*. Harper & Row.

Menninger, K., & Tiedemann, K. (1973). *Whatever became of sin?* Hawthorn Books.

Merton, T. (1974). *New seeds of contemplation* (Rev. ed.). Norton.

Molendijk, T. (2018). Toward an interdisciplinary conceptualization of moral injury: From unequivocal guilt and anger to moral conflict and disorientation. *New Ideas in Psychology*, *51*, 1–8.

Peterson, C., & Seligman, M. (2004). *Character strengths and virtues: A handbook and classification*. Oxford University Press.

Rambo, L. (1993). *Understanding religious conversion*. Yale University Press.

Richardson, F., Fowers, B., & Guignon, C. (1999). *Re-envisioning psychology: Moral dimensions of theory and practice*. Jossey-Bass.

Rieff, P. (1959). *Freud: The mind of a moralist*. University of Chicago Press.

Rieff, P. (1966). *The triumph of the therapeutic*. Harper Collins.

Rizzuto, A. (1979). *The birth of the living God: A psychoanalytic study*. University of Chicago Press.

Rizzuto, A. (1991). Religious development: A psychoanalytic point of view. *New Directions for Child Development*, *52*(Special Issue: Religious Development in Childhood and Adolescence), 47–60.

Seligman, M. (2018). PERMA and the building blocks of well-being. *The Journal of Positive Psychology*, *13*(4), 333–335. https://doi.org/10.1080/17439760.2018.1437466

Seligman, M., & Csikszentmihalyi, M. (2000). Positive psychology: An introduction. *American Psychologist*, *55*, 5–14.

Sperry, L. (1999). The somatic dimension in healing prayer and the conversion process. *Journal of Christian Healing*, *21*(3 & 4), 47–62.

Sperry, L. (2003). *Handbook of diagnosis and treatment of DSM-IV-TR personality disorder* (2nd ed.). Brunner/Mazel.

Sperry, L. (2007). *Ethical and professional practice in counseling and psychotherapy*. Allyn & Bacon.

Sperry, L. (2012). *Spirituality in clinical practice: Theory and practice of spiritually oriented psychotherapy* (2nd ed.). Routledge.

Sperry, L. (2016). *Handbook of diagnosis and treatment of DSM-5 personality disorders* (3rd ed.). Brunner-Routledge.

Sperry, L. (2021a). Collaborative healing of clergy sexual abuse and sacred moral injury. *Journal of Christian Healing*, *37*(2), 5–13.

Sperry, L. (2021b). Moral injury in Christian organizations: Sacred moral injury. In J. Peteet, S. Moffic, A. Hankir, & H. Koenig (Eds.), *Christianity and psychiatry* (pp. 113–127). Springer.

Sperry, L. (2023). Psychotherapy alone is insufficient: Treating clergy sexual abuse and sacred moral injury. *Spirituality in Clinical Practice*, *10*(4), 350–357.

Sperry, L. (2024a). Spiritually integrative psychotherapy: An impending paradigm shift in theory and practice. In L. Miller (Ed.), *The Oxford handbook of psychology and spirituality* (2nd ed., pp. 314–332). Oxford University Press.

Sperry, L. (2024b). The moral domain, moral injury, and the healing process. *Journal of Christian Healing*, *40* (1), 5–14.

Svoboda, E. (2022, September 19). Moral injury is an invisible epidemic that affects millions. *Scientific American*. www.scientificamerican.com/article/moral-injuryis-an-invisible-epidemic-that-affects-millions/

Svrakic, D., Whitehead, C., Przybeck, T., & Cloninger, C. R. (1993). Differential diagnosis of personality disorders by the seven factor model of temperament and character. *Archives of General Psychiatry*, *50*, 991–999.

Taylor, C. (1997). *Philosophical arguments*. Harvard University Press.

Wilber, K. (1977). *The spectrum of consciousness*. Quest.

Wilber, K. (1995). *Sex, ecology, spirituality: The spirit of evolution*. Shambala.

Wilber, K. (1999). *Integral psychology: Consciousness, spirit, psychology, therapy (A synthesis of premodern, modern, and postmodern approaches)*. Shambala.

Wilber, K., Engler, J., & Brown, D. (1986). *Transformation of consciousness: Conventional and contemplative perspectives on development*. Shambala.

Winnicott, D. (1960). *The maturational processes and the facilitatory environment*. Hogarth Press.

Worthington, E., Kurusu, T., McCullough, M., & Sandage, S. (1996). Empirical research on religion and psychotherapeutic processes and outcomes: A 10 year review and research prospectus. *Psychological Bulletin*, *119*(3), 448.

Chapter 3

Developmental Models of the Spiritual Dimension

Chapter 2 introduced the five dimensions of human experience as well as six perspectives or frames of reference for understanding the spiritual dimension and the process of spiritual development. This chapter describes seven additional perspectives. Unlike the perspective in Chapter 2, these perspectives represent stage models of human development that directly or indirectly address the spiritual dimension and the process of spiritual development. The next section provides a general introduction to these stage models, including critiques of stage theories in general. Subsequent sections then describe each of these eight. New to this edition is a description of a promising research-based model, the Religious/Spiritual Stress and Resilience Model.

Stage Models and Human Development

Foundational to theory and practice in spiritually integrated psychotherapy are developmental theories or models rooted in four traditions: (1) psychodynamic theory—Freud, Erikson, and Jung; (2) structural-developmental theory—Piaget, Kohlberg, Fowler, Kegan, and Helminiak; (3) transpersonal theory—Wilberr; and (4) spiritual traditions—Keating. A fifth tradition appears to be emerging. It involves empirically based models such as the Religious/Spiritual Stress and Resilience Model (Lefevor et al., 2021).

This chapter describes representative theories or stage models in all four traditions. Among the psychodynamic theories, Erikson's stage model has some relevance for spiritually integrated psychotherapists in that it is a relational model of the development of virtues. For Erikson an individual's ego develops through eight stages during the human life cycle. At each stage the ego must integrate somatic, psychological, social, moral, and cultural factors in order to achieve a stable sense of self. In this model, a developmental crisis precedes the next stage, and resolution of this crisis

DOI: 10.4324/9781003425991-4

requires the individual to synthesize both positive and negative elements, i.e., generativity vs. stagnation.

Rather than based on the life cycle, the structural-developmental theories are based on formal structures which develop according to a predictable, universal, sequential, and hierarchal pattern. Each stage represents increasingly complex and differentiated ways of cognitively structuring one's experience of reality. Piaget was the first of the structural-developmentalists and established a developmental paradigm for identifying stages of cognitive or intellectual development in children and adolescents. Kohlberg, Fowler, Kegan, and Helminiak have elaborated stage models of moral, faith, self, or religious development based on Piaget's paradigm. Not surprisingly, three of these stage models, i.e., those developed by Kohlberg, Fowler, and Kegan, have had particular appeal for professionals involved in Christian spiritual formation.

It should be noted that Kohlberg's and Fowler's stage models have generated considerable research, as well as considerable criticism and controversy. It is beyond the scope of this chapter to systematically review this research or the criticism and controversy. Rather, since the purpose of presenting these stage models is to suggest their clinical utility understanding the spiritual dimension and spiritual development, critiques specifically related to clinical utility will be briefly noted.

Because of such criticisms and the increasing appeal of Eastern religions and the recovery of the Christian contemplative tradition, there is mounting interest in the writings of Ken Wilber, from the transpersonal tradition, and Thomas Keating from the Christian spiritual tradition. As will become evident, both of these spiritual theorists and writers have complementary models of the spiritual dimension and spiritual development.

Models Relating to Spiritual Development

Historical Models

From the beginning spiritual writers have attempted to describe the process of spiritual development. The spiritual life was viewed as an "ascent" to God and the metaphors "ladder" and "stages" were often used to describe the process of spiritual growth. For instance, the John Climacus, a seventh-century monk, described the spiritual life as consisting of 30 steps in his classic book the *Ladder of Divine Ascent*. On the other hand, Origen of Alexandria viewed the spiritual life as passing through three stages beginning with purification from sin which led to illumination by grace of God which finally led to union with God (Cunningham & Egan, 1996). In the Christian spiritual tradition this three-stage approach to spiritual development—purgative, illuminative, and unitive—came to be

Table 3.1 Summary of the "Three Ways" of Spiritual Growth

Purgative: The beginner undergoes a progressive purgation or purification of all attachments which hinder total surrender to God. Prayer is largely discursive, and spiritual practices include fasting and almsgiving. The outcome is elimination of vice.

Illuminative: The proficient moves from discursive to affective prayer, i.e., more heart centered. Growth in virtue movement away from the darkness of sin leads to "illumination." The outcome is growth in virtue.

Unitive: The virtues and prayers of the illuminative way have created a heart open and docile to the promptings and actions of the Spirit. A state of union or "spiritual marriage" between the self and God occurs. The outcome is increased spiritual gifts.

known as the Three Ways, also designated as beginner, proficient, and the perfect (O'Keefe, 1995; Sperry, 2024). Table 3.1 contains a capsule summary of the stages in the Three Ways.

It is noteworthy that the ways of purgation and illumination reflect the moral dimension in that they "presuppose that any growth in prayer and holiness requires a moral conversion and vice versa. For the person to grow in holiness he or she must grow as a person of virtue. To become holy, one must become truly good" (O'Keefe, 1995, p. 49). O'Keefe contends that the Three Ways require both religious and moral conversion. Gelpi (1998) would add that intellectual, affective, and sociopolitical conversion are also required for full ongoing conversion or transformation.

Presumably, spiritual growth reflects an individual's health and well-being. In my clinical experience, this has been borne out. Specifically, it is my observation that the ways or stages of spiritual growth are related to scores on the Level of Personality Functioning Scale (LPFS), which is a measure of impairment in terms of identity, self-direction, empathy, and intimacy (American Psychiatric Association, 2022, pp. 895–898). I have also observed that the stage of spiritual growth is also related to the duration of an individual's response to distress and upset. For instance, individuals with higher stages of spiritual growth have relatively shorter distress than those with lower levels. In other words, the stage of spiritual growth and these two clinical indicators rather accurately reflect an individual's overall mental health and well-being.

Specifically, those at the purgative stage tend to function relatively well in non-stressful situations, but poorly when under moderate stress during which they can exhibit a range of negative affects. Their LPFS level is likely in the range of 1–2. Their experience of distress and upset usually lasts for hours. Those at the illuminative stage function quite well in non-stressful situations and reasonably well when under moderate stress during which they can exhibit a range of negative affects. Their experience of distress

Table 3.2 Stage of Spiritual Growth, LPFS, and Duration of Distress

Spiritual Growth	*LPFS*	*Duration of Distress*
(Pre-purgative)	1–3	Several hours or days
Purgative	1	Hours
Illuminative	0–1	Minutes to an hour
Unitive	0	Momentary

typically lasts for minutes to an hour. Their LPFS level is likely in the range of 0–1. Finally, those at the unitive stage function well in all situations and their experience of distress and upset is very short-lived and momentary. Accordingly, their LPFS level is likely to be 0. Table 3.2 portrays the relationship of these three factors.

Contemporary Models

In order to understand the process of spiritual development over the life span it is useful to recognize how major domains of human development such as cognitive, psychosocial, and moral undergird and find expression in specifically spiritual experience and content (Sperry, 2012). For example, Erikson's stages of psychosocial development provide a useful perspective for recognizing how religious content is woven into major life processes such as identity formation and interpersonal intimacy, as well as growth in virtue and religious sentiment. Furthermore, Piaget's theory of cognitive development forms a heuristic basis for understanding how object permanence, symbolic representation, logical thinking, and formal operational thought are involved in increasingly advanced cognitive abilities for representing the presence of an unseen God, and how concepts of moral development may be affected by the religious context in which they arise, as well as in symbolizing objects of faith, thinking about religious questions, and conceptualizing the complex interactions between faith and life experiences, as has been articulated in both Kohlberg's theory of moral development and Fowler's theory of faith development.

Stage Models Addressing the Spiritual Dimension

Although the spiritual and religious dimension interacts with development processes differentially for individuals and groups, it is clear that spirituality and religion play a significant part, in casual and consequential ways, in the lives of many individuals. While this resultant interaction usually has developmentally beneficial repercussions, sometimes it is negative or mixed.

Table 3.3 Stage Models Addressing the Spiritual Dimension

1. Stages of Psychosocial Development
2. Stages of Moral Development
3. Stages of Faith Development
4. Stages of Self-Development
5. Stages of Spiritual Development
6. Stages of Spiritual Growth
7. Stages of the Spiritual Journey

The following sections briefly describe several stage theories of development that have direct or indirect bearing on spiritual development. We begin with Erikson's stages of psychosocial development (1984), then describe Kohlberg's model of moral development, which is followed by Fowler's model of faith development (1981) and Kegan's theory of self-development (1983) plus three others. Table 3.3 list these seven models.

Stages of Psychosocial Development

As noted above, Erikson's stages of psychosocial development provide a useful perspective for recognizing how religious and spiritual content is woven into major life processes such as identity formation and interpersonal intimacy. It is interesting to note that Erikson recognizes the domain of character in his system. He does this by specifying the specific virtue associated with each stage. Surprisingly, theorists in the fields of moral psychology and moral philosophy do not appear to have recognized the importance of Erikson's insight regarding the process of the development of virtue.

The eight stages of psychosocial development with their associated virtues are:

1. **Trust vs. mistrust:** At birth, infants are dominated by biological needs and drives. The quality of their relationship with caregivers will influence the extent to which trust (or mistrust) in others and the world in general is sensed. The virtue of *hope* is associated with this stage.
2. **Autonomy vs. doubt and shame:** Social demands in early childhood for self-control and bodily regulation, i.e., toilet training, influence feelings of self-efficacy vs. self-doubt. The quality or virtue of *will*, the will to do what is expected and expectable, emerges at stage two.
3. **Initiative vs. guilt:** During the preschool period children begin actively to explore and intrude upon their environment. The virtue of purpose—the courage to pursue personally valued goals in spite of risks and possible failure—now ascends.

4. **Industry vs. inferiority**: The social context in which the first three crises are negotiated is predominantly the home and immediate family. In stage four, however, children begin school or formal instruction of some sort. Mastery of the tasks and skills valued by one's teachers and the larger society is now the focal concern. The quality or virtue of *competence* is said to develop.
5. **Identity vs. diffusion**: Adolescence is the pivotal time when adolescents actively attempt to synthesize their experiences in order to formulate a stable sense of personal identity. While this process is psychosocial in nature—a social fit or "solidarity with group ideals" must occur—Erikson emphasizes the role of accurate self-knowledge and reality testing. Individuals come to view themselves as products of their previous experiences; a continuity of experience is sensed. Positive resolutions of prior crises—being trusting, autonomous, willful, and industrious—facilitate identity formation, whereas previous failures may lead to identity diffusion. The virtue of *fidelity*, i.e., the ability to maintain commitments in spite of contradictory value systems, emerges during adolescence.
6. **Intimacy vs. isolation**: In young adulthood one must be willing and able to unite one's own identity with another's. Since authentic disclosure and mutuality leave one vulnerable, a firm sense of identity is prerequisite. The quality or virtue of *love* ascends during this stage.
7. **Generativity vs. stagnation**: This stage associated with middle adulthood is the time in the life span when one strives to actualize the identity that has been formed and shared with selected others. The generation or production of offspring, artifacts, ideas, products, and so forth is involved. The virtue of *care* now emerges: generative adults care for others through parenting, teaching, supervising, and so forth, whereas stagnating adults are absorbed in their own personal needs.
8. **Integrity vs. despair**: The final stage focuses on the perceived completion or fulfillment of one's life cycle. The last virtue to emerge is *wisdom*. The wise person understands the relativistic nature of knowledge and accepts that one's life had to be the way it was.

Stages of Moral Development

As noted in the introduction, Kohlberg proposed a stage model of moral reasoning based on the structural-developmental paradigm established by Piaget. Kohlberg's intent was to describe the developmental process of moral reasoning rather than moral action. He recognizes that the theoretical link between moral reasoning and action is elusive, i.e., individuals can exhibit the same action for different reasons.

He proposed three levels of moral reasoning—pre-conventional, conventional, and post-conventional—and predicted that the relationship between moral reasoning and action would be strongest at the post-conventional level where actions are theorized to be mediated by rational principles. Unfortunately, data does not consistently support this prediction. So why bother to describe this stage model? First, these stages of moral development serve as benchmarks for comparing other stage theories and even some perspectives, i.e., the stage theories of faith, self, and religious development and the conversion theory perspective. Second, character development is being rediscovered today. Training programs, some of which are based on this stage model, are being utilized in public education, in community development circles, and in some spiritual formation programs. And third, the moral dimension, which involves the character and ethics perspectives, i.e., becoming a virtuous therapist, is emphasized in this text.

This model describes three levels with six stages. They are:

Pre-Conventional Stages

In these stages morality is externally based. And there is a decided emphasis on external control.

1. Punishment and obedience orientation. Right and wrong are decided on whether one obeys authority or whether one gets punished for one's actions.
2. Instrumental relativist orientation. Right and wrong are decided upon whether one gets a reward, i.e., by others, society, or God, for what one does.

Conventional Stages

In these stages the emphasis is on pleasing others or maintaining standards.

3. Interpersonal concordance: Also called "good boy," "nice girl" orientation. Right and wrong are based on what a "good" person would do under the circumstances; motives and intentions are taken into account in efforts to please others.
4. Social system maintenance: Also called the law and order orientation. Right and wrong are based on maintaining the social system and living within reasonable, established rules; showing respect for higher authority and doing one's duty are important.

Post-Conventional Stages

In these stages moral reasoning is based on an understanding of abstract moral principles upon which more concrete rules and laws are based.

There is an acknowledgment of conflict and internal choice among alternatives exists.

5. Social contract orientation. Right and wrong are based on agreed upon social contracts. Concern about the common good makes contractual laws obligatory and binding. At this stage an individual's moral judgment reflects and values the implicit or explicit will of the majority.
6. Universal ethical principles orientation. Right and wrong are based on internalized standards regardless of conformity or non-conformity with social mores. Personal commitment rather than social consensus informs one's choice among moral principles, and conduct is dictated by a self-selected ideal irrespective of the reaction of others.

Critique of Moral Development Theory and Research

It is interesting to note that much of the research and writing on moral development for the past 30 years has been based on the work of Kohlberg and Gilligan with little or no awareness of the significant limitations of their theories. Unfortunately, much of this work appears to be based on flawed empirical responses from Kohlberg's stages 3 and 4. Even by his own measure, almost no one attains the highest stage of moral development, and on the newer scoring system the highest stage has not been empirically confirmed (Flanagan, 1991).

Criticism of this moral development theory has intensified (Shweder & Haidt, 1993). Recently, Flanagan (1996) remarked that Kohlberg's theory was "a dismal failure, an utterly degenerate research program despite many true believers" (p. 138). Even staunch advocates of Kohlberg's approach now concede that moral sensitivity, motivation, and character must be studied as well as moral judgment (Rest et al., 1997). Finally, neither Kohlberg nor his followers have successfully demonstrated that moral thinking produces morally correct action. In fact, research conducted on the cognitive processes of morally exemplary individuals indicated that they scored primarily at the level of conventional morality, a finding that seriously challenges the value of the testing and moral education programs inspired by Kohlberg (Colby & Damon, 1992).

Carol Gilligan's work on moral development also appears to suffer significant limitations. In her book, *In a Different Voice*, Gilligan (1982) challenged Kohlberg's model of moral development and proposed two key ideas. The first was that there are two basic moral perspectives, one based on justice and the other on caring. The second was that men mostly prefer the justice perspective while women mostly prefer the care perspective. These ideas resulted in a vigorous debate about the adequacy of the care/justice hypothesis and the widespread impression that Gilligan had demonstrated distinct gender differences in moral thinking. Despite her caveats, her book was read not as a hypothesis about a different voice but rather as proof of her discovery of a different voice. In the subsequent debate, empirical evidence was advanced that men and women do *not* in fact score differently on moral reasoning, and that whether an individual utilizes a care or justice perspective may relate more to the nature of the problem presented than with gender. The data also indicated that men and women switch readily from one perspective to another, with only very small numbers of either gender using one perspective exclusively (Kerber, 1986; Walker, 1991).

Gilligan's original position and subsequent hypotheses rest on theories of childhood development which have been criticized by a number of female researchers (Flanagan & Jackson, 1987; Friedman, 1993; Larrabee, 1993; Tanner, 1996). Nevertheless, the popularity of Gilligan's model has neither been diminished by its many critics, nor dimmed by her inability to verify a distinct moral developmental pattern for females, a project she posited was essential before any further comparisons between the moral experience of men and women could be made (Gilligan, 1988).

Stages of Faith Development

For James Fowler (1981), faith is directed toward a person's object(s) of ultimate concern, irrespective of the specific content of faith. Fowler (1981) conceptualizes faith structurally, rather than in terms of specific beliefs, but recognizes that lived faith expresses itself in specific belief. In this sense, faith represents how individuals develop cognitively and spiritually in dealing with ultimate, transcendental reality and meaning. Understood in this way, faith is clearly relevant to the spiritual dimension in psychotherapy and counseling since it represents the inner orientation to questions of meaning and value; that is, to questions that for many people are associated predominantly with spirituality and religion.

Fowler (1981) describes faith development in six stages, with a pre-faith stage representing an emergent stage in which a fund of trust and mutuality is built up during the first years of life. The six stages are:

1. **Intuitive-projective faith** (ages 3–7), which is a fantasy-filled, imitative phase in which the child can be powerfully and permanently influenced by the visible faith of primally related adults. Imagination predominates in this stage. For example, a child may imagine a world of kind angels and feel trusting toward reality, or a child may imagine a punitive God and develop guilt and fear.
2. **Mythic-literal faith** (ages 7 to puberty), in which individuals begin to take on for themselves the stories, beliefs, and observances that

symbolize belonging to their community. Beliefs and symbols are understood literally, and anthropomorphic stories are the major way of understanding faith content.

3. **Synthetic-conventional faith:** From adolescence to early adulthood, faith is presumably structured in interpersonal but mostly conformist terms, with authority as important. Beliefs and values (ideology of clustering values) are felt deeply but are largely unexamined. Fowler maintains that this stage is typical of adolescents and normative for adults.
4. **Individuative-reflective faith:** The stage of faith in which the self and one's beliefs begin to take on a personalized system of explicit meanings to which one is personally committed. Symbols are translated into concepts for self-examination and critical reflection, although there is still much unconscious material.
5. **Conjunctive faith**, which involves the integration into self of much that was suppressed or unrecognized in the interest of stage 4's self-certainty and conscious adaptation to reality. Sensitive to paradox and ready for closeness to that which is different, one strives to establish syntheses of opposites and sees the possibility of an inclusive community of being. People in this stage are ready to exert themselves energetically for their beliefs.
6. **Universalizing faith** involves looking beyond the constraining paradoxes and the specific content of one's particular faith to seek a future order of relating justly and lovingly to others. People at stage 6 exhibit qualities that shake our usual criteria of normalcy: heedless to self-preservation; vivid attention to transcendent moral and religious actuality; devotion to universalizing compassion; enlarged vision of universal community. The rare person in stage 6 resembles in many respects such individuals as Mohandas Ghandi and Mother Teresa, for whom the final challenge of integrity was a lifelong journey.

Critique of Faith Development Theory and Research

Given that Fowler's model is based on Kohlberg's research, it should not be surprising that the Faith Development model would be subject to criticism. Ford-Grabowsky's critique of Fowler's model of faith development is trenchant. Ford-Grabowsky (1987) argued that masculine and cultural biases resulted in Fowler's focus on cognition to the neglect of religious sentiments and to focus on the positive aspects of development to the neglect of deception and sin as stumbling blocks to the development of faith. Johnson (1989) has leveled a more basic criticism of stage theories. She contends that because stage theories do not address the matter of character and virtue—and focus rather on ego development—they have limited value in understanding the process of spiritual growth and development, at least from a Christian perspective. Finally, others have criticized the basic structural-developmental premise that these stages are universal and invariant.

Implications of the Faith Development Model for Clinical Practice

Fowler's developmental scheme has several implications for the spiritual dimension in counseling. By outlining cognitive, affective, and behavioral elements of religious development at different life stages, Fowler provides the counselor with a way of understanding typical and problematic spiritual development. Spiritual belief is a process of growth in the multiple dimensions of faith, of transforming religious meaning, not clinging to a particular symbolization or formulation of content. Thus, faced with issues involving the spiritual dimension, the developmentally aware counselor may help a client examine and transform literal and symbolic formulations of religious meanings and at the same time retain the essential reality of religious meaning behind the words and symbols. In this way, the counselor helps the client personalize and individualize faith meanings without breaking from the authentic core of one's religious roots. For clients who are concerned about remaining faithful to their religious tradition and overcoming the restraints and problems associated with specific symbols or formulations of earlier stages of believing, the counselor who understands the developmental dynamics of faith may be able to help the client to consider alternative perspectives that are still essentially congruent with the client's core spirituality/religiousness. For example, for a client whose disturbance involves a connection between the power of God and the symbol of a stem father, the counselor may help the client rethink and feel God's power as a supporting, transforming care linked to people who symbolize human care irrespective of gender.

Stages of Self Development

Although much has been written about the development and dynamics of self, i.e., Object Relations Theory and Self Psychology, there have been relatively few efforts to articulate a stage model of self-development. Even though Jane Loevinger (1976) has extensively researched ego development and devised a theoretically derived and data-based theory of the stages of ego development, it was Robert Kegan (1983) who proposed a stage theory of self-development that is highly regarded by spiritual directors and spiritually oriented psychotherapists. The appeal of Kegan's model for contemporary spirituality is that it addresses the two basic human desires expressed in all spiritual literature: the desire for attachment or relationship as well as for separation or autonomy. Furthermore, this theory is particularly attractive to therapists and spiritual directors since Kegan addresses the functions of attachment in women as well as in men (Conn, 1989; Liebert, 1992).

In the book, *The Evolving Self*, Kegan describes a constructive-developmental approach to human development in which the basic dynamic is meaning-making activity. Meaning making unifies and generates thought and feeling as well as self (subject) and other (object). For Kegan, emotion is the experience of defending, surrendering, and reconstructing a center of meaning. Human activity involves creating the other, i.e., differentiation, as well as relating to it, i.e., integration. Self-other relations emerge from the ongoing process of development, which involves a succession of increasing differentiations of the self from the world. The result of this process is a more complex object of relation.

Basic to every stage of development, including infancy, is meaning-making evolution. Fusion, differentiation, and belonging are activities that recur in new forms at each phase of development as a person makes the meaning of "self" and "other" again and again. Each stage of development can surrender its controlling independence for freely chosen interdependence, which involves balancing the universal longing for both autonomy and attachment. Unlike other stage theories, Kegan describes the necessity for development beyond the stage of autonomous self-direction wherein control is favored over mutuality which inhibits intimacy. For Kegan, the most mature stage is one in which the self-surrenders its controlling independence for freely chosen interdependence and relates to others with mutuality and equality. From this perspective, spiritual maturity becomes a matter of freely surrender oneself and risking a genuinely mutual relationship with others and with God.

The theory of the evolving self specifies five stages of development. They are:

1. **Impulsive Stage:** This self evolves from the "Incorporative" which is undifferentiated and controlled by reflexes; Kegan labels it Stage "0." The impulsive self is embedded in and subjected to impulses and perceptions which are unorganized and constantly changing. The result is that the impulsive self can rapidly alternate between extremes of emotion. It cannot tolerate ambivalence.
2. **Imperial Stage:** With the emergence of concrete operational thinking the child creates an interior world and objectifies impulses and perceptions. The result is that the self is no longer controlled by impulses and perceptions and can actively and purposefully explore its environment.
3. **Interpersonal Stage:** This self is able to relate to others by coordinating its needs with the needs of others and by exhibiting some measure of empathy. Nevertheless, this is a pre-identity stage which means

relationships are characterized by clinging fusion, i.e., this self is unable to separate itself from its relationships. Although feelings of mutuality are all important to this self, it fears the loss its own self and the experience of nothingness.

4. **Institutional Stage:** A coherent sense of identity is achieved which means this self is able to separate itself from its relationships and can experience a sense of self ownership. Nevertheless, control and independent strength constitute its main agenda or organization, and these outweigh the pull of attachment and intimacy. Furthermore, this self is unable to fully and critically reflect on this organization.
5. **Interindividual Stage:** This self is no longer constrained by its organization, but is free to relate to others fully as a "universal" person with others. At this stage the self becomes capable of surrendering its controlling autonomy and independence for freely chosen interdependence, and thereby relate to others with mutuality and equality. This self is capable of genuine intimacy with self and others and can tolerate inner emotional conflict. Accordingly, this self is capable of and disposed to the transforming union of divine love.

Stages of Spiritual Development

Extending the tradition of the structural theories of human development, Helminiak (1987) has described what he calls the stages of spiritual development in his book, *Spiritual Development: An Interdisciplinary Study*. His basic assumption is that spiritual development is not a separate line of development alongside physical, emotional, intellectual, moral, ego, or faith development. Rather, spiritual development embraces all these dimensions of human development. Spiritual development is best conceptualized as human development when it is characterized by four factors: integrity or wholeness, openness, self-responsibility, and authentic self-transcendence. It is the ongoing integration of the human spiritual principle into the very structures of the personality until the personality becomes the adequate expression of the fully authentic person. Helminiak describes five distinct developmental stages in this process of integration.

1. **Conformist Stage.** This is the beginning point of spiritual development. It is characterized by a deeply felt and extensively rationalized worldview, accepted on the basis of external authority and supported by approval of one's significant others.
2. **Conscientious Conformist Stage.** This stage is characterized by beginning to assume responsibility for the awareness that because of unthinking adherence to an inherited worldview one has actually abdicated

responsibility for one's life. At this stage individuals begin to learn that their lives are what they decide to make of them.

3. **Conscientious Stage.** This is the first true stage of spiritual development. It is characterized by the achievement of significant structuring of their life according to their own understanding of things, by optimism regarding their newly accepted sense of responsibility for themselves and their world, and by commitment to their principles.
4. **Compassionate Stage.** At this stage individuals learn to surrender some of the world they have so painstakingly constructed for themselves. Their commitments are no less intense, but they are more realistic, more nuanced, and more supported by deeply felt and complex emotion. They become more gentle with themselves and with others.
5. **Cosmic Stage.** As this final stage unfolds, their habitual patterns of perception, cognition, interrelation, and all others become more fully authentic. They become more fully open to all that is, ever willing to change and adjust as circumstances demand, alive and responsive to the present moment, in touch with the depths of their own selves, aware of the furthest implications of their spiritual nature, in harmony with themselves and with all else—and all this not as a momentary, passing experience but as an enduring way of being, permeating the very structure of their concrete selves. There is a profound merging, insofar as it is possible, between spirit and self. It is that state of full integration when the personality is the adequate instrument of the authentic person. It becomes a way of life that has been variously described by the great spiritual traditions as mysticism, samadhi, satori, kensho, moksha, cosmic consciousness, or enlightenment.

Stages of Spiritual Growth

Ken Wilber (1999) has proposed a stage theory of spiritual development from a much different perspective than the one articulated by Helminiak. It is an integrative theory of consciousness that Wilber contends embraces the essential truths of Eastern and Western thinking, from ancient wisdom traditions to modern science. He calls this theory the Full Spectrum Model of the stages of human growth and development. Over the past two decades this generic model has undergone changes and modifications. Three renderings of it follow.

The Evolutionary Spectrum Model

The first is the evolutionary model of consciousness. Wilber describes the evolving structures of consciousness which make up what he calls the spectrum or the Great Chain of Being. There are six major increasingly differentiated levels of consciousness from lowest to highest (Wilber, 1983a/1996). These six levels are:

1. **Reptilian consciousness** is the most primitive level of consciousness. It is characterized by immersion in nature, immediate fulfillment of instinctual needs, and the absence of any consciousness of self.
2. **Typhonic consciousness** is the level of consciousness involving the development of a body-self distinct from other objects. It is characterized by the inability to distinguish the part from the whole, and images in the imagination from external reality.
3. **Mythic membership consciousness** is the level of consciousness that is socially determined. It is characterized by an unquestioned assimilation of the values and ideas of one's social group, and involves the phenomena of over-identification and conformity to the group's value systems. In short, one's identity and self-worth is drawn from one's family, ethnic, or religious community.
4. **Mental egoic consciousness** involves the development of full reflective self-consciousness, beginning with the capacity for logical reasoning at about eight years of age and arriving at abstract thinking around 12 or 13. This level of consciousness is characterized by the sense of personal responsibility and feelings of guilt regarding one's attitudes and behavior.
5. **Intuitive consciousness** is the level of consciousness that is beyond rational thinking. It is characterized by harmony, cooperation, forgiveness, negotiation to resolve differences, and mutuality rather than competitiveness. It involves a sense of oneness with others and of belonging to the universe.
6. **Unitive consciousness** is that level of consciousness that reflects the experience of transformative union as well as the process of infusing the experience of divine love into all one's faculties and relationships.

The Developmental Spectrum Model

This developmental model is a subset of the evolutionary model of consciousness. Each stage consists of developmental tasks which require new abilities and levels of adaptation. As these tasks are met the individual psychic organization becomes more differentiated. Failure to adequately address such tasks results in fixation or interferes with full consolidation of the next stage. Wilber indicates the correspondence of his seven stage model to various other models and constructs (Wilber, 1983b/1996, pp. 246–248). The seven stages are:

1. **Archaic:** This stage includes the material body, sensations, perceptions, and emotions. It is equivalent to Piaget's stage of sensorimotor

intelligence, Maslow's physiological needs, and Loevinger's autistic and symbiotic stages.

2. **Magic**: This stage includes simple images, symbols, and the first rudimentary concepts, or the first and lowest mental productions. They are "magical" in the sense that they display condensation, displacement, and "omnipotence of thought." It is equivalent to Freud's primary process and Piaget's preoperational stage of thinking, and is correlated with Kohlberg's pre-conventional morality, Loevinger's impulsive and self-protective stages, and Maslow's safety needs.
3. **Mythic**: This stage is more advanced than magic, but not yet capable of clear rationality or hypothetico-deductive reasoning. It is equivalent to Piaget's stage of concrete operational thinking, Loevinger's conformist and conscientious-conformist stages, Maslow's belongingness needs, and Kohlberg's stages of conventional morality.
4. **Rational**: This stage is equivalent to Piaget's stage of formal operational thinking and is correlated with Loevinger's conscientious and individualistic stages, Kohlberg's post-conventional morality, and Maslow's self-esteem needs.
5. **Psychic**: "Psychic" does not necessarily refer to "paranormal," but rather to "psyche" as a higher level of development than the mind per se. Its cognitive structure has been called "vision logic" or integrative logic, and is correlated with Loevinger's integrated and autonomous stages, and Maslow's self-actualization needs.
6. **Subtle**: This stage involves archetypal meaning and the "illumined mind." It is essentially the transpersonal structure of life, where intuition is in its highest sense. It is the beginning of Maslow's self-transcendence needs.
7. **Causal**: This level is the endpoint of all growth and development. It is "Spirit" in the highest sense, and Tillich's "Ground of Being" or Spinoza's "Eternal Substance."

The Transpersonal Spectrum Model

Wilber contends that these seven stages of the Developmental Spectrum Model can be further reduced to three general realms: the pre-personal, i.e., pre-conventional, the personal, i.e., conventional, and the transpersonal, i.e., post-conventional. Here it will be referred to as the Transpersonal Spectrum Model. Recall that Kohlberg also uses the designations pre-conventional, conventional, and post-conventional.

There is widespread agreement among transpersonal philosophers and psychologists that these three stages or realms are the most basic and useful way of differentiating reality (Cortright, 1997; Walsh, 2000). Wilber has linked his spectrum model of consciousness to spectra of psychopathology and psychotherapy in addition to development. Movement through these three basic stages is from lesser to greater consciousness and from fragmentation to wholeness. This third rendering of the spectrum model can be summarized as:

1. **Pre-Personal Level:** This is a primitive level of development, and so developmental failures involve more primitive psychopathology such as psychosis, severe personality disorders like narcissistic and borderline disorders, and neurosis. Standard psychotherapeutic methods such as dynamic psychotherapy and what Wilber calls "structure-building therapy" can be useful interventions at this level.
2. **Personal Level:** While the individual at this level may lead a conventional daily life they are far from being happy and enlightened. Anxiety and worry about the meaning of life, the future, relationships, and matters of conscience are common concerns. Wilber describes typical psychopathology at this stage to include "cognitive script pathology," "identity neurosis," and "existential pathology" for which he recommends transactional analysis, cognitive therapy, introspection, and philosophical analysis.
3. **Transpersonal Level:** At this level the self has developed full self-consciousness, has gone beyond any psychic wounds and defenses, and has actualized or is actualizing much of its finite potential. The spiritual traditions refer to psychopathology here as the "perils of the path" (Cortright, 1997, p. 69). Predictable perils include "spiritual emergencies," "dark night of the soul," "psuedo-nirvana," and "failure to integrate." Treatment or interventions at this level include structure-building therapy, meditation and other spiritual practices, and spiritual direction (Wilber, 1999).

Stages of the Spiritual Journey

As described by Thomas Keating (1998), a Trappist monk and noted authority on contemplative prayer, self-transformation is a spiritual journey. A spiritual journey is basically a journey of self-discovery since the encounter with God is also an encounter with one's true self. Like Wilber, Keating (1995) has attempted to integrate basic insights from the ancient spiritual tradition with the insights of contemporary psychology. Even though Keating has intimate knowledge of the Eastern religious and spiritual traditions, he has developed a model that is primarily based within the Christian contemplative tradition. Like Wilber, the domain of consciousness is a core consideration for Keating. Accordingly, Keating relates his Stages of the Spiritual Journey—at least as it has been articulated in the Christian tradition—to Wilber's Evolutionary Spectrum Model. Table 3.4 illustrates this comparison.

Table 3.4 Comparison of Stages of Consciousness and Stages of the Spiritual Journey

Stages of Consciousness	*Stages of the Spiritual Journey*
Unity Consciousness	Unity
Unitive Consciousness	Transforming Union Dark Night of the Spirit
Intuitive Consciousness	Intermediate Contemplative Prayer Dark Night of the Soul
Mental Egoic Consciousness	Initial Contemplative Prayer
Mythic Membership Consciousness Typhonic Consciousness Reptilian Consciousness	

Derived from the writings of Wilber, 1983/1996, and Keating, 1998

These six stages refer to different levels of relating to God (Keating, 1992, p. 142). Although Keating has not systematically articulated these stages, they can be described in the following way.

1. **Initial Contemplation:** This stage corresponds to Wilber's mental egoic stage of consciousness in which an individual is capable of full reflective self-consciousness. For this stage Keating indicates a number of prayer forms and spiritual practices called "*lectio divina*." These include contemplative prayer which is praying or communing beyond words, thoughts, and feelings. Contemplative prayer is a "process moving from the simplified activity of waiting upon God to the ever-increasing predominance of the gifts of the Spirit as the source of one's prayer" (Keating, 1998, p. 145). Centering prayer, a passive form of contemplative prayer is commonly practiced at this stage.
2. **Dark Night of the Senses:** This dark "night" refers to a stage or period of spiritual dryness and desolation in which the individual feels abandoned by God and is unable to pray and receive spiritual consolations as before. The goal of this stage is the purification of one's motivation, a time of passive purification. In the spiritual literature this is also called the Dark Night of the Soul.
3. **Intermediate Contemplation:** This stage corresponds to Wilber's intuitive stage of consciousness in which an individual can experience a sense of oneness with others and of belonging to the universe. Keating designates this stage as "stages of prayer" and indicates representative prayer forms that foster and maintain a sense of oneness and belonging: the prayer of full union, the prayer of union, the prayer of quiet and infused recollection.

4. **Dark Night of the Spirit:** refers to the purification of the unconscious beyond the dark night of the senses, and aims to eliminate the remaining remnants of the false self, particularly spiritual pride. "The final purgation of spiritual pride is traditionally as the dark night of the spirit" (Keating, 1995, p. 98).
5. **Transforming Union:** The full and ongoing sharing of God's life and loving presence sharing in all five dimensions of human experience. Unlike previous, occasional experiences of unity and God's presence, daily life is experienced with "the invincible conviction of continuous union with God" (Keating, 1998, p. 101). This stage involves a restructuring of consciousness in which the divine reality is perceived to be present in oneself and in all that is. While relatively few achieve this stage, Keating indicates that it should be regarded as the normal Christian life.
6. **Unity:** In this stage the individual is nearing the completion of the spiritual journey. It is also called the stage of perfect wisdom, the kind of wisdom that finds happiness in persecution for the sake of the Kingdom of God. Individuals have "moved beyond self-interest to such a degree that they no longer have a possessive attitude toward themselves... they become sources of diving life and peace for others" (Keating, 1998, p. 112).

The Stages of Consent on the Spiritual Journey

The stages of the spiritual journey correspond to the passage of human life from birth to death. The spiritual journey requires a series of "consents" that most spiritual seekers were unable to make in childhood, adolescence, and early adulthood for various reasons, including unhealed emotional damage. Keating describes four such stages of consent (Keating, 1998). The four stages are:

First Consent: Associated with childhood, this is the consent to accept the basic goodness of one's being as a gift from God and to be grateful for it.

Second Consent: Associated with early adolescence, this the consent to accept the full development of one's being by activating one's talents and creative energies and assume responsibility for oneself and one's relationships.

Third Consent: Associated with early adulthood, this is the consent to accept the fact of our non-being and the diminutions of self that occur through illness, old age, and death.

Fourth Consent: This is the consent to be transformed. The transforming union requires consent to the death of the false self. Many, even those advanced on the spiritual journey, are more afraid of the death of the false self than of physical death.

The Dynamics of the Spiritual Journey

Briefly stated, Keating's perspective on the spiritual dimension is that one's inmost center is the divine ground of one's being from which the true self unfolds. Because of the human condition living out of the power of the true self is greatly compromised. In response to the traumas and pain associated with birth and infancy, individuals develop a false self which represses the true self and hides its potential. The false self remains operative when individuals are emotionally dominated by external events or unconscious defenses instead of acting with freedom. Through spiritual practices and centering prayer individuals are able to break through these unconscious barriers and recover their true selves. In other words, the spiritual journey involves the dismantling of the false self and the recovery of the true self. The remainder of this section elaborates the dynamics of the spiritual journey as interpreted from the psychological and spiritual perspectives by Keating.

Keating's formulation of the early life development of the false self and the reclamation of the true self as the basis for personal transformation on the spiritual journey is both original and compelling. He develops an integrative formulation of spiritual growth which incorporates insights from developmental psychology, depth psychology, family systems theory, transpersonal psychology, anthropology, the neurosciences, as well as from the contemplative tradition and mysticism (Keating, 1995).

The ability to truly love oneself and others requires a considerable degree of self-sacrifice and self-denial. Such love is easier spoken about than put into practice. This is because of a flaw in human nature inclining one to selfishness. Religious traditions refer to this flaw as original sin, and Keating (1999a) calls it the "human condition." Because of the human condition, one's best actions are marred by selfish motives, though these tend to be unrecognized. The writings of St John of the Cross describe the spiritual journey which begins when the individual responds to the call to move away from self-love toward a truly disinterested love; that is, a love which seeks the best for the other and neither clings nor manipulates. Everyone begins the spiritual journey distorted and in need of healing. The journey is about accepting a transforming love that deactivates one's limited and imperfect human ways of thinking, loving, and acting, and changes them into divine ways.

Human ways of thinking, loving, and acting are limited and imperfect because they are subject to the distortions of the *false self*. This false self must be transformed in the *true self*. The false self is described by Keating (1999b) as the self we think we are as compared to the true self, which is the self we actually are. The false self seeks fame, power, prestige, and wealth. It emerges from what could be called the human condition. All individuals are born into life and into a particular culture with three basic instinctual needs: (1) the need for love and affection; (2) the need to survive; and (3) the need for power and control.

The need for affection affects how individuals believe they are perceived by others, and how individuals desire to belong and to feel valued, needed, and loved by others. The basic instinct to survive affects how individuals perceive the trustworthiness of reality, as well as their sense of security or threat in a given environment. The need to exercise power in one's life affects how individuals treat others, and the extent to which they attempt to control other people's lives. These instinctual needs are natural, good, and essential. Yet, when they are not satisfied, they become demands.

Happiness is equated with the prompt and constant fulfillment of these demands, clustered by a complex of emotions for achieving one's needs and wants. This complex of emotions can be likened to a computer program in which a single action can trigger a whole series of responses which are designed to achieve happiness through the satisfaction of our demands. Keating (1999a) calls this phenomenon "emotional programs." Eventually these emotional programs for happiness become exaggerated into centers of motivation that function below the level of conscious awareness. Thus, what may be intended as a completely selfless action is actually driven by an unconscious selfish motive.

The false self is formed by compensatory behavior, through which individuals seek to protect themselves from real or imagined deprivations in regard to the needs for affection, survival, or control. The false self seeks happiness in overcompensating these needs. When one's instinctual needs are not being fulfilled, we try to make sure they will be through our behavior. This then becomes an ingrained pattern of behavior which severely limits one's freedom. Certain emotions which Keating calls "afflictive emotions" are created by one's emotional program (Keating, 1995). Afflictive emotions include anger, fear, and discouragement, emotions which are spontaneous reactions to the failure to acquire things perceived to be good and difficult to attain, or to the failure to avoid things perceived to be evil and difficult to avoid.

Basically, the false self is a constellation of energies involving the basic needs for affection, survival, and control. To the extent to which individuals feel deprived of something believed necessary for their happiness, they are likely to feel upset and disconcerted. Until the false self is addressed individuals are essentially victims of their beliefs and emotions.

Unless and until these needs are met, individuals experience themselves as out of balance, and their emotional programs for happiness attempt to compensate. Emotional programs cause problems only when they surreptitiously influence one's behavior to overcompensate. In such circumstances even when one's intention is to help another, the other is subtly manipulated to satisfy one's own needs.

Another determinant of the false self is what Keating (1999b) calls "cultural conditioning." Culture refers to any social group to which one belongs or has belonged in the family and community. Cultural conditioning begins very early in life and involves the processes of identification and over-identification with the groups that provide for our needs for security, affection, and control. Conformity with group norms ensures both acceptance and socialization. Accordingly, individuals acquire their preconceived ideas, values, biases, and prejudices. The result is that emotional programs are established by early childhood and tend to be relatively resistant to modification by logic or reason. They are largely non-rational and because they remain at a pre-conscious level, individuals are unaware of their operative functioning. They are addictive, because whenever the perceived needs are met, needs for bigger and better things arise. They are insatiable since no symbol can ever fully satisfy our thirst for happiness.

> The combination of these two forces—the drive for happiness in the form of security… affection… power and control, and over-identification with the particular group to which we belong—greatly complicates our emotional program for happiness. In our younger days, this development is normal. As adults activity arising from such motivation is childish.
>
> (Keating, 1999a, p. 15)

In short, the false self is programmed for human misery.

As noted earlier, emotional programming is like a computer program with unlimited memory. These programs store every emotional experience from the womb to the present moment, irrespective of our ability to remember or recall such experiences. While the event may be forgotten, the emotional responses are not. They can very easily be retrieved in a situation similar to the one that triggered the emotional response in the first place. Thus, when any event resembling those once felt to be harmful, dangerous, or rejecting occurs, the same feelings surface, usually disproportionate to the situation. Even though one may not have experienced serious trauma, nearly everyone has experienced early childhood losses and conflicts, which typically result in the emotional wounding and sense of unfulfillment carried into adulthood. Predictably, individuals compulsively enact a pattern of seeking approval, security, and a sense of well-being from others or from situations, even though these are never fully satisfying.

When individuals decide to seriously commit themselves to the spiritual journey, they do not begin with a clean slate or new tape. Much reprogramming is required. Initially, this involves ascertaining the content of that tape by listening to it, and then attempting to remove any aspects that are obstacles on the spiritual journey. We are dealing with subtle forces that are very powerful. To dismantle the false self-system requires more than good resolutions. Spiritual practices and disciplines are necessary to help in facing the shadow side of personality. As these obstacles are gradually brought into the light, individuals begin, or continue, the process of deep healing and transformation. Such healing is not merely superficial nor external but is the beginning of a transformation of the entire personality.

Unless the entire array of one's pre-conceived values and ideas are directly examined and squarely confronted, the prospect of genuine spiritual growth is compromised. Until these hidden motivations are faced, individuals cannot act out of the true self but will continue filtering reality through their own needs and wants, which is, of course, the false self.

It is absolutely essential to realize that the false self can operate in a very subtle manner. As soon as it thinks it may come under attack, it camouflages itself and hides its true nature. The naked false self is totally self-centered and can array itself in religious and spiritual guises that are eminently acceptable and difficult to discern. Individuals can appear to be leading exemplary lives observing the externals of etiquette and religiosity. The false self will utilize spiritual disciplines and religious vestiges to subtly feed its needs for acceptance, security, and power.

Coming to grips with the false self requires a conscious plan and deliberate effort. Psychotherapy alone may not be sufficient. Nevertheless, the first step is to accept the reality of the false self and begin to recognize its operational patterns. Failure to do so obviates one's good intentions and efforts involving spiritual practices. That is because the false self acts like an electronic air cleaner, filtering out what it does not want to see or hear. It sees and hears what suits it and dismisses whatever challenges it with anger and immediate rationalizations.

Curiously, a major deterrent to recognizing the operation of the false self is the subtle manner in which it adapts itself to the spiritual life. It will still seek happiness through the emotional programs of esteem, power, and security; and it will seek to remain in control of the relationship with God. Furthermore, it will seek esteem in spiritual ways, but will react in anger when one's talents or personal holiness is not recognized. Service to others will be about power over them rather than about self-sacrifice or self-giving. It is only by examining one's reactions to others' lack of gratitude or lack of notice that one begins to glimpse one's true motivation. In short, the false self is very extraordinarily subtle, and unless it is faced head on it will continue to influence one's thoughts and actions.

What can be done to reverse the effects of the false self? Centering prayer is the method Keating advocates for dismantling the false self. He notes that this form of prayer can heal the emotional wounds and can open the individual to greater interior freedom and union with God. As a result of the deep rest of body, mind, and spirit, experienced in the regular practice of centering prayer, the individual's defense mechanisms loosen, and the undigested material of early life emerges from the unconscious in the form of primitive feelings or a barrage of images or commentaries. Another effect of this process of dismantling of the false self is an increase in self-consciousness. Furthermore, one's "idea [representation] of God becomes more expanded and profound" (Keating, 1995, p. 102).

> Our awareness during prayer becomes a channel of evacuation similar to the evacuation channels of the physical body… Early emotional traumas were never fully digested, integrated or evacuated because as infants and children we could not articulate our pain… They can only be dissipated by acknowledging or articulating them.
>
> (Keating, 1995, pp. 78–79)

Keating calls this process "unloading the unconscious" and indicates that it can occur both during the time of contemplative prayer and outside the time of prayer. As noted earlier, he calls this process Divine Therapy. By such means the roots of self-centeredness are healed and the emotional programming of the past is erased and replaced. "The *practice of virtue* is the traditional term for erasing the old programs and writing new programs…" (Keating, 1992, p. 16).

In contrasting Divine Therapy with traditional psychotherapy, Keating notes that in Divine Therapy it is:

> not a question of analyzing or discovering what the original difficulty was that might have caused the emotional damage. It is simply a process of unloading the emotional garbage of a lifetime… normally, if we can put up with the purging process, it heals our deepest wounds and uncovers the Divine presence that was present within us all along.
>
> (Keating, 1999b, p. 25)

He suggests that spiritually integrated psychotherapy or counseling may be indicated if the individual becomes "stuck" in or becomes too distraught or otherwise cannot tolerate the purging process.

In short, Keating offers a compelling restatement of the ancient description of the spiritual journey in contemporary psychological language. Not surprisingly, practicing clinicians and spiritual guides have found Keating's formulation clinically useful in conceptualizing their practice of spiritually integrated psychotherapy. Table 3.5 summarizes Keating's conceptualization of the process and dynamics of spiritual transformation.

Table 3.5 The Process and Dynamics of Self-Transformation

1. The true self, which is centered in God, is the basic core of one's goodness. While God and the true self are intimately related, the true self is not God.
2. The human condition, also called original sin, is the universal experience of achieving reflective self-consciousness without certitude of personal union with God. This gives rise to a sense of incompletion, alienation, and guilt, includes all of one's emotional damage from early life experiences and self-serving habits woven into one's personality, is culturally conditioned, and its constellation is one's emotional program, called the false self. The false self motivates all one's basic drives for security and survival, affection and esteem, and power and control. It blocks awareness of the true self.
3. Dismantling the false self requires spiritual practices and purification—called unloading the unconscious, the process of surfacing previously unconscious emotional programming from early life in the forms of primitive feelings or images. This unloading begins when one regularly practices forms of meditation like centering prayer. This self-directed process is called Divine Therapy. It can be facilitated by spiritual guidance and/or psychotherapy, particularly if the individual gets "stuck" or is overwhelmed by the process.
4. An increasing awareness of one's true self, along with a deep sense of spiritual peace and joy accompanying this process, balances the psychic pain of the disintegrating and dying of the false self. This is self-transformation.

The Religious/Spiritual Stress and Resilience Model

Psychotherapists and other mental health professions can cause or compound harm by dismissing or downplaying clients' efforts to discuss their religious or spiritual beliefs. These experiences may constitute microaggressions. As with other forms of microaggression the therapeutic alliance and treatment outcomes can be negatively affected, particularly among clients with specific identities (Trusty et al., 2022). While many sexual and gender minorities consider themselves religious or spiritual, the impact of their religiousness or spirituality on their health and well-being is not well understood. The impact of such microaggressions on clients' health and well-being is now only beginning to be studied. Some initial research suggests that spiritual resilience may foster stress-related growth that emerges through a process of lived transformation and results in increased self-awareness, self-understanding, and a revised construction of identity (Nelson-Becker & Thomas, 2020).

Until recently no research was based on a theoretical and developmental model involving the constructs of religious and spiritual stress and resilience. The Religious/Spiritual Stress and Resilience Model (RSSR) is a research-based model for understanding how religion and spirituality positively and negatively impact the health of sexual and gender minorities (Lefevor et al., 2023). This model bridges existing theorizing on minority stress, structural stigma, and religious and spiritual health pathways to articulate the circumstances under which sexual and gender minorities likely experience religion and spirituality as health promoting or health damaging. Conceptually, the RSSR is a descriptive model in which the relationship between religion, spirituality, and health is mediated by stress and resilience processes and moderated by variables unique to the religious and spiritual experiences of these minorities. The RSSR is based on five empirical assertions regarding the relationship between religiousness/spirituality and health among these minorities.

1. Minority stress and resilience processes influence health.
2. Religion and spirituality influences general resilience processes.
3. Religion and spirituality influences minority-specific stress and resilience processes.
4. These relationships are moderated by several variables relevant to religion and spirituality, like congregational stances on same sex sexual behavior and gender expression, an individual's degree of SGM and religious or spiritual identity integration, and how the individual engages with religion and spirituality.
5. Relationships among minority stress and resilience, religion and spirituality, and health are bidirectional.

(Lefevor et al., 2023)

Lefevor et al. (2023) report on their meta-analysis of 73 studies and conclude that religiousness/spirituality has a small but positive relationship with health among sexual minorities. Moderator analyses suggest that the strength of the relationship between religiousness/spirituality and health depends on three factors: (1) the sexual minority individual's degree of sexual identity integration; (2) the individual's specific religious/spiritual beliefs, practices, and motivations; and (3) the extent to which their environmental circumstances support the individual's sexual and/or religious identities (Lefevor et al., 2023).

This model is unique in that these findings have important implications for the practice of spiritually integrated psychotherapy.

Concluding Note

This chapter has described eight developmental stage models that directly or indirectly address the spiritual dimension. By and large, those models were single dimensional models in that these models focused on a single dimension or aspect of one dimension, i.e., Kohlberg's stage of moral development and the moral dimension. A notable exception was Wilber's Spectrum Model which is more multidimensional in scope. Chapter 2 has described other perspectives, i.e., non-stage theories and models, of the process of spiritual development. While most of these have focused on a single or dual dimensions, one, namely conversion theory, is multidimensional. Table 3.6 compares the various models and perspectives described in both Chapters 2 and 3.

Presumably each of these stage models can contribute something to one's understanding and appreciation of the process of spiritual development. What potential clinical value do these various stage models offer for the practice of spiritually integrated psychotherapy and counseling? Table 3.7 indicates some key insights from these stage models that are applicable in incorporating the spiritual dimension in a clinical setting.

Finally, it is noteworthy that the Religious/Spiritual Stress and Resilience Model is timely given the increased awareness of microaggressions in the therapeutic process, and because this model is empirically derived.

Table 3.6 Comparison of Single and Multidimensional Models and Perspectives

Dimensions of Experience	*Single Dimensional Models and Perspectives*	*Dimensions of Transformation*	*Spectrum Model of Development*
Spiritual	Self-Transformation Perspective Spiritual Development Model Transpersonal Perspective Self-Transcendence Perspective	Religious	Spiritual
Psychological	Faith Development Model Self-Development Model Object Relations Perspective	Intellectual Affective	Cognitive Affective
Social	Psychosocial Development Model	Sociopolitical	Interpersonal
Moral	Moral Development Model Ethical Perspective Character Perspective	Moral	Moral
Somatic		Somatic	

Table 3.7 Stage Models and the Spiritual Dimension

Stage Model	*Key Insights Regarding the Spiritual Dimension*
Psychosocial Development	Development is relational; and there is a developmental sequence to the acquisition of virtues
Moral Development	Moral reasoning does not necessarily produce moral actions; women's moral reasoning can differ from men's moral reasoning
Faith Development	Belief is a process of growth in the transforming of religious meanings rather than the clinging to a particular formulation of the content of a belief or doctrine
Self-Development	Spiritual maturity = freely surrendering oneself and risking a genuinely mutual relationship with others and God
Spiritual Development	Spiritual development = process of developing integrity, wholeness, self-responsibility, and self-transcendence
Spiritual Growth	Depending on the definition of spirituality, spiritual growth may occur before, alongside, or after psychological development, but always requires spiritual disciplines
Spiritual Journey	Dismantling the false self and recovering the true self is the road map of the spiritual journey; spiritual growth requires meditation/contemplation and spiritual practices

References

American Psychiatric Association. (2022). *Diagnostic and statistical manual of mental disorders*, Fifth edition, Text revision. American Psychiatric Association.

Colby, A., & Damon, W. (1992). *Some do care: Contemporary lives of moral commitment*. Free Press.

Conn, J. (1989). *Spirituality and personal maturity*. Paulist.

Cortright, B. (1997). *Psychotherapy and spirit: Theory and practice in transpersonal psychotherapy*. State University of New York Press.

Cunningham, L., & Egan, K. (1996). *Christian spirituality: Themes from the tradition*. Paulist Press.

Erikson, E. H. (1984). Reflections on the last stage—and the first. *The Psychoanalytic Study of the Child*, *39*(1), 155–165.

Flanagan, O. (1991). *Varieties of moral personality: Ethics and psychological realism*. Harvard University Press.

Flanagan, O. (1996). *Self-expression: Mind, morals, and the meaning of life*. Oxford University Press.

Flanagan, O., & Jackson, K. (1987). Justice, care, and gender: The Kohlberg-Gilligan debate revisited. *Ethics*, *97*, 622–637.

Ford-Grabowsky, M. (1987). Flaws in faith-development theory. *Religious Education*, *82*(1), 81–83.
Fowler, J. (1981). *Stages of faith: The psychology of human development and the quest for meaning*. Harper & Row.
Friedman, M. (1993). *What are friends for? Feminists perspectives on personal relationships and moral theory*. Cornell University Press.
Gelpi, D. (1989). Conversion: Beyond the impasses of individualism. In D. Gelpi (Ed.), *Beyond individualism* (pp. 1–30). Notre Dame University Press.
Gelpi, D. (1998). *The conversion experience: A reflective guide for RCIA participants and others*. Paulist Press.
Gilligan, C. (1982). *In a different voice: Psychological theory and women's development*. Harvard University Press.
Gilligan, C. (1988). Remapping the moral domain: New images in self and relationship. In C. Gilligan, J. Ward, & J. Taylor (Eds.), *Mapping the moral domain: A contribution of women's thinking to psychological theory and education* (pp. 3–19). Harvard University Press.
Helminiak, D. (1987). *Spiritual development: An interdisciplinary study*. Loyola University Press.
Johnson, S. (1989). *Christian spiritual formation in the church and classroom*. Abingdon Press.
Keating, T. (1992). *Open mind, open heart*. Continuum.
Keating, T. (1995). *Intimacy with God*. Continuum.
Keating, T. (1998). *Invitation to love: The way of Christian contemplation*. Continuum.
Keating, T. (1999a). *The human condition: Contemplation and transformation*. Paulist Press.
Keating, T. (1999b). Practicing centering prayer. In G. Reininger (Ed.), *The diversity of centering prayer* (pp. 16–26). Continuum.
Kegan, R. (1983). *The evolving self: Problem and process in human development*. Harvard University Press.
Kerber, L. (1986). On in a different voice: An interdisciplinary forum. *Signs*, *11*(2), 304–333.
Larrabee, M. (Ed.). (1993). *An ethics of care: Feminists and interdisciplinary perspectives*. Routledge.
Lefevor, G. T., Davis, E. B., Paiz, J. Y., & Smack, A. C. P. (2021). The relationship between religiousness and health among sexual minorities: A meta-analysis. *Psychological Bulletin*, *147*(7), 647–666. https://doi.org/10.1037/bul0000321
Lefevor, G. T., Etengoff, C., Davis, E. B., Skidmore, S. J., Rodriguez, E. M., McGraw, J. S., & Rostosky, S. S. (2023). Religion/spirituality, stress, and resilience among sexual and gender minorities: The religious/spiritual stress and resilience model. *Perspectives on Psychological Science*, *18*(6), 1537–1561.
Liebert, E. (1992). *Changing life patterns: Adult development in spiritual direction*. Paulist.
Loevinger, J. (1976). *Ego development: Conceptions and theories*. Jossey-Bass.
Nelson-Becker, H., & Thomas, M. (2020). Religious/spiritual struggles and spiritual resilience in marginalised older adults. *Religions*, *11*(9), 431.
O'Keefe, M. (1995). *Becoming good, becoming holy: On the relationship of Christian ethics and spirituality*. Paulist Press.

Rest, J., Edwards, L., & Thoma, S. (1997). Designing and validating a measure of moral judgement: Stage preference and stage consistency approaches. *Journal of Educational Psychology*, *89*, 5–28.
Shweder, R., & Haidt, J. (1993). The future of moral psychology: Truth, intuition, and the pluralist way. *Psychological Science*, *4*(6), 360–374.
Sperry, L. (2012). *Spirituality in clinical practice: Theory and practice of spiritually oriented psychotherapy* (2nd ed.). Routledge.
Sperry, L. (2024). Spiritually integrative psychotherapy: An impending paradigm shift in theory and practice. In L. Miller (Ed.), *The Oxford handbook of psychology and spirituality* (2nd ed., pp. 314–332). Oxford University Press.
Tanner, K. (1996). The care that does justice: Recent writings in feminist ethics and theology. *Journal of Religious Ethics*, *24*, 171–191.
Trusty, W. T., Swift, J. K., Black, S. W., Dimmick, A. A., & Penix, E. A. (2022). Religious microaggressions in psychotherapy: A mixed methods examination of client perspectives. *Psychotherapy*, *59*(3), 351–362. https://doi.org/10.1037/pst0000408
Walker, L. (1991). Sex differences in moral reasoning. In W. Kurtines & J. Gewirtz (Eds.), *Handbook of moral behavior and development* (pp. 333–364). Lawrence Erlbaum.
Walsh, R. (2000). *Essential spirituality: The 7 central practices to awaken heart and mind*. Turner Publishing Company.
Wilber, K. (1983a). *Up from Eden: A transpersonal view of human evolution*. Quest Books.
Wilber, K. (1983b). *Eye to eye: The quest for the new paradigm* (3rd ed.). Shambala.
Wilber, K. (1999). *Integral psychology: Consciousness, spirit, psychology, therapy (A synthesis of premodern, modern, and postmodern approaches)*. Shambala.

Chapter 4

Spiritual Dynamics, Crises, and Emergencies in Psychotherapy

Many believe that the spiritual life and journey is a stress protector and a health-enhancer, and many recent books and articles herald the heath advantages of participation in religious activities and spiritual practices. In other words, the spiritual journey is considered a safe path. Actually, the spiritual journey involves a number of dangers and risks. One of these is a sense of exaggerated self-importance or ego-inflation, particularly the belief that one is holier and better than others. But there are a number of spiritual crises and spiritual emergencies that can be experienced on the spiritual journey, and clinicians are faced with the prospects of differentiating these from major psychopathology. Furthermore, when individuals seek psychotherapy, their spiritual and religious issues predictably reflect their unique personality dynamics. This chapter describes the *Diagnostic and Statistical Manual of Mental Disorders, Fifth Edition, Text Revision* (American Psychiatric Association, 2022) diagnostic category relevant to religious and spiritual problems, as well as detailing the most common spiritual crises and spiritual emergencies noted in psychotherapy clients. It then describes the importance of differential diagnosis and provides useful criteria for differentiating spiritual crises and emergencies from severe psychopathology. Finally, it discusses the unique religious and spiritual dynamics and issues operative in individuals seeking psychotherapy and counseling.

DSM-5-TR

The American Psychiatric Association's *Diagnostic and Statistical Manual of Mental Disorders, Fifth Edition, Text Revision* (DSM-5-TR; American Psychiatric Association, 2022) contains one diagnostic designation regarding religious and spiritual matters. It is the code "Religious or Spiritual Problem" (Z65.8) for specifying a religious or spiritual problem. This diagnostic code and category focuses more on "spiritual crises" as brief reactive responses to specific religious and spiritual experiences. "This category can be used when the focus of clinical attention is a religious or

DOI: 10.4324/9781003425991-5

spiritual problem. It includes distressing experiences that involve the loss or questioning of faith, problems associated with conversion to a new faith, or questioning of spiritual values than may not necessarily be related to an organized church or religious institution" (American Psychiatric Association, 2022, p. 834). Moral injury might also be included in this category (Sperry, 2021). Parenthetically, the conditions described in the subsequent sections on "Spiritual Crisis" and "Spiritual Emergency" could likewise be coded as Z65.8.

Spiritual Crisis

Crisis is commonly defined as an emotionally significant event or radical change of status in a person's life; an unstable or crucial time or state of affairs in which a decisive change is pending. During a crisis an individual's sense of coherence and faith in the continuity of life is shaken, or even shattered, by the stress of a life event. Furthermore, the core elements of an individual's being and connectedness to others are often stretched to the breaking point in a crisis situation. Crises can be of varying degrees of severity, with some being of relatively brief duration while others are longstanding or intermittent. If one assumes that the spiritual dimension is central to all other dimensions of human experience, then it follows that all or most crises are essentially spiritual crises. There are critical transition points in the spiritual life and individuals are greatly influenced by various life events which must be integrated into one's:

> belief structures or they become split off from one's very being resulting in unhealthy rebellion, denial, or apathy. Many honest seekers have turned away from the church and formal religion or, at least, have been puzzled by how their spiritual lives have not fit into the neat pattern so often presented of the faith journey.
>
> (McBride, 1998, p. 4)

McBride (1998) describes, in considerable detail, the issues and dynamics associated with several life crises that involve the spiritual dimension. Table 4.1 is a list of such crises. McBride's book length description of these various crises is important for a number of theoretical and clinical reasons. A significant theoretical reason is that McBride demonstrates the breadth and depth of scientific literature related to this DSM category.

Spiritual Emergencies

Spiritual emergency is a term for describing "how the self becomes disorganized and overwhelmed by an infusion of spiritual energies or new realms of experience which it is not yet able to integrate" (Cortright, 2019,

Table 4.1 Common Spiritual Crises

- Trauma
- Relationships and family problems
- Disillusionment with the Church
- Belief transition
- Denominational identity
- Losses
- Physical illness
- Extremes of thinking or living
- Psychological disturbance
- Religious burnout
- Ethical conflicts
- Personal identity
- The crisis of working with people in crisis

p. 156). The subtitle of the classic text in this area, *Spiritual Emergency* (Grof & Grof, 1989) is quite apt in elucidating the meaning of spiritual emergencies: "When Personal Transformation Becomes a Crisis."

Crises arising when the process of growth and change becomes chaotic and overwhelming are not uncommon and have been described in the sacred literature of all ages as a result of meditative practices and as signposts of the "mystical path" (Grof & Grof, 1989, p. x). Individuals experiencing such episodes believe their sense of self-identity is fragmenting, that their old beliefs and values no longer hold true, and that the ground beneath their personal reality is radically changing. New realms of spiritual experiences can appear suddenly and dramatically leading to immense confusion, anxiety and, sometimes, impaired functioning. Such individuals, who may have no obvious personal vulnerability or family history of mental illness, may wonder if they are experiencing psychosis or psychotic-like symptoms.

Traditionally, psychiatry has not differentiated mysticism from psychosis. As a result, such transformational crises and non-ordinary states of consciousness tend to be treated with psychotropic medication and hospitalization. Not surprisingly, then, mental health professionals are likely to misdiagnose.

There are ten common spiritual emergencies described in Grof and Grof's classic text (1989). Six of these are quite well known to the American public since they have been highlighted in various popular movies and television series. In this book, these ten are presented in the order of their everyday familiarity to most Americans and mental health professionals. Table 4.2 lists these ten spiritual emergencies.

1. **Peak Experiences.** These are also called episodes of unitive consciousness, and sometimes are misdiagnosed as depersonalization or derealization. In these states, individuals report a sense of becoming one with

Table 4.2 Spiritual Emergencies

- Peak Experiences
- Near Death Experiences
- Possession States
- Past-Life Experiences
- Experiences of UFO Encounters
- Communicating with Spirit Guides and Channeling
- The Crisis of Psychic Openings
- Psychological Renewal Through Return to the Center
- The Awakening of Kundalini
- Shamanic Crisis

other persons, nature, or the entire universe. Time and space seem to be transcended and the feelings range from profound peace to ecstatic rapture.

2. **Near Death Experiences.** Because these experiences have been well publicized in the past two decades, they are less likely to be misdiagnosed as delusional disorders as in the past. Typically, the experience involves passage through a tunnel or tube toward a source of light. During this passage the individual describes being unconditionally loved, forgiven, and accepted, and then returns to live according to this higher vision. This experience may be profoundly disturbing and difficult to integrate or appreciate as a second chance to live a more spiritually balanced life.
3. **Possession States.** This phenomenon can be diagnosed as a dissociative identity disorder, as schizophrenia or as a conversion disorder. In it the individual has the distinct impression of being invaded and controlled by an evil entity and engages in bizarre vocalizations and behaviors including contortions and wild spasms. Accurate differential diagnosis is important here. Traditionally, psychology has formulated this phenomenon as an invasion of the ego with id impulses and energies, resulting in a diagnosis of psychosis. It may well be that in some situations this psychological explanation is accurate while in other instances the phenomenon is entirely spiritual in original, and in still other instances there is a mixture of psychosis and possession.
4. **Past-Life Experiences.** Commonly misdiagnosed as hallucinations or delusions, this phenomenon occurs during an altered state of consciousness triggered by regressive therapies such as the breathwork in rebirthing, primal therapy, or in hypnotherapy. It is one of the most dramatic of the spiritual emergencies, particularly when the process occurs in an uncontrolled manner. Typically, it is associated with intense emotional catharsis and physical sensations and the convincing sense of personally remembering and reliving an event previously experienced. After the

process is completed, significant improvement or resolution of present day-symptoms associated with the past-life experience is usually reported.

5. **Experiences of UFO Encounters.** This phenomenon is usually diagnosed as hallucinations or delusions associated with schizophrenia or other psychoses. It is usually experienced as encounters and, sometimes, abduction by what appear to be extraterrestrial beings and spacecraft. Individuals who report these experiences believe them to have actually happened. Such close encounters raise serious concerns about the relationship of consciousness to "objective reality" as well as the personal and collective unconscious. Though it is highly unlikely that such close encounters are "real," some sort of inner experience has occurred, which presents a challenge in differentiating pure psychopathology from unconscious imagery and the archetypal realm of the collective unconsciousness.
6. **Communicating with Spirit Guides and Channeling.** Most likely to be diagnosed as dissociative identity disorder or schizophrenia, this phenomenon involves contact with a suprahuman entity by a channeler or medium either while in a trance or telepathically. Such an experience is very troublesome in that the experience of seeing spirits and hearing voices can lead to serious philosophical confusion in someone with a conventional scientific worldview.
7. **The Crisis of Psychic Openings.** Likely to be misdiagnosed as hallucinations or delusions, or as a depersonalization or dissociative disorder, this phenomenon involves an influx of information from non-ordinary sources such as telepathy, clairvoyance, indiscriminate verbalizations, out-of-body travel, or precognition. It precipitates a spiritual emergency when the individual has no conceptual framework in which to make sense of these experiences, i.e., seeing subtle beings or hearing others' thoughts. As their ordinary self/other boundaries fragment, individuals may believe that their very self is also fragmenting.
8. **Psychological Renewal Through Return to the Center.** Not surprisingly, this experience has been diagnosed as psychoses, such as schizophrenia or bipolar disorder. In it individuals experience a death followed by a regression to the beginning of their lives wherein a clash between the cosmic forces of good and evil is reenacted. A sacred marriage with a divine or mythic figure symbolizing the balancing of masculine and feminine of one's personality may occur. Then, as experience begins to subside, there may be a vision of a transformed universe in which the individual is given the task of bringing about world renewal. Finally, as the intensity of the process recedes the realization that the drama was an inner, psychological transformation rather than an outer reality allows the individual to return to ordinary consciousness.

9. **The Awakening of Kundalini.** This is the most commonly experienced and widely known form of spiritual emergency. Since it tends to be misdiagnosed as mania, an anxiety disorder or conversion disorder, it is essential that clinicians are aware of its manifestations. Kundalini is a form of creative cosmic energy residing in the body's energy centers or chakras. These may be activated by meditation or other spiritual practices releasing new levels of consciousness which can have a spiritual purification function. This is called Kundalini awakening. The energy flow may be gentle or overwhelmingly intense, resulting in visions, widening of consciousness, clairvoyant perception, or frightening involuntary spasms, jerking, or repetitive movements.
10. **Shamanic Crisis.** This crisis tends to be misdiagnosed as schizophrenia or depression. It is a dramatic episode of consciousness that resembles what anthropologists have called "shamanic illness," the initiation experience of shamans. Americans reporting such crises indicate experiencing similar emotional and physical torture, death, rebirth, and a sense of connectedness to animals, plants, or the whole of nature.

Differential Diagnosis

As individuals are encouraged to discuss spiritual matters, a clinician's skill in differentiating health from pathological religious experiences becomes important. Two common differential diagnostic considerations are: differentiating psychosis from "mystical voices and visions" and other "spiritual emergencies," and differentiating clinical depression from the "dark night of the soul."

Differentiating spiritual emergency from psychosis can be quite challenging. Cortright (2019) indicates that it is essential that three sets of criteria be employed to make this determination adequately and accurately. The three sets of criteria are: (1) criteria for spiritual emergencies; (2) criteria for psychosis; and (3) criteria for spiritual experience with psychotic features.

The criteria for making the DSM-5-TR diagnosis of brief psychotic disorder (F23) are rather straightforward, i.e., one or more of the following: delusions, hallucinations, disorganized speech, or grossly disorganized or catatonic behavior. Three criteria for spiritual emergency have been proposed by Grof and Grof (1989). They are: (1) changes in consciousness in which there is significant transpersonal emphasis; (2) the individual's capacity to view the condition as an inner psychological process and approach it in an inner way; and (3) the capacity to form an adequate therapeutic alliance and maintain a spirit of cooperation. Finally, criteria for spiritual experience with psychotic features when elements of both spiritual emergency and psychosis appear to be present have been described by Lukoff (1985). The criteria are: (1) ecstatic mood; (2) sense of newly gained knowledge; (3) if present, delusions with mythological themes; and (4) no conceptual disorganization.

Barnhouse (1986) provides specific criteria for differentiating the hallucinations of the psychotic individual from the voices and visions related to mystical experiences in the non-psychotic. She suggests asking in detail what the individual:

> thinks an appropriate response to the voices and visions might be. Psychotic responses are highly idiosyncratic, usually having to do with the self, others being involved only in a paranoid way. Normal responses are in the direction of healthier self-understanding, better relations with others or constructive action of some sort.
>
> (p. 102)

Differentiating clinical depression from the "dark night" of the spiritual seeker can also be challenging. Both may include such features as hopelessness, helplessness, emptiness, loss of self-confidence, and decreased motivation. May (2023) offers three differentiating criteria: functioning, sense of humor, and compassion. In the dark night impairment of work and relationships is not noted as it is in major depression. A healthy sense of humor is retained in the dark night as contrasted with anhedonia in major depression and the cynical, bitter humor of dysthymia. Finally, May notes that compassion for others is enhanced during the dark night, which contrasts with the self-absorption observed in clinical depression.

Spiritual Dynamics and Personality Styles

Personality may be thought of as the stable and enduring patterns that influence an individual's perceptions, thoughts, feelings, and actions. Such patterns define us as the unique individuals we are. Those patterns that are healthy and adaptive are designated as personality styles. Those that are overly rigid, maladaptive, and affect others negatively are called personality disorders. To keep matters in perspective, the distinction between a trait and a personality disorder needs to be made. Any person can manifest one or more of the traits or features of any of the personality styles without possessing the extremely rigid, compulsive, and maladaptive or disordered pattern of that style.

The disordered pattern, originally called the character neurosis, is rigid and maladaptive and negatively impacts others. That is, others experience varying degrees of anger and suffering as a result of relating to individuals with disordered personalities. Most individuals have a mix of two or more personality patterns that makes them unique (Sperry, 2016).

Where an individual resides on the continuum between personality styles and personality disorders is, in part, a function of early life experiences, but is largely a matter of day-to-day decisions. Just as virtues and vices are outcomes of a lifetime of positive or negative habits and disciplines which are related to moment-to-moment choices involving moral actions, so too is one's personality. The biblical correlate of the personality disorder would be a "hardened heart," while a healthy personality would correspond to a "heart of flesh."

The more rigid and disordered personalities are, the more they adopt rigid conceptual categories and ideologies, and "need" simple answers to complex problems and issues. Not surprisingly, they adopt rigid behavior patterns, particularly compulsive behaviors. Fortunately, psychotherapy and spiritual growth can transform these disordered patterns into healthier styles, at least in some instances.

What follows is a description of the unique religious and spiritual dynamics associated with six personality styles. When individuals with these personality styles seek advice and counsel on spiritual matters in the course of psychotherapy or counseling, it is useful when the clinician has some understanding of how they image God or the higher power in their lives, as well as how they are likely to engage in prayer and spiritual practices, and other religious and spiritual features. Accordingly, following a concise summary of the psychological dynamics of each style (based on Sperry, 2016), there is a brief description of the image of God, prayer style, and other religious and spiritual features associated with each personality style (based on Sperry, 2000, 2012).

The Spiritual Dimension and the Narcissistic Personality

Narcissistic personalities usually exhibit tremendous potential and great things are expected of them. While some of these individuals can be extremely effective personalities, eventually, and inevitably, problems arise. For one, their unceasing need for admiration and the exploitative nature of their relationships become irritating. And, as time goes by, their personal presence seems less than genuine, having a gamey quality to it. In their striving for success, they easily and readily manipulate others. Typically, it is significant stressors such as the onset of physical aging, career setbacks, and the increasing experience of the emptiness in their relationships that precipitates crises, which they may interpret in spiritual and religious terms.

Narcissists believe they must rely on themselves rather than on others for the gratification of their needs. They live with the conviction that it is unsafe to depend on anyone's love or loyalty. Instead, they pretend to be self-sufficient. But, in the depths of their being they experience a sense of deprivation and emptiness. To cope with these feelings and assuage their insecurity, narcissistic individuals become preoccupied with establishing their power, appearance, status, prestige, and superiority. At the same time, they expect others to recognize their entitlement and specialness, and meet their needs. What is particularly striking is their interpersonal exploitativeness. Narcissistic individuals live under the illusion that they are entitled to be served, that their own desires take precedence over those of others, and that they deserve special consideration in life.

Religious and Spiritual Dynamics

The religious and spiritual dynamics of narcissistic personalities are rather predictable and unique and are reflected in their image of God, their prayer style, and other religious and spiritual patterns (Sperry, 2000, 2012).

Image of God

Because of their self-absorption, self-deceiving narcissists must creatively distort the precept to love God and neighbor to fit their pathological perspective. For them, God—and everyone else—exists for one purpose: to love and take care of them. Their basic spiritual deficit is a lack of awareness of grace and an incapacity for gratitude. Not surprisingly, they imagine God as an all-giving father, and they perceive faith as magical entreaty.

Prayer Style

Consequently, they believe God will do exactly as they ask in their prayers, with no regard to the kind of claim God has on them. For them, there is only one kind of prayer: the prayer of petition or demand. Prayer as praise, self-examination, forgiveness, or thanksgiving has little meaning for them. Some narcissistic personalities may have intense mystical leanings that pull them in the direction of mystical experience, including the occult. This is understandable in light of their sense of specialness and grandiosity. However, they are more likely to experience a hypomanic state of self-exaltation than a true mystical state. When prayers are not answered as they expect, they become narcissistically wounded and feel deeply rejected. As a result, they may reject God, becoming an atheist for an instant or forever, because God has let them down.

Other Religious and Spiritual Features

Spirituality provides a ready-made forum to reinforce and reconfirm their grandiose self. For the narcissistic personality, the notion of vocation as a "call" from God or as a sign of "being set apart" serves as further reinforcement and confirmation of their belief in their inherent specialness and superiority over others. The roles of minister, spiritual guide, or teacher provides a forum to exhibit that special call. Thus, the spiritual forum is first and foremost a performance where the audience or spiritual directee "mirrors," i.e., admires and praises, this personality. Essentially, the narcissist believes that the actual purpose of spiritual activity is "worship" of themselves!

Narcissistic individuals are also likely to be insensitive to the suffering and needs of others. While they may help others in need and engage in acts of charity, they will do it only if their charitable deeds are noticed by others. If their efforts do not bring attention to them, they won't make a donation, extend a helping hand, lend a listening ear, or for that matter, continue it when the attention and praise of others stops.

Narcissism and Evil

Evil behaving individuals attack others instead of facing their own failures and construct layers of self-deception to avoid the pain of self-examination, and too often wreak havoc in the lives of others. Human evil has been described as that which kills the spiritual and has been linked to narcissism. Various psychological definitions of evil have been proposed. Zimbardo defines it as consisting of "intentionally behaving in ways that harm, abuse, demean, dehumanize, or destroy innocent others—or using one's authority and systemic power to encourage or permit others to do so on your behalf" (Zimbardo, 2007, p. 5). Scott Peck's definition is similar. He defines evil as the use of "power to destroy others for the purpose of defending or preserving the integrity of one's sick self" (Peck, 1983, p. 241). Of particular note is that Peck contends that the central defect in human evil is not a lack of conscience, but rather a particular variant of the narcissistic personality disorder which is called malignant narcissism. He characterizes malignant narcissism in the following manner. It is a consistent destructive pattern of scapegoating behaviors, along with excessive intolerance to criticism and other forms of narcissistic injury, abrogation of responsibility, and intellectual deviousness.

The Spiritual Dimension and the Obsessive-Compulsive Personality

Obsessive-compulsive individuals seem to be naturally attracted to religious and spiritual practices. This is probably because obsessive-compulsive individuals tend to be preoccupied with rules and duties. Rules provide a sense of orderliness in their lives as well as a measure of control. While obsessive-compulsivity is not necessarily synonymous with a conservative ideology, it certainly is not inconsistent with it. Following rules and the established order is comforting to this personality, as it confirms their view that the world functions best when there is order rather than chaos, and life is gentle and predictable rather than harsh and unpredictable.

Individuals with obsessive-compulsive personality are also individuals who are unable to express warmth and caring except in limited situations. They tend to believe that any spontaneous expression of emotion could be dangerous, and that the extreme expression of emotion represents "craziness." Therefore, they keep their feelings under control. Even their cognitive processes are attenuated and rigid, lacking a sense of playfulness and flexibility.

Interpersonally, they are often polite and loyal, although somewhat rigid and stuffy in their dealings with others. While they are likely to show respect and deference—even to the point of obsequiousness—to superiors, they tend to show relatively little interest in collegiality with peers and those who report to them. They seldom delegate responsibilities for fear that the task will not be done properly. Accordingly, they are firm believers in the dictum: "If you want it done right, do it yourself."

In Western culture, a certain degree of compulsivity in one's work is highly esteemed and rewarded by others. But for individuals with obsessive-compulsive personality such cultural reinforcement becomes a burden and an invitation to workaholism. When these individuals are not working, they believe they are not being responsible and thus have no self-worth. Therefore, they must always be doing something. They must take work home with them, and even when they are on vacation, at the very least, they must stay in touch with their office by text or email. Since many obsessive-compulsives have also internalized the theologically ridiculous dictum "idleness is the devil's workshop," they also feel morally obliged to work compulsively.

They are inclined to be overconscientious and excessively moralistic and inflexible about matters of ethics, law, or values. Although they may generally seem to be mild mannered individuals, they can become quite self-righteous and unpleasant when a pet idea or ideology of theirs is attacked. They may find it difficult to be generous in donating money, time, or gifts to others when little or no personal gain will result. And they find it difficult to relinquish worn-out and worthless objects even when these objects have no actual or sentimental value to them. Generosity is not a high priority for them: they believe in conserving everything they can. They may have large collections of books or records or whatever. They seem to have literally internalized the belief that it's better to save things for a rainy day than to be unprepared and unprotected.

Not surprisingly, these individuals experience excessive guilt feelings because of their internalized sense that they must assume tremendous amounts of responsibility for life. As a result, they are chronically anxious and tense, and seldom are able to look and feel relaxed. They are seldom spontaneous and almost never euphoric, and they cannot live in the present because of their fear of what the future may hold for them. So, they are always prepared—like good Boy Scouts and Girl Scouts—for the expected and unexpected. Since they secretly doubt their ability to deal with the enormity of life, they reduce life to its smallest pieces. They believe that by managing these small pieces, they will eventually control the whole. Of course, it won't happen this way because life cannot be controlled. But they religiously cling to this fiction. Thus, their lives tend to be characterized by a quiet sort of desperation, drabness, and worry.

Religious and Spiritual Dynamics

The religious and spiritual dynamics of obsessive-compulsive personalities are rather predictable and unique and are reflected in their image of God, their prayer style, and other religious and spiritual patterns (Sperry, 2000, 2012).

Image of God

These individuals typically image God as a taskmaster, judge, or police officer. Because of their early life expectation or demand—from parents or caretakers—to be responsible and perfect, these individuals come to believe that God holds these same expectations of them. The belief is that God expects great things of them and will judge them accordingly. Certain scriptures further reinforce this expectation. For instance, "Be perfect, as your heavenly Father is perfect," and the parable of the talents tends to be interpreted literally by these individuals.

Prayer Style

It should not be surprising that the prayer style of obsessive-compulsive individuals tends to focus on their own faults, failings, and need for forgiveness. They will hear and say the words "Lord, I am not worthy that you should come under my roof but speak the words and I shall be healed," but they can only allow themselves to believe the first part: "Lord, I am not worthy." They find it almost impossible to believe that they can be healed and be worthy. Rather, they easily believe and feel that they are sinful and are not, and cannot become, lovable. The words: "You are my beloved in whom I am well pleased" seem directed at others but could never refer to them. Parenthetically, one of the markers that pastoral psychotherapists look for as the obsessive-compulsive personality grows and matures is their increasing acceptance of their status as God's "beloved."

Other Religious and Spiritual Features

Spiritually oriented obsessive-compulsive personalities are likely to believe they were meant to do something important with their lives. They often report that when they were teens or young adults, they experienced a "call" to do something important spiritually or religiously with their lives. Since obsessive-compulsive personalities believe that they must always do what is right and what is expected of them, they look outside themselves for a sense of direction or confirmation. This confirmation may come in a scripture passage they read or in talking to a revered spiritual person, and they conclude that God has somehow clarified the direction.

In spiritual circles, these individuals are more likely to be viewed by others as spiritual or religious overachievers rather than as friendly and caring persons. They tend to be somewhat emotionally immature and are seldom satisfied with their lives. Although they may extol the virtue of living in the moment, they seldom, if ever, take the time to smell the roses. Their interpersonal relationships tend to be predictably remote and lacking in all but superficial intimacy. Yet, they have some capacity for deeper intimate sharing and risk-taking if they can let down their intellectual defenses.

Under moderate levels of stress, these individuals can become overly obsessive regarding religious matters. This may be manifested by guilt feelings, complaining, or scrupulosity. They may find themselves overwhelmed with anxiety or depressive feelings. Then a recurrent thought or scriptural passage convinces them that they are spiritually lost because they "sinned" and cannot be forgiven. As a result, they become agitated and depressed and refuse all measure of reassurance and comfort. They may even become irrational, clinically depressed, and preoccupied with suicidal thoughts.

The Spiritual Dimension and the Passive-Aggressive Personality

The predominant feature that characterizes the passive-aggressive personality is resistance to demands for performance in their work, their relationships, as well as their spiritual beliefs and behaviors. Passive-aggressive personalities follow a strategy of negativism, defiance, and provocation, and are unable to make up their minds as to whether to adhere to the demands of others or to resist their demands. Consequently, their behavior is characterized by both passivity and aggressiveness. They appear to be ambivalent about nearly everything and cannot decide whether to be independent or dependent, or whether to respond to situations actively or passively. They constantly struggle with the dilemma of whether to be submissive or assertive. They resolve this dilemma with a compromise: they express their anger and resistance indirectly through procrastination, dawdling, stubbornness, inefficiency, and forgetfulness.

The passive-aggressive's resistance often reflects hostilities that they are afraid to show openly, but instead have displaced on others. An aura of agreeableness and cordiality usually masks their negativistic resistance. They may smile when they "agree" to do something but under their breath they express their true thoughts and feelings.

These individuals were likely to have experienced being cut off and displaced from their parents' affection at the time of birth of a younger sibling which contributed to their ambivalence of feelings and behavior. Often, these individuals were "chosen" to play a peacemaking role in conflicted families. Therefore, they became fearful of commitments, unsure of their own desires, competencies, the reactions of others, and afraid to express feelings directly. Indecisiveness, contradictory behavior, and fluctuating attitudes were practiced and reinforced. As children, and then as adults, they developed a pattern of shifting rapidly and erratically from one type of behavior to the next, while refusing to acknowledge their own responsibility for their difficulties.

Their basic stance toward life is one of non-cooperation. Because they firmly believe that life has not and cannot be fair, and that other persons have failed to cooperate with them, they feel justified in not only being uncooperative, but in making everyone else's life miserable. Because of their ambivalent self-image, they feel misunderstood, cheated, and unappreciated by life. Subsequently, they easily adopt the role of martyr or "injustice collector" to prove their distress and disaffiliation with others. Furthermore, they are convinced that nothing has ever or will ever work out for them. Needless to say, their selective memory screens out all the past successes they have experienced. Yet, they are resentful and envious of others. If things are going too well for themselves or others, they will make sure that they spoil it. By "snatching defeat out of the jaws of victory" they recreated their expected disillusionment. Consequently, these individuals learned to appear agreeable and show good intentions, but not necessarily enact them. Over time, they established a characteristic personality pattern marked by irresponsibility, uncooperativeness, and lack of commitment.

Religious and Spiritual Dynamics

The religious and spiritual dynamics of passive-aggressive personalities are intimately related to their pattern of ambivalence and negativity This pattern is reflected in their image of God, prayer life, and other religious and spiritual features (Sperry, 2000, 2012).

Image of God

They tend to hold harsh and unloving images of God, and their pessimistic spiritual outlook mirrors the rest of their rather unhappy, unproductive lives. Not surprisingly, obedience is not their strong suit, as they basically distrust and resent authority. Unfortunately, there is one "obedience" to which they are "faithful": that is, not to appear angry or show negative affect. They are exasperating to other members of the community as well as to leaders, particularly because they are never at a loss to "excuse" their own shortcomings in their ministry or blame these shortcoming or failures on others.

Prayer Style

Among the various personality types, the prayer life of passive-aggressive personalities is quite unique. While other personality types may storm heaven with all kinds of petitions or demands of God in their prayers, the passive-aggressive personality's prayer life is remarkable in that hardly exists. While in public liturgical settings they may go through the motions of ritual of praying and may fool ministry peers, superiors, or parishioners, in private they may not even try. After all, they find it very difficult to trust God to meet their needs, so they don't even try.

Other Religious and Spiritual Features

Consistent with their overall pessimism, procrastination, and disorganization in their lives, these personalities tend to be so devoid of faith that their lives are not in any way meaningful in the present, and so devoid of hopefulness about anything working out for them in the future that they seldom make efforts to grow spiritually. If they have begun spiritual direction, they are likely to be early dropouts. If they start reading a religious inspirational book, they are unlikely to finish it. One might surmise that they would surely become atheists, but that requires more courage and resoluteness than they believe they are capable of. So, instead of leaving the ministry they stay, and make their lives and the lives of those around them miserable. Over time, these individuals have a reputation of being "spiritual sourpusses." In short, these individuals lead lives of quiet desperation; more specifically, lives of quiet spiritual desperation.

The Spiritual Dimension and the Borderline Personality

The borderline personality is easily recognized by a pattern of emotional instability and relational extremes. Impulsive, unpredictable, and intense verbal outbursts and threats, as well as physical displays of temper or self-damaging acts, including suicide attempts and self-mutilation, are characteristic of this personality. Surprisingly, this emotional lability tends to be short-lived. After that the person calms down and tends to behave as if nothing unusual had happened. Characteristically unstable in relationships, the borderline individual sometimes over idealizes another person, viewing that individual as incapable of any wrong—yet when frustrated with that person, he or she devalues that individual in the next instant. Because of their personality dynamics these individuals tend to be perpetual "spiritual seekers." They are highly attracted to religious organizations and spiritual practices in hopes of obtaining healing and "salvation." Not surprisingly, they are also attracted to psychotherapy, and are particularly fascinated with depth psychologies, such as Jungian analysis, which they imagine can make them whole and complete persons.

Experienced religious and spiritual leaders are likely to have considerable experience with this personality. It would not be unusual for a church community or large meditation group to have a borderline personality. Religious organizations with an emphasis on love and acceptance can expect to attract individuals who struggle with feelings of emptiness and isolation. Initially, the borderline personality may appear guarded in such a setting. As the organization persists in love and acceptance, however, the borderline personality will form intense attachments. This individual may give glowing testimony to the group's concern and hospitality, and they will predictably respond by giving even more of themselves. As the demands of the borderline personality increase, the organization begins to feel controlled, manipulated, or trapped and predictably withdraws from these individuals. In response to what they perceive as a rejection and the possible loss of the relationship, they may offer to do anything, or accept nearly any humiliation or abuse to save the relationships and avoid the dread and pain of rejection. In anticipation of the threat of rejection, borderlines utilize a variety of psychological defensive maneuvers, particularly the primitive defense of "splitting." Since they have difficulty tolerating both negative and positive feelings simultaneously for the same person, they tend to view others as either "all good" or "all bad." Not surprisingly, those deemed "bad" become targets for the borderline's emotional outbursts.

Overwhelming personal charm is another defense they utilize. To win and maintain the emotional support of others they may lavish these individuals with gifts, time, or praise. Similarly, borderline females may use flattery or seductiveness to secure the attention of male leaders or those who are otherwise influential in the religious organization or spiritual group. When others do not respond as they expect, borderlines will experience feelings of abandonment and worthlessness.

Religious and Spiritual Dynamics

In terms of religious beliefs and spiritual behavior, borderline personalities are considerably ambivalent in their beliefs, feelings, relationships, and behaviors. This theme is reflected in their image of God, prayer life, and other religious and spiritual features (Sperry, 2000, 2012).

Image of God

Predictably, borderline personalities tend to be as confused about the nature and presence of God as they are about their own identity and purpose in life. Not surprisingly, borderline personalities have difficulty maintaining constancy in their spiritual lives. As in other relationships, they are likely to view God as "all good" and themselves as "all bad." As such, they have difficulty dealing with their feelings toward God. Not surprisingly, their image of God can be as variable as their moods. When they are elated, God is imaged as kindly and beneficent, but when they are angry and depressed, God is imaged as a tyrant and source of all their problems. Because of their propensity to project blame outside themselves, they will harbor rageful thoughts and feelings against God and their religious organization even though they are extremely hesitant about admitting they harbor such thoughts and feelings.

Prayer Style

Borderline personalities tend to use spiritual discipline in a self-centered fashion. Prayer becomes a tool for getting God's attention. Their prayers tend to be exclusively prayers of petition: "Oh, God, get me that pastorate, so I can really love you," or "God, make the pastor care as much about me as I do about him." In a childlike fashion, they may make all kinds of promises if their prayers are answered. When their prayers go unanswered, they are crushed and conclude that they will never be acceptable and lovable in God's eyes. God hates them they contend because unanswered prayers mean that God has rejected them.

Other Religious and Spiritual Features

Normally mild-mannered, higher functioning borderline personalities are occasionally observed to engage in vengeful behaviors, such as vitriolic character assassinations and summarily firing a parish council member over what others would consider a trivial matter. What accounts for such un-Christian-like actions? James Masterson, MD has studied the moral thinking process and behaviors of borderline individuals and indicates that they utilize the "talionic principle" in guiding their moral behavior. The talionic principle or "*lex talionis*" is the principle of retributive justice based on the Mosaic law of "eye for an eye, tooth for a tooth." This revengeful, retribution-based moral code, which is more primitive than the Christian moral code of forgiveness, is consistent with the primitive splitting defense so characteristic of this personality disorder. In the movie *Fatal Attraction*, the borderline personality disordered character played by Glenn Close "gets even" with the character played by Michael Douglas by pouring acid on his car, disclosing their affair to Douglas' wife, and then cooking his daughter's pet rabbit on the family's stove. These vengeful behaviors are in retribution for Douglas' rejection of her. Needless to say, borderline personalities have difficulty with the concept of forgiveness. There are some profound implications of this avenging belief with regard to the borderline personality's participation in both psychotherapy and spiritual direction which are discussed in the treatment section.

Furthermore, their spiritual perception is greatly dependent on relational experiences with others. To the extent to which they regularly experience rejection they find it difficult, if not impossible, to tolerate a relationship with God. Predictably, they will idealize a minister or spiritual leader as a kindly, loving substitute father figure. However, whenever this idealized individual fails to live up to their private expectations or because of some minor shortcoming, the idealized individual becomes the target of the borderline personality's rage and is immediately devalued. Since they have not learned to integrate opposite perceptions and feelings, such as love and hate, they are perpetually in turmoil, the kind of turmoil that affects most others around them.

Here is where relatively healthy religious groups and organizations have the potential for being the instrument of deep healing for the borderline personality. For it is only in such a context of a sustained and consistent atmosphere—a holding environment—of love and concern that borderline personalities can ever experience God's love in a sustained way. The challenge, of course, is for such religious organizations to set realistic limits for such personalities and maintain these limits in the face of the borderline's instability. Unfortunately, there are relatively few religious and spiritual communities that can consistently provide the kind of "holding environment" that borderline personalities need. Unless these individuals are fortunate enough to have this sustained experience, it is unlikely that they will achieve a sufficient degree of healing and wholeness to function adequately.

It is for this reason that borderline individuals, even highly functioning ones, are likely to be ineffective as ministers or spiritual guides. They are very likely to fail at all but the least stressful of ministries, which are those that have minimal work expectations and deadlines and even fewer interpersonal demands. Since the majority of ministry positions today are high-stress, high-demand positions that require considerable interpersonal skills, borderline personalities are a poor fit for most religious organizations. Nevertheless, borderline individuals are very attracted to the spiritual life in hopes that it can make up for the early trauma and deprivations they experienced.

The Spiritual Dimension and the Depressive Personality

DSM-IV-TR (American Psychiatric Association, 2000) includes an investigational diagnosis called Depressive Personality Disorder that has considerable face validity and clinical utility in understanding and treating a growing number of individuals today. Central to this disorder is a persistent and pervasive feeling of dejection, gloominess, joylessness, and unhappiness. Individuals with this disorder lack a sense of humor, are overly serious and seem to be incapable of relaxation and enjoyment. They view both the present and the future negatively. They judge others as harshly as they view themselves and tend to focus on others' failings rather than their positive attributes. They may exhibit a wry sense of humor, or they may be openly cynical. In short, pervasive pessimism is a guiding factor in their lives. Unfortunately, it was no longer included in DSM-5 or DSM-5-TR, but depressive personalities were included in PDM-2 (Lingiardi & McWilliams, 2017).

Individuals with this personality style also tend to be quiet, passive and introverted. They tend to be followers rather than leaders and will often allow others to make a wide range of decisions for them. To the extent to which they have histories of early abuse, they tend to be ambivalent about authority figures. Though they may appear friendly and gregarious, they also fear isolation and being alone. They may experience periods of clinical depression and anxiety. Such episodes of depression are usually precipitated by a real loss or abandonment, such as divorce or the death of a spouse.

The depressive personality shares some common features with dysthymic disorder and major depressive disorder. Dysthymic disorder is characterized as a chronic form of depression that last two years or longer, and has less severe depressive symptoms than major depressive disorders. While depressive personality disorder is a chronic disorder (actually, it is a life-long condition), it emphasizes cognitive (self-critical, negativistic, and pessimism), intrapersonal (unhappiness, brooding, inadequacy, and worthlessness), and interpersonal (judgmental and critical of others, and blaming) dimensions, which dysthymic disorder does not.

The depressive personality, according to Weiser (1994), is relatively common in spiritual circles. Weiser notes that individuals with depressive personalities, especially those with compulsive features, are increasingly attracted to religious and spiritual training programs, and are prime candidates for acceptance. To the extent that such programs encourage and support dependence and compliance rather than independence, they can expect to attract certain personality types. Such individuals are likely to be dutiful, obedient, and loyal and can be expected to ascribe to traditional beliefs and values and orthodox practice. They may have a history of volunteer activity and tend to be cooperative rather than competitive. Interestingly, they are likely to be viewed as psychologically healthy individuals simply because they are not a threat to others. They are unlikely to be creative, visionary, or propose new ideas or new programs.

Religious and Spiritual Dynamics

In terms of religious and spiritual dynamics, these individuals appear to be orthodox in their beliefs, and loyal followers despite their ambivalence. This theme is reflected in their image of God, prayer life, and other religious and spiritual features (Sperry, 2000, 2012).

Image of God

Depressive personalities tend to view God as all powerful and as well as merciless at times, and themselves as insignificant and not likely to experience his mercy. So, God is imaged as a blend of Rescuer and Punisher. When prayers are not "answered" or they are not otherwise "rescued," they are likely to fear that God has abandoned them.

Prayer Style

Just as they depend on others to take care of them, they depend on God to take care of their needs. Not surprisingly, petitionary prayer predominates with these individuals: "God help me... protect me... take care of me... comfort me..." When their prayers are not answered as they would like, they easily lose faith and fear being abandoned by God. At such times they turn to others for consolation and comfort.

Other Religious and Spiritual Features

Because of their sense of inadequacy and limited experience in taking responsibility for themselves, they tend to seek out religious counselors repeatedly. They may shift their dependency to spiritual directors or counselors and make numerous telephone calls to them for reassurance between interviews. If the counselor is away on a vacation, they may feel devastated by their sense of abandonment. Not surprisingly, they may have two or more counselors at once without telling them about each other. Interviews and telephone calls are ways of reducing anxiety about the fear of separation.

The Spiritual Dimension and the Hypomanic Personality

The hypomanic personality has been a part of the psychiatric and psychoanalytic literature for nearly a century (Aktar, 1992). Recently, interest in this personality style has been revived due to the clinical and research focus on both the personality disorders and the so called bipolar-spectrum disorders. Unlike hypomania, which is an episode of an elevated mood that must last at least four days, hypomanic personality refers to a style of personality—both character and temperament—that is stable, fixed, and enduring rather than episodic. Currently, hypomanic personality disorder is not included as a distinct and separate diagnostic entity in DSM-5-TR, but it is included in the *Psychodynamic Diagnostic Manual (PDM-2)* (Lingiardi & McWilliams, 2017) and the International Classification of Diseases (ICD-10-CM; CDC, 2023).

The hypomanic personality is consistently described in the literature as being characterized by high energy, needing little sleep, success-oriented, work addiction, playfulness, and talkativeness, but also by defective empathy, impulsivity, disregard of limits, meddlesomeness, and a corruptible conscience. Aktar (1986, 1992) has succinctly described the clinical features of the hypomanic personality.

He notes that their self-concept is grandiose and overconfident. There is a sense of specialness that they share with narcissistic personalities. Moreover, they tend to be cheerful and optimistic most of the time, and they have little doubt about their capacity to make things happen. Nevertheless, they are given to self-doubt and find being alone difficult. Their cognitive style is characterized as glib, articulate, and knowledgeable. They have a penchant for recalling trivia and enjoy punning and the playful use of language. Thus, although they may have a breadth of knowledge, they may often lack depth in most areas. In terms of interpersonal relationships, they quickly and easily develop a broad network of friends and acquaintances, yet they exhibit empathic deficits. They also have a tendency to over idealize others, which can easily switch to contempt. Typically, they foster one or two extremely dependent relationships with individuals who serve and care for them. With regard to love and sexuality they tend to be seductive and flirtatious and are fond of gossip and sexual innuendo.

Hypomanic personalities may be sexually precocious and promiscuous. Sustaining a commitment to an intimate partner may be difficult, and they find equality in such relationships disquieting, preferring to be the dominant individual instead. In terms of social adaptation, they tend to be successful in their endeavors because of their energetic, workaholic style, and because of their capacity to be decisive and daring. In the process they may display questionable judgment in social and financial matters. Not surprisingly, they gravitate toward leadership positions. Unfortunately, they become inordinately dependent upon praise and acclaim.

Religious and Spiritual Dynamics

The religious beliefs and spiritual dynamics of the hypomanic personality are unique. These individuals embody a unique image God, manifest a particular style of prayer, and manifest predictable religious behaviors. These religious and spiritual dynamics reflect their basic spiritual deficit which is a lack of awareness of grace and an incapacity for gratitude (Sperry, 2000, 2012).

Image of God

Hypomanic personalities tend to image God as an all-giving father whose only purpose is to love and care for them. As an all-giving father, God looks down on them with great favor. He will make all their grand plans materialize. And God is there to admire their many accomplishments. Because God is all giving, they assume that God will answer all their prayers. In short, God's purpose is to serve them. They are on earth, not to serve God or others, but are instead privileged to be the recipient of others' service. Not surprisingly, they understand faith as their response to an all-giving God, i.e., faith is the assurance that their needs and wants will be met, that their various projects will be blessed and flourish (Sperry, 2000, 2012).

Prayer Style

Like narcissists, the hypomanic personality believes God will respond exactly as they request in their prayer, irrespective of the claim God has on them. For them, there is only one type of prayer: petitionary prayer. Prayer of praise and thanksgiving may be for other people, but not for them. In the prayers of hypomanic personalities, bad things may happen to good people, but certainly not to special people like them.

Other Religious and Spiritual Features

Because of their self-preoccupation and the belief that God's purpose is to serve them, they are likely to be insensitive to the suffering and needs of others. While they can and do engage in acts of charity, it is for one of two reasons. First, the act is related to the accomplishment of one of their grand plans; that is what is important, not the disadvantaged little people that receive some benefit from it. Second, the charitable act is performed because they will be noticed by others. However, if their charitable efforts fail to bring attention to themselves, they are less likely to make a donation or lend a listening ear or a helping hand. And, when the attention and praise of others stops, so will their charitable behavior (Sperry, 2000).

With regard to ethics and moral standards, these individuals tend to be enthusiastic about ethical and moral matters but can cut ethical corners and can be corrupted. In their enthusiasm, they tend to set high standards for themselves and others, though they may fall considerably short of them. Because of their fascination with all aspects of life, they can become particularly enamored of new trends in psychology, philosophy, and theology.

Concluding Note

The chapter has explored spiritual crises, spiritual emergencies, religious and spiritual disorders and problems, and related spiritual issues. Also described were the most common personality styles/disorders and their characteristic God representations, prayer styles, and other spiritual behaviors. The first four chapters of the book focused on the theory underlying spiritually integrated psychotherapy, while Chapters 5–13 focus on the practice of spiritually integrated psychotherapy.

References

Aktar, S. (1986). Hypomanic personality disorder. *Integrative Psychiatry*, 6(1), 37–52.

Aktar, S. (1992). Hypomanic personality disorder. In *Broken structures: Severe personality disorders and their treatment* (pp. 177–200). Jason Aronson.

American Psychiatric Association. (2000). *Diagnostic and statistical manual of mental disorders*, 4th edition, Text revision. American Psychiatric Association.

American Psychiatric Association. (2022). *Diagnostic and statistical manual of mental disorders*, 5th edition, Text revision. American Psychiatric Association.

Barnhouse, R. (1986). How to evaluate patients' religious ideation. In L. Robinson (Ed.), *Psychiatry and religion: Overlapping concerns* (pp. 89–106). American Psychiatric Press.

CDC. (2023). *International classification of diseases, Tenth revision, Clinical modification (ICD-10-CM)*. CDC.

Cortright, B. (2019). *Psychotherapy and spirit: Theory and practice in transpersonal psychotherapy*. Dev Publishers.

Grof, S., & Grof, C. (Eds.). (1989). *Spiritual emergency: When personal transformation becomes a crisis*. Tarcher/Putnam.

Lingiardi, V., & McWilliams, N. (Eds.). (2017). *Psychodynamic Diagnostic Manual* (2nd ed.). Guilford Press.
Lukoff, D. (1985). The diagnosis of mystical experiences with psychotic features. *Journal of Transpersonal Psychology*, *17*(2), 155–181.
May, G. (2023). *Care of mind, care of spirit: A psychiatrist explores spiritual direction*. Balaji Publications.
McBride, J. (1998). *Spiritual crisis: Surviving trauma to the soul*. Haworth Press.
Peck, S. (1983). *People of the lie: The hope for healing human evil*. Simon & Shuster.
Sperry, L. (2000). *Ministry and community: Recognizing, healing, and preventing ministry impairment*. Liturgical Press.
Sperry, L. (2012). *Spirituality in clinical practice: Theory and practice of spiritually oriented psychotherapy* (2nd ed.). Routledge.
Sperry, L. (2016). *Handbook of diagnosis and treatment of DSM-5 personality disorders: Assessment case conceptualization and treatment*. Routledge.
Sperry, L. (2021). Moral injury in Christian settings: Sacred moral injury. In J. Peteet, S. Moffic, A. Hankir, & H. Koenig (Eds.), *Christianity and psychiatry* (pp. 113–127). Springer Nature.
Weiser, C. (1994). *Healers, harmed & harmful*. Fortress Press.
Zimbardo, P. (2007). *The Lucifer effect: Understanding how good people turn evil*. Random House.

Chapter 5

The Practice of Spiritually Integrated Psychotherapy

Psychotherapy has undergone considerable changes recently because of the ongoing changes and developments in psychotherapy. This chapter begins with an overview of eight elements that reflect current theory, research, and practice, and their evolution. They include: clinical outcomes, empirically supported treatments, practice-based evidence, the therapeutic alliance, client factors, therapist effects, competencies, and mechanisms of change. Similar changes are occurring in spiritually integrated psychotherapy. It then discusses current terminology in spiritually integrated psychotherapy. Finally, it describes developments in psychotherapy competencies as well as spiritual and religious competencies. This discussion serves as an introduction and overview of Chapters 6–9.

Recent Developments in Psychotherapy

A remarkable evolution in the theory, research, and practice of psychotherapy has been underway since the 1990s and has steadily influenced the development of spiritually integrated psychotherapy (Richards et al., 2023). As a result, both conventional and spiritually integrated psychotherapy have become more focused, effective, and accountable.

In 2005 the American Psychological Association formally embraced evidence-based practice in psychology. Evidence-based practice can be defined as "the integration of best research evidence with clinical expertise and patient values" (Institute of Medicine, 2001, p. 147). It is broader than the concept of empirically supported treatment (described below) in that it explicitly considers client values and clinical expertise, i.e., utilizing clinical skills and past experience to rapidly identify the client's health status, diagnosis, risks and benefits, and personal values and expectations. Presumably, then, competent and well-informed clinicians would develop and maintain enhanced therapeutic alliances, utilize best practices information, implement treatment tailored to match client diagnoses, need, and preferences, and monitor clinical outcomes (DeLeon, 2003).

DOI: 10.4324/9781003425991-6

This section overviews eight elements that reflect current theory, research, and practice, and their evolution. They include: clinical outcomes, empirically supported treatments, practice-based evidence, the therapeutic alliance, client factors, therapist effects, competencies, and mechanisms of change.

Clinical Outcomes

Outcomes have become the coin of the realm in psychotherapy today. While processes are still considered important, the culture of accountability and the empirically based treatment movement has made clinical outcomes a central consideration in psychotherapy practice. Outcomes refer to the effects or endpoints of specific interventions or therapeutic processes. Two types of outcomes can be distinguished: immediate or formative outcomes and final or summative outcomes. Outcomes can be assessed in a pre-post-treatment fashion or in an ongoing fashion, i.e., by monitoring outcomes at each session. Research points to better outcomes when clinicians engage in ongoing monitoring than with pre-post assessment or no formal assessment of outcomes (Lambert et al., 2003).

Empirically Supported Treatment

In the 1990s the call for accountability in health care quickly was operationalized as "evidence-based practice" (EBP). Basic to EBP were "empirically based treatments" (EBTs) provided in the context of "randomized clinical trials" (RCTs) and treatment manuals. Manualized treatment, as it is known, involves structured treatment interventions that are performed according to specific guidelines which increase the probability that the interventions are consistently followed across settings, therapists, and clients.

However, the Clinical Psychology Division of the American Psychological Association preferred the term "empirically supported treatment" (EST) to EBP. EST refers to interventions for which empirical research has provided evidence of their effectiveness. As health care cost were spiraling upward, therapists practice patterns were portrayed as the basic cause of waste, inefficiency, and escalating costs. As a result, health care systems and managed care plans moved to standardize care and specify rules for the provision of that care. The expectation was that clinicians—including psychotherapists—would only provide encounter-based, as opposed to relationship-based, services, and be able to demonstrate that services provided were evidence-based and cost-effective. This was the beginning of what has been called the "EST movement in psychotherapy" (Reed et al., 2002).

Psychology had already embraced evidence-based assessments and treatments as part of its long-held commitment to research on assessment and psychotherapy. In 1995 an APA task force was formed to address ESTs in psychotherapy. This EST task force identified both "well-established treatments" and "probably efficacious treatments." Not surprisingly, most were short-term behavioral and cognitive-behavioral approaches, while longer-term, more complex approaches such as psychodynamic interventions were not well represented (APA Division of Clinical Psychology, 1995).

The EST movement has significantly impacted psychotherapy practice. It provided managed care and insurance companies with considerable leverage in controlling costs by restricting the practice of psychological health care. It also prompted local, state, and federal funding agencies to require the use of ESTs. The result is that ESTs are becoming established as the standard of care in psychotherapy. This conclusion is problematic as it is based on a questionable assumption. The assumption is that the provision of EST represents a necessary and sufficient condition for a positive therapeutic outcome.

Practice-Based Evidence

To make outcome research more relevant to clinical practice, a methodology called "practice-based evidence" (PBE) was developed as an alternative to EBT based in RCT settings with manualized treatment. Instead, research studies would be undertaken in the context of routine practice settings. Thus, research would no longer focus on validating specific treatment packages, but focus on whether treatment as usual provides benefits to the types of clients seen at a specific treatment site by specific therapists (Sanders et al., 2015). This approach is in line with the American Psychological Association's official stance on EBP, which encourages practice-based studies and the evaluation of outcomes in routine practice (APA Presidential Task Force on Evidence-Based Practice, 2006).

A major advantage of this approach is that it can study the effectiveness of spiritually integrated therapy without the use of manualized treatment. Thus, the therapeutic efforts of specific therapists are studied, instead of the treatment modality as a whole. It also allows therapists to be involved in the formulation of research questions relevant to their clinical or administrative needs, increasing the likelihood that the research will have an impact on practice. PBE and RCTs are not mutually exclusive but have the potential to answer different questions and to examine the outcomes and processes of psychotherapy from different perspectives (Captari et al., 2022).

The Bridges group was mentioned in Chapter 1. They have funded a number of PBE studies that include the routine monitoring of treatment processes and outcomes of spiritually integrated treatment approaches as they naturally occur in actual mental health treatment settings. It is noteworthy that Bridges does not fund RCTs of spiritually integrated treatment (Richards et al., 2015, 2023).

Therapeutic Alliance

The APA Task Force on Empirically Supported Therapy Relationships (ESR) was formed in 1999 in reaction to the earlier task force on empirically supported interventions. ESR emphasized the person of the therapist, the therapy relationship, and the non-diagnostic characteristics of the patient (Norcross, 2002). The therapeutic relationship and its associated "common factors" are often consistently the single most important variable in the extensive literature on psychotherapy outcome research, to the near exclusion of therapist factors (Wampold & Imel, 2015). An earlier meta-analysis by Lambert (1992) had found that specific techniques—those that were the focus of the studies underlying the EST Task Force report—accounted for no more than 15% of the variance in therapy outcomes. In contrast, the therapy relationship and factors common to different therapies accounted for 30% of the variance in therapy outcomes. Therapeutic alliance is a type of therapeutic relationship which encompasses three factors: the therapeutic bond between client and therapist, the agreed-upon goal/s of treatment, and an agreement about methods to achieve that goal/s. The therapeutic alliance is described in more detail in Chapter 6.

Following the ESR task force report it became increasingly clear that an either-or stance, ESTs or empirically supported relationships, was untenable. Instead, there was increasing acceptance that both ESTs and empirically supported relationships were operative in treatment outcomes.

Client Factors

That "both-and" understanding would soon be found to be shortsighted. A subsequent meta-analysis of the elements accounting for psychotherapy change (Lambert & Barley, 2001) found that the largest element accounting for change (40%) was due to extra-therapeutic factors, also referred to as "client resources" or "client." This finding was essentially the same as previously reported (Lambert, 1992). The client element includes several factors such as motivation and readiness for change, capacity for establishing and maintaining relationships, access to treatment, social support system, and other non-diagnostic factors.

Therapist Effects

Until very recently, psychotherapy research and training programs have emphasized common factors and treatment factors but not therapist factors. It was assumed that therapists were basically the same and they did not need to be the focus of research or training. This understanding was dubbed the myth of uniformity (Wampold & Imel, 2015). But the reality is that some therapists are better, meaning that they are more effective than other therapists. The question is how and why they are different (Castonguay & Hill, 2017).

Highly effective therapists demonstrate what is called therapist expertise (Sperry & Carlson, 2014) or high-level "therapist effect" (Sperry, 2022).

Therapist effect refers to the impact of a given therapist on a client's treatment outcome when compared to the outcomes of another therapist (Sperry, 2021). This effect is identified when a therapist consistently achieves better outcomes with clients than other therapists, regardless of the presenting issues or the treatment delivered. From a research perspective, therapist effect represents the amount of variance attributable to who the therapist is rather than to treatment effect (Wampold et al., 2017).

While in the past it was assumed that treatment effects were higher than therapist effects, currently "the preponderance of the evidence indicates that there are important therapist effects (in the range of 3 percent to 7 percent of the variability in outcomes) accounted for by therapists" (Wampold & Imel, 2015, p. 176). Of surprise to many, "therapist effects generally exceed treatment effects, which at most account for one percent of the variability in outcomes" (Wampold & Imel, 2015, p. 176).

Highly effective therapists tend to have sophisticated interpersonal skills and easily form strong therapeutic alliances, induce clients to accept treatment, and work therapeutically with them. They develop accurate case conceptualizations which form the basis for planning, tailoring, and implementing appropriate interventions, and then monitor treatment progress, usually with outcome measures (Sperry, 2022).

Therapist effect has also been identified in trainees. Recent research indicated that, after accounting for effects related to therapeutic orientation and clinical experience, some therapists-in-training had consistently more favorable client outcomes, while other trainees had less favorable outcomes (Edmondstone et al., 2023). This and other research recommend that training programs intentionally emphasize therapist effect and expertise. This means identifying strategies for fostering therapist expertise so that trainers, supervisors, and therapists themselves can focus on improving clinical outcomes (Wampold & Imel, 2015).

Therapist Effect in Spiritually Integrated Psychotherapy

There is no question that therapist effect makes a difference in conventional psychotherapy. Presumably, it can also make a difference in spiritually integrated psychotherapy. However, there has been relatively little research on therapist effect in comparison to the research on spiritually oriented treatments, i.e., treatment effects. In many respects, spiritually integrated psychotherapy is at least a decade or two behind in researching therapist effect (Sperry, 2016).

For spiritually integrated psychotherapy to fully develop and mature as a field, some significant challenges must be addressed. The first is to accept that therapist effects explain more variance than treatment effects. The second is to make therapist effect an integral part of clinical research in spiritually integrated psychotherapy. The third is for psychotherapy training programs to intentionally ground teaching and supervision in research on both treatment effects and therapist effects. Only when all three challenges are met will spirituality integrated psychotherapy continue to grow and flourish (Sperry, 2016).

Psychotherapy Competencies

In addition to the focus on these five elements is the role of competencies. Competency represents a paradigm shift in psychotherapy training and practice, and, not surprisingly, has effected and will continue to effect change. Requirement standards are beginning to be replaced with competency standards, core competencies are replacing core curriculums, and competency-based licensure is on the horizon. The shift to psychotherapy competency is also an accreditation standard in psychiatry training programs that now requires that trainees demonstrate competency in three psychotherapy approaches. Training programs in clinical psychology programs have solidly embraced competencies, and marital and family therapy and professional counseling programs are poised to follow suit. Because competencies involve knowledge, skill, and attitudinal components, competency-based education is very different in how psychotherapy is taught, learned, and evaluated (Sperry & Sperry, 2023).

Six essential psychotherapy competencies have been described. They are: (1) articulate a conceptual framework for psychotherapy practice; (2) develop and maintain an effective therapeutic alliance; (3) develop an integrative case conceptualization and treatment plan based on an integrative assessment; (4) implement interventions; (5) monitor treatment progress and outcomes and plan for termination process; (6) practice in a culturally sensitive and ethically sensitive manner (Sperry, 2021, 2022).

Competencies: American Psychological Association

Research indicates that clients want to have their spiritual and religious concerns addressed in psychotherapy. For the most part, these issues are neither discussed nor included in assessment or treatment planning. While medicine, psychiatry, and the counseling professional require some training in spiritual and religious issues, psychologists receive little or no training in this area, in part because there is no agreed-upon set of spiritual competencies or training guidelines (Vieten & Lukoff, 2022).

Many of the proposed spiritual and religious competencies were based on literature reviews, theory, and clinical expertise. In contrast, Vieten and colleagues developed a set of empirically based spiritual and religious competencies for the field of psychology including attitudes, knowledge, and skills in the spiritual and religious domains (Vieten et al., 2013). Table 5.1 summarizes these competencies.

Table 5.1 Spiritual and Religious Competencies for Psychology

Attitudes

1. Demonstrate empathy, respect, and appreciation for clients from diverse backgrounds and affiliations.
2. View and appreciate spirituality and religion as important aspects of human diversity.
3. Be aware of how one's own background and beliefs influence one's clinical practice.

Knowledge

4. Learn how diverse beliefs and practices are important to one's clients.
5. Understand that spirituality and religion are different but overlapping constructs.
6. Understand and recognize the difference between spirituality and psychopathology
7. Recognize that spirituality and religiousness develop and change over the life span.
8. Recognize how spiritual and religious resources and practices may support psychological well-being and recovery from psychological disorders.
9. Recognize how spirituality and religion can negatively impact psychological health.
10. Identify legal and ethical issues related to spirituality and religion that may surface in working with clients.

Skills

11. Conduct empathic and effective psychotherapy with clients from diverse spiritual and religious backgrounds, affiliations, and levels of involvement.
12. Inquire about spiritual and religious background, experience, practices, attitudes, and beliefs as a standard part of understanding a client's history.
13. Help clients explore and access their spiritual and religious strengths and resources.
14. Identify and address spiritual and religious problems in clinical practice and make referrals when necessary.
15. Stay abreast of research and developments related to clinical practice and engage in ongoing assessment of one's own spiritual and religious competence.
16. Acknowledge the limits of one's qualifications and competence and seek consultation, further training, or appropriate referral.

Summarized from Vieten et al., 2013; Vieten & Lukoff, 2022

Practice guidelines tend to be based on empirically based competencies. In the field of psychology such guidelines have been developed for several forms of multicultural diversity. However, no practice guidelines for spiritual and religious diversity have yet to be promulgated, although an APA Division 36 task force has been established for this purpose (Vieten & Lukoff, 2022).

Competencies: American Counseling Association

The Association for Spiritual, Ethical, and Religious Values in Counseling (ASERVIC), a division within the American Counseling Association, articulate a set of competencies for counseling practice involving spiritual issues (Miller, 1999). Later ASERVIC provided the revision: "Competencies for Addressing Spiritual and Religious Issues in Counseling" (Cashwell & Watts, 2010). It consists of 13 competencies of which the first five are cognitive competencies, e.g., "can describe the similarities and differences between spirituality and religion," while the last five are clinical competencies. These involve assessment, diagnosis, goals setting, and the utilization of spiritually sensitive treatment interventions. Table 5.2 summarizes these competencies. It is anticipated that an ASERVIC Task Force will provide an update to these competencies in 2025.

Core Clinical Competencies in Spiritually Integrated Psychotherapy Practice

The lists of spiritual and religious competencies offered by APA and ACA are comprehensive and cover attitudes, knowledge, and skills. However, the everyday practice of spiritually integrated psychotherapy involves primarily core clinical competencies. Table 5.3 provides a list of such core clinical competencies for actual practice. These practice-based competencies were derived from Aten and Leach (2009), Sperry and Sperry (2023), and Sperry (2016).

Mechanisms of Change in Psychotherapy

For decades the question has been asked: "How does psychotherapy work to effect change?" In technical terms the question involves both the basic target of change and the mechanisms of change in the psychotherapeutic process. Specifying the target and the mechanisms of change began in research and practice in Era III and continues to expand in Era IV.

The Special Interest Group on Convergence in Psychotherapy of the Society for the Exploration of Psychotherapy Integration identified

Table 5.2 Spiritual and Religious Competencies in Counseling (ASERVIC)

1. Describes S/R, including the basic beliefs of various spiritual systems, major world religions, agnosticism, and atheism.
2. Recognizes that client's S/R beliefs (or absence) are central and can influence psychosocial functioning.
3. Explores his/her own attitudes, beliefs, and values about S/R.
4. Evaluates the influence of his/her S/R beliefs and values on the client and the counseling process.
5. Can identify the limits of his/her understanding of the client's S/R perspective and is acquainted with S/R resources.
6. Responds to client communications about S/R with acceptance and sensitivity.
7. Uses S/R concepts consistent with client's S/R perspectives acceptable to the client.
8. Recognizes S/R themes in client communication and address these when relevant.
9. Assesses client's S/R perspective by gathering information from the client and/or other sources.
10. Makes a diagnosis and recognizes client's S/R perspectives can a) enhance well-being; b) contribute to client problems; and/or c) exacerbate symptoms.
11. Sets goals with the client that are consistent with the client's S/R perspectives.
12. Able to a) modify therapeutic techniques to include client's S/R perspectives, and b) utilize S/R practices when appropriate and acceptable to client.
13. Can therapeutically apply theory and current research supporting the inclusion of a client's S/R perspectives and practices.

Summarized from Cashwell & Watts, 2010

Table 5.3 Core Clinical Competencies in Spiritually Integrated Psychotherapy Practice

1. Develop a therapeutic alliance that is sensitive to spiritual dimension.
2. Maintain the therapeutic alliance and deal with spiritual transference–countertransference, alliance ruptures, ambivalence, and resistance.
3. Assess and diagnose, including the spiritual dimension.
4. Incorporate the spiritual dimension in the case conceptualization.
5. Incorporate the spiritual dimension in treatment planning and mutual goal setting.
6. Implement spiritual and psychological interventions.
7. Refer to or consult with religious/spiritual resources, if indicated.
8. Monitor and evaluate overall treatment progress and outcomes on all dimensions, including the spiritual dimension.
9. Incorporate spiritual dimension in the termination process.

"pattern" as the basic target of change, with the basic goal of psychotherapy being to replace entrenched maladaptive patterns with more adaptive ones. Such patterns are encoded in long-term memory, within neural networks and pathways that are influenced by the strength and number of synapses (Smith, 2022, 2024).

Contemporary neuroscience has identified two mechanisms by which maladaptive patterns can be modified: "extinction" and "memory reconsolidation." Extinction influences the cortex to inhibit expression of the maladaptive pattern. Memory reconsolidation involves a process wherein memories are available to be altered for a short time after they are activated and recalled. When originally created a memory is stored in neural pathways, and when that memory is retrieved it can be modified (Lane et al., 2015). In psychotherapy, the process of memory reconsolidation reprograms information so that a healthier response and pattern is retained. This information is stored in neural networks as a result of new, corrective experiences or cognitions (Ecker & Vaz, 2022; Lane et al., 2015). These mechanisms are widely represented in the brain and are generalizable to the full range of psychotherapy interventions.

Based on the science of memory reconsolidation as well as extinction, change mechanisms can be precisely defined. Then, psychotherapeutic techniques can be focused on the process of shifting and changing the maladaptive pattern to a more adaptive pattern. Presumably, this involves three processes. First is the activation of the maladaptive pattern and its emotional component. Second is the provision of disconfirming information and extinction of negative emotion. Third is learning a more adaptive patterns and its transmission from consciousness to limbic memory. All three processes are facilitated by a positive and supportive therapeutic relationship (Smith, 2022, 2024).

Terms and Designations

As a field or specialty evolves a consensus slowly develops regarding terminology and the definitions of key constructs. In the interim confusion about terms and designations is common. This is currently the situation in spirituality and psychotherapy. As noted in Chapter 1 there is not yet a consensus on the definition of general terms such as spirituality nor is there consensus about the relationship of spiritual dimension and the psychological dimension. More specifically, there is no consensus on the meaning of the designation psychospiritual problem and interventions, but increasing consensus on the designations of the practice of psychotherapy that is sensitive to the spiritual dimension. This section addresses both of these considerations.

Psychospiritual Problem and Interventions

The terms "psychological," "spiritual," and "psychospiritual" seem like useful designations for describing the kind of problems and interventions employed in the practice of spiritually integrated psychotherapy. At first glance it would seem relatively easy to classify interventions as either "psychological," "spiritual," or "psychospiritual." For example, there would be no question that cognitive restructuring should be classified as a psychological intervention, or that prayer is a spiritual intervention or practice. But what constitutes a psychospiritual intervention? While some would insist that mindfulness is a psychospiritual intervention (Mijares & Khalsa, 2005), others consider it a psychological intervention (Segal et al., 2002), and still others classify it as a spiritual intervention (Aten et al., 2011). The point is that there is no consensus among professionals about the meaning of the term "psychospiritual."

A review of the professional literature over the past 40 years indicates that the term psychospiritual was used more often in the 1980s and early 1990s than in the present. Take, for example, the initial proposal for adding a new diagnostic category to DSM-IV (American Psychiatric Association, 1994) that addressed religious and spiritual concerns. The proposed name for the category was "Psychoreligious and Psychospiritual Problems" (Lukoff et al., 1992). DSM leadership voted against this terminology and instead chose the more conventional designation "Religion and Spiritual Problems" (American Psychiatric Association, 1994). In DSM-5 the designation was changed to "Religious and Spiritual Problems" (American Psychiatric Association, 2013).

It is probably no coincidence that recent textbooks and professional books, book chapters, and articles on spirituality and spiritually integrated psychotherapy do not use the term "psychospiritual," and if it is mentioned in passing, it is not formally defined. In short, because there is no consensus on the meaning of the designation "psychospiritual" its usage is of questionable value, at least at this time.

Psychotherapy Sensitive to the Spiritual Dimension

Currently the terms spiritually oriented, spiritually accommodative, spiritually informed, and spirituality integrated psychotherapy are often used synonymously. While there is some overlap among them, there are also differences. Typically, spiritually accommodative approaches combine a manualized treatment with practices and beliefs from a specific religious tradition. In contrast, spirituality oriented approaches are less standardized and more inclusive which increases their applicability to a fuller range of spiritual beliefs and religious traditions (Schlosser & Safran, 2009). An example of spirituality accommodative psychotherapy is Christian-accommodative cognitive-behavioral therapy. In this widely used and researched approach, Christian images, prayer, biblical examples, and religiously focused cognitive disputation may be utilized with Christian clients (Johnson & Ridley, 1992; Propst et al., 1992). Examples of spirituality integrated psychotherapy include theistic integrative psychotherapy which addresses spiritual issues from a theistic perspective (Richards, 2009), and spiritually oriented psychotherapy which is grounded in a biopsychosocio-spiritual model, as well as attachment theory and God image research (Sperry, 2013).

As spiritually integrated psychotherapy has continued to evolve over the recent past, the following definition of it has emerged. It reflects the importance of the essential psychotherapy competencies and distinguishes it from pastoral counseling and spiritual direction.

> Spiritually integrated psychotherapy is a broad designation that refers to approaches provided by therapists that integrate the essential psychotherapy competencies as well as spiritual resources in addressing spiritual issues and struggles to resolve psychological and relational problems. Although it can also foster spiritual change and growth, spiritually integrated psychotherapy accomplishes this as a by-product that accompanies psychological change. It is distinct from pastoral counseling and spiritual direction in its treatment focus and training.
>
> (Sperry, 2024, p. 11)

Rather than being a new treatment approach, spiritually integrated psychotherapy integrates or weaves greater sensitivity and explicit attention to the spiritual dimension into the therapeutic process (Richards et al., 2023). Accordingly, spirituality can be interwoven into virtually any psychotherapeutic approach whether dynamic, cognitive-behavioral, existential-humanistic, or family systems. As the result of this integration, the "character of each of these forms of psychotherapy will be deepened and enriched, and psychotherapy as a whole will be transformed" (Pargament et al., 2005, p. 161).

Concluding Note

Psychotherapy is a rapidly changing field. The culture of accountability, the evidence-based treatment movement, and the competency movement have and will continue to require that psychotherapy practice be accountable, effective, and competent. Spiritually integrated psychotherapy is also evolving. It is no longer sufficient for clinicians to demonstrate some sensitivity to a client's religious and spiritual issues while adapting a conventional psychotherapeutic approach. Increasingly, clinicians working with clients with spiritual and religious issues will be expected to attend to all five elements: clinical outcomes, evidence-supported treatments, the therapeutic alliance, client factors, and therapist factors throughout all phases of the therapeutic process from assessment and establishing a therapeutic alliance to termination.

References

American Psychiatric Association. (1994). *Diagnostic and statistical manual of mental disorders*, 4th ed. American Psychiatric Association.

American Psychiatric Association. (2000). *Diagnostic and statistical manual of mental disorders*, 4th ed., *Text revision*. American Psychiatric Association.

American Psychiatric Association. (2022). *Diagnostic and statistical manual of mental disorders*, 5th ed., Text revision. American Psychiatric Association.

APA Division of Clinical Psychology. (1995). Training in and dissemination of empirically validated psychological treatments: Report and recommendations. *Clinical Psychologist*, *48*, 3–27.

APA Presidential Task Force on Evidence-Based Practice. (2006). Evidence-based practice in psychology. *The American Psychologist*, *61*(4), 271–285.

Aten, J., & Leach, M. (Eds.). (2009). *Spirituality and the therapeutic process: A comprehensive resource from intake to termination*. American Psychological Association.

Aten, J. D., McMinn, M. R., & Worthington, E. L. Jr. (2011). *Spiritually oriented interventions for counseling and psychotherapy*. The American Psychological Association.

Captari, L. E., Sandage, S. J., & Vandiver, R. A. (2022). Spiritually integrated psychotherapies in real-world clinical practice: Synthesizing the literature to identify best practices and future research directions. *Psychotherapy*, *59*(3), 307–320. https://doi.org/10.1037/pst0000407

Cashwell, C., & Watts, R. (2010). The new ASERVIC competencies for addressing spiritual and religious issues in counseling, *Counseling and Values*, *55*, 2–5.

Castonguay, L. G., & Hill, C. E. (Eds.). (2017). *How and why are some therapists better than others? Understanding therapist effects*. American Psychological Association. https://doi.org/10.1037/0000034-003

DeLeon, P. H. (2003). Remembering our fundamental societal mission. *Public Service Psychology*, *28*, 13.

Ecker, B., & Vaz, A. (2022). Memory reconsolidation and the crisis of mechanism in psychotherapy. *New Ideas in Psychology*, *66*, 100945.

Edmondstone, C., Pascual-Leone, A., Soucie, K., & Kramer, U. (2023). Therapist effects on outcome: Meaningful differences exist early in training. *Training and Education in Professional Psychology*, *17*(2), 149–157. https://doi.org/10.1037/tep0000402

Institute of Medicine. (2001). *Crossing the quality chasm: A new health system for the 21st century*. Institute of Medicine.

Johnson, W. B., & Ridley, C. R. (1992). Brief Christian and non-Christian rational-emotive therapy with depressed Christian clients: An exploratory study. *Counseling and Values*, *36*(3), 220–229.

Lambert, M. (1992). Psychotherapy outcome research: Implications for integrative and eclectic therapists. In J. Norcross & M. Goldfried (Eds.), *Handbook of psychotherapy* (pp. 94–129). Basic Books.

Lambert, M., & Barley, D. E. (2001). Research summary on the therapeutic relationship and psychotherapy outcome. *Psychotherapy: Theory/Research/Practice/Training*, *38*, 357–361.

Lambert, M., Whipple, J., Smart, D., Vermeersch, D., Nielsen, S., & Hawkins, E. (2003). Is it time for clinicians to routinely track patient outcomes? A meta-analysis. *Clinical Psychology: Science and Practice*, *10*, 288–301.

Lane, R. D., Ryan, L., Nadel, L., & Greenberg, L. (2015). Memory reconsolidation, emotional arousal, and the process of change in psychotherapy: New insights from brain science. *Behavioral and Brain Sciences*, *38*, 1–64.

Lukoff, D., Lu, F., & Turner, R. (1992). Toward a more culturally sensitive DSM-IV: Psychoreligious and psychospiritual problems. *The Journal of Nervous and Mental Disease*, *180*(11), 673–682.

Miller, G. (1999). The development of the spiritual focus in counseling and counselor education. *Journal of Counseling & Development*, *77*, 498–501.

Norcross, J. (2002). Empirically supported therapy relationship. In J. Norcross (Ed.), *Psychotherapy relationships that work: Therapist contributions and responsiveness to patients* (pp. 3–16). Oxford University Press.

Pargament, K. (2007). *Spiritually integrated psychotherapy: Understanding and addressing the sacred*. Guilford.

Pargament, K., Murray-Swank, N., & Tarakeshwar, N. (2005). An empirically based rationale for a spiritually integrated psychotherapy. *Mental Health, Religion & Culture*, *8*(3), 155–165.

Propst, L. R., Ostrom, R., Watkins, P., Dean, T., & Mashburn, D. (1992). Comparative efficacy of religious and nonreligious cognitive-behavioral therapy for the treatment of clinical depression in religious individuals. *Journal of Consulting and Clinical Psychology*, *60*(1), 94–103. https://doi.org/10.1037/0022-006X.60.1.94

Reed, G. M., McLaughlin, C., & Newman, R. (2002). American Psychological Association policy in context: The development and evaluation of guidelines for professional practice. *American Psychologist*, *57*, 1041–1047.

Richards, P. S. (2009). Toward religious and spiritual competence for psychologists: Some reflections and recommendations. *Professional Psychology: Research, and Practice*, *40*, 389–391.

Richards, P. S., Pargament, K. I., Exline, J. J., & Allen, G. E. K. (2023). Introduction: Bringing spiritually integrated psychotherapies into the health care mainstream. In P. S. Richards, G. E. K. Allen, & D. K. Judd (Eds.), *Handbook of spiritually integrated psychotherapies* (pp. 3–29). American Psychological Association. https://doi.org/10.1037/0000338-001

Richards, P. S., Sanders, P. W., Lea, T., McBride, J. A., & Allen, G. E. (2015). Bringing spiritually oriented psychotherapies into the health care mainstream: A call for worldwide collaboration. *Spirituality in Clinical Practice*, *2*(3), 169–179.

Sanders, P. W., Richards, P. S., McBride, J. A., Lea, T., Hardman, R. K., & Barnes, D. V. (2015). Processes and outcomes of theistic spiritually oriented psychotherapy: A practice-based evidence investigation. *Spirituality in Clinical Practice*, *2*(3), 180–190. https://doi.org/10.1037/scp0000083

Schlosser, L., & Safran, D. (2009). Implementing treatments that incorporate client's spirituality. In J. Aten & M. Leach (Eds.), *Spirituality and the therapeutic process: A comprehensive resource from intake to termination* (pp. 193–216). American Psychological Association.

Segal, Z., Teasdale, J., & Williams, M. (2002). *Mindfulness-based cognitive therapy for depression*. Guilford Press.

Smith, J. (2022, April 26). Why understanding neurobiology of maladaptive patterns is vital to psychiatry? *Psychiatric News*. https://doi.org/10.1176/appi.pn.2022.05.5.28

Smith, J. (2024). Knowledge of memory reconsolidation can improve psychodynamic technique. *Psychodynamic Psychiatry*, *52*(1), 8–12. https://doi.org/10.1521/pdps.2024.52.1.8

Sperry, L. (2013). Distinctive approaches to religion and spirituality: Pastoral counseling, spiritual direction, and spiritually integrated psychotherapy. In K. I. Pargament, A. Mahoney, & E. P. Shafranske (Eds.), *APA handbook of psychology, religion, and spirituality (Vol. 2): An applied psychology of religion and spirituality* (pp. 223–238). American Psychological Association. https://doi.org/10.1037/14046-011

Sperry, L. (2016). Therapist effects and spiritually oriented psychotherapy. *Open Theology*, *2*(1), 286–295.

Sperry, L. (2021). *Pattern focused therapy: Highly effective CBT practice in mental health and integrated care settings*. Routledge.

Sperry, L. (2022). *Highly effective therapy: Effecting deep change in counseling and psychotherapy* (2nd ed.). Routledge.

Sperry, L. (2024). The moral domain, moral injury, and the healing process. *Journal of Christian Healing*, *40*(1), 5–14.

Sperry, L., & Carlson, J. (2014). *How master therapists work: Effecting change from the first through the last session and beyond*. Routledge.

Sperry, L., & Sperry, J. (2023). *Core competencies in counseling and psychotherapy: Becoming a highly competent and effective therapist* (2nd ed.). Routledge.

Vieten, C., & Lukoff, D. (2022). Spiritual and religious competencies in psychology. *American Psychologist*, *77*(1), 26–38. https://doi.org/10.1037/amp0000821

Vieten, C., Scammell, S., Pilato, R., Ammondson, I., Pargament, K. I., & Lukoff, D. (2013). Spiritual and religious competencies for psychologists. *Psychology of Religion and Spirituality*, *5*(3), 129–144. https://doi.org/10.1037/a0032699

Wampold, B. E., & Imel, Z. E. (2015). *The great psychotherapy debate: The evidence for what makes psychotherapy work*. Routledge.

Wampold, B. E., Baldwin, S. A., Holtforth, M., & Imel, Z. E. (2017). What characterizes effective therapists? In L. G. Castonguay & C. E. Hill (Eds.), *How and why are some therapists better than others? Understanding therapist effects* (pp. 37–53). American Psychological Association.

Chapter 6

Therapeutic Relationship

Effective therapy typically begins with the establishment of an effective therapeutic relationship, also called a therapeutic alliance. The therapeutic alliance can have a profound effect on the treatment process and outcomes. Research consistently demonstrates that the therapeutic relationship is the best predictor of therapeutic outcome (Horvath & Symonds, 1991; Orlinsky et al., 2004). Research also indicates that incorporating spiritual issues in the treatment process can facilitate or complicate the relationship-building process (Morrison & Borgen, 2010). Accordingly, relationship building and maintenance are critical in the practice of spiritually integrated psychotherapy. In addition, resistance and countertransference are not uncommon in spiritually integrated psychotherapy and are essential in fostering client progress and reducing premature termination. This chapter focuses on the development and maintenance of an effective relationship, more formally referred to as the therapeutic alliance. It begins with a discussion of establishing an effective therapeutic relationship. Then, it describes the importance of maintaining that relationship, and discusses the ways in which resistance and countertransference are present in spiritually integrated psychotherapy, and strategies for dealing with these processes. One of these is motivational interviewing. Finally, it illustrates key points in a case example.

Establishing an Effective Therapeutic Alliance

The therapeutic alliance begins with the first contact between client and therapist and continues until the last contact. Although initial interactions are especially important, as first impressions usually are, the development of the therapeutic alliance is intertwined with all aspects of the treatment process, and it evolves and changes over time. An effective therapeutic alliance may develop as early as the first session but must be in place by the fifth session if treatment is to be successful (Orlinsky et al., 2004; Sperry

DOI: 10.4324/9781003425991-7

et al., 1996). Needless to say, every client–therapist contact, either positive or negative, influences the development and maintenance of the therapist alliance.

A clinically useful view of the therapeutic alliance operationalizes it with three factors: bond, goals, and tasks (Bordin, 1979). Important to the formation of a strong therapeutic bond is that clients feel understood, safe, and hopeful. It also means that they are more likely to take the risk of disclosing painful affects and intimate details of their lives, as well as risk thinking, feeling, and acting in more adaptive and healthier ways. Besides the therapeutic bond, clinicians need to attend to mutually agreed upon therapeutic goals and tasks or methods. This entails a recognition of the client's explanatory model and expectations for treatment goals and methods and the way treatment will be provided (Sperry, 2022; Sperry et al., 2003). Such expectations are influenced by cultural factors and norms. Among some cultures, it is customary for family members to accompany the designated client to appointments. Since there may be the unspoken expectation that family members be included in the treatment process, effective clinicians will inquire about such expectations. Similarly, there may be "silent expectations" about the type of intervention utilized. Sometimes, the silent expectation is that healing requires some measure of touch or contact. Some clients prefer action-oriented approaches over strictly talk-oriented approaches. In short, an effective therapeutic alliance involves a "meeting of hearts" and a "meeting of minds" between therapist and client (Sperry & Sperry, 2023).

The Therapeutic Alliance with Couples

Just as in individual therapy, the working alliance in couple and family therapy (CFT) involves the creation of a strong emotional bond as well as negotiation of goals and tasks with the therapist. However, family members often vary in the degree to which they like and agree with the therapist about treatment goals and tasks. Moreover, each person observes and is influenced by how others in the family feel about the therapy and by how the couple or family unit as a whole is responding to what is taking place in treatment (Friedlander et al., 2006). This means that at any point in treatment there are at least two therapeutic alliances that interact systemically. For example, the degree to which the female partner likes the therapist and is engaged in the treatment may either facilitate or hinder the other partner's willingness to trust the therapist. The female partner's involvement also depends on the marital bond, her sense of safety, and whether she agrees with the other partner about the problems, goals, or need for treatment (Friedlander et al., 2006).

Therapist and Therapeutic Alliance

Clinical lore holds that therapists who embody the core conditions of effective treatment, empathy, respect, and acceptance (Rogers, 1961), and who demonstrate active listening and responding, facilitate the development of an effective alliance. In such a relationship, clients will feel accepted, supported, and valued, and believe that their therapist cares about them and is worthy of their trust. As a result, they become hopeful and confident that treatment will be successful.

Research has validated some of the clinical lore of the therapist's contribution to the alliance but does not support Rogers' claim that the three core conditions are the necessary *and* sufficient conditions for therapeutic change (Norcross, 2002). However, there is increasing support for the premise that specific therapist attributes and skill sets are positively related to an effective therapeutic alliance (Orlinsky et al., 2004; Sperry & Sperry, 2023). Therapists in an effective alliance present in a warm and friendly manner and are confident and experienced. They are interested in and respectful toward the client, and they relate with honesty, trustworthiness, and openness. During treatment they remain alert and flexible and provide a safe environment in which clients can discuss their issues. They are supportive, use active and reflective listening, affirm the client's experience, and demonstrate an empathic understanding of each client's situation (Sperry, 2022). Furthermore, they attend to the clients' experiences and facilitate the expression of affect, to enable a deep exploration of concerns. They provide accurate interpretations of the client's behavior and are active in treatment and draw attention to past therapeutic successes (Ackerman & Hillensroth, 2003; Orlinsky et al., 1994, 2004; Sperry & Sperry, 2023).

In short, the development of a good therapeutic alliance is essential for the success of psychotherapy regardless of the approach. The therapist's ability to incorporate the client's needs, expectations, and abilities into a therapeutic plan is essential in building the alliance. Because the therapist and client often judge the quality of the alliance differently, active monitoring of the alliance throughout therapy is needed. Responding nondefensively to a client's hostility or negativity is critical to establishing and maintaining a strong alliance (Sperry, 2022). Finally, the clients' evaluation of the quality of the alliance is the best predictor of outcome; nevertheless, the therapist's input has a strong influence on the client and is therefore critical (Horvath et al., 2011).

Spirituality and Relationships

As a preface to discussing how spirituality can and does influence therapeutic relationships, some preliminary considerations should be noted.

First, relationships between individuals and spiritual beings bear many of the characteristics of human relationships, yet they possess unique aspects that can serve as resources in ways that human relationships cannot. For example, a personal relationship between self and spiritual beings may be the only relationship in which there are no secrets, and can be counted upon to be available, to provide a continuous source of meaning, and to witness what is just and unjust (Griffin & Griffin, 2002).

A second consideration is that many spiritual traditions stress the value of relationships: with the divine, with the broader world, with neighbors, and with the self. "Furthermore, many spiritual teachings and traditions embrace the idea that people are made for intimate relationship and communal living and are made more whole by connections characterized by trust, integrity, and respect" (Young et al., 2009, p. 175). In such traditions, the individual's relationship to the divine is considered the agent of transformation, whereas in psychotherapy, the therapist–client relationship is considered the catalyst for change. It is noteworthy that both perspectives emphasize the quality of the relationship. Accordingly, experiencing the transformative power of a relationship with the divine can greatly facilitate the therapist–client relationship (Young et al., 2009).

Third, the client–therapist relationship may be best viewed as a sacred resource. Consequently, "the sacred qualities of the connection between client and therapists may be among the most critical of therapeutic ingredients" (Pargament, 2007, p. 269). In short, the therapeutic relationship can and does reflect a client's previous spiritual experiences, and an effective therapeutic relationship is most likely to occur in the context of trust, respect, and empathy. Research is beginning to confirm these observations (Pargament & Exline, 2021).

Research on Spiritual Factors and the Therapeutic Alliance

Research demonstrates the importance and value of the therapeutic alliance for all clients, particularly those with a spiritual orientation (Young et al., 2009). One recent study reports on the influence of spiritual factors on the therapeutic alliance, particularly with regard to therapeutic empathy (Morrison & Borgen, 2010). The importance of therapeutic empathy cannot be underestimated given that the quality of the therapeutic alliance predicts both commitment to therapy, i.e., premature termination rates, and treatment outcomes. Because the therapist's capacity to empathically connect with clients is essential for developing and maintaining an effective therapeutic alliance, empathic deficits and even brief empathic "pauses" can easily strain or rupture the alliance (Sperry, 2022).

Research has demonstrated that therapists' spiritual and religious beliefs can positively and negatively influence their therapeutic empathy. Using the critical incident technique Morrison and Borgen (2010) identified 14 helping and 3 hindering categories of Christian spiritual and religious beliefs that influence a therapist's empathy toward clients. As predicted, the helping categories (e.g., empathy for the client because God cares for the client, and relationship to faith leading naturally to an empathic relationship with the client) did foster the therapeutic alliance.

Of particular value for clinical practice were the hindering categories. The first category involved client actions which were contrary to the therapist's belief system. Examples of this category include the therapist's inability to empathize with clients who were about to make decisions contrary to the therapist's spiritual beliefs, and the therapist's inability to empathize in response to a client harming others that contradicted the religious beliefs of the therapist. Instead of responding empathically, therapists were more likely to challenge or confront the client's behavior. The second category involved instances where empathy was limited because of the therapist's own blind spots or biases. Examples of this category include prejudice against a religious group that is legalistic because of the therapist's own negative experience of legalism, and the therapist's inability to empathize with client problems that are considered unacceptable in the context of the therapist's faith, such as sexual disorder involving deviance. The third category involved incidents where empathy was hindered with clients who were of the same faith or denomination as the therapist. Examples of this category include the therapist's inability to empathize because of the therapist's frustration with a client who avoids responsibility by spiritualizing problems, or because of the therapist's expectation that clients should hold the same view of religious issues as the therapist (Morrison & Borgen, 2010).

The results of this study underscore the importance of fostering empathy with spiritually oriented clients. Fostering empathy and an atmosphere that respect clients' spiritual beliefs and practices while exploring spiritual themes related to their therapeutic issues is essential in developing and maintaining an effective therapeutic relationship (Kelly, 1995).

In addition, research also finds that clients' capacity to form therapeutic relationships appears to be related to their attachment style. Those with secure attachment more easily form such bonds, while those with insecure attachment have more difficulty in forming therapeutic alliances with therapists early in the therapeutic process. It may require more time and patience on the therapist's part to develop the therapeutic alliance (Eames & Roth, 2000). Clients may need "to have a corrective emotional experience in counseling, which involves therapists treating clients in a manner that is unlike that which they would normally experience from others" (Young et al., 2009, p. 177).

In short, it is advisable for therapists to assess spiritually oriented clients to determine if there are experiences that would make the formation of a therapeutic alliance difficult and then endeavor to address those factors. Effective therapists will address clients' spirituality and spiritual concerns with an attitude of patience and openness, and they assist clients in maximizing the benefits of their spiritual beliefs and practices as an adaptive resource in the treatment process.

Maintaining an Effective Therapeutic Alliance

Because of its impact on the treatment process and outcomes, establishing an effective therapeutic relationship is a critical challenge for the therapist (Sperry, 2022). As noted in the previous chapter, a specific set of competencies and skills are necessary for developing such a relationship. Maintaining an effective therapeutic relationship is an equally critical therapeutic challenge for therapists, and it too requires a specific set of specific competencies and skills. Needless to say, therapist competency and capability in dealing with these challenges and impasses is essential to the competent practice of psychotherapy. This chapter addresses these impasses.

Just as there are "treatment promoting factors" as described in Chapter 3, there are also "treatment interfering factors." Treatment interfering factors, also called impasses, are factors that arise within and between sessions that impede the progress of therapy. Four categories of treatment interfering factors can be noted in clinical situations: client, therapist, client–therapist relationship, and treatment process. This chapter deals directly with two specific interfering factors in the client–therapist relationship. These interfering factors are: resistance and ambivalence, and transference–countertransference enactments. Each of these factors and strategies for resolving them are discussed in separate sections. Finally, a case example illustrates the recognition and resolution of one of these interfering factors.

Resistance and Ambivalence

Resistance to change, including resistance to the therapeutic relationship, is a problem that complicates psychotherapy, particularly for trainees. It is one of the most important yet least understood concepts in psychotherapy. Resistance is usually understood as a client's outright refusal to engage in activities inside or outside of session, such as coming late for sessions, or failing to self-monitor thoughts, feelings, and behaviors. In fact, ambivalence is the most common presentation of resistance. Ambivalence is typically manifested as defensive avoidance or a repetitive pattern of interpersonal behaviors that cause distress or result in limited gratification, and is described as "resistant ambivalence" (Engle & Arkowitz, 2006). It reflects discrepancies among self-schemas relevant to change, i.e., schemas associated with movement toward change and those associated with movement away from change. Most often clients are not fully aware of their self-schemas and the discrepancies among them that cause resistant ambivalence (Arkowitz et al., 2007).

Since resistant ambivalence is also an interpersonal phenomenon, it is best understood in the interpersonal context in which it occurs. When it occurs in a therapeutic setting, it is essential that the therapist views it as a temporary state rather than a personality trait. Resistant ambivalence is operative when the following elements are observed:

- The client believes or agrees that the anticipated change is in his or her own best interest.
- The client has sufficient information and the capacity to make the change happen.
- The client demonstrates initial movement toward change with words and other behaviors.
- The client, at the same time, demonstrates movement away from change with words and other behaviors.
- The client experiences a negative emotional reaction to the failure to change.

(Engle & Arkowitz, 2006)

Spirituality and Resistance

There are various ways in which resistance or ambivalent resistance is present in spiritually integrated psychotherapy. For instance, clients may use spirituality to avoid relating to others. Or they may engage in spiritual pursuits to avoid other responsibilities. Or they may avoid addressing psychological problems by use of spiritual solutions (sometimes referred to as "spiritual bypass"). Or it may present as rigidity or delimiting beliefs. In such instances, therapeutically confronting the client's resistance, ambivalence, or avoidance may be indicated (Young et al., 2009).

Resistance to Discussing Spirituality

Reluctance to discuss spirituality is not always an indication of resistance. At times, it may be clear to a therapist that a spiritual issue may be underpinning a client's presenting concerns although the client may be reluctant to address his or her spirituality. This presents a therapeutic and relational challenge. It may be that the client does not feel sufficiently safe and ready to discuss the matter. Here is a strategy for beginning to deal with such reluctance or avoidance. Explore clients' feelings about discussing their spiritual beliefs. Explain the value of including spirituality in psychological treatment. Address how clients' psychological issues are related to their spiritual perspective. In this process, utilize empathic responding and attunement in assisting clients in exploring the link between their spirituality and psychological difficulties (Young et al., 2009). Undoubtedly, this process involves clarifying and summarizing content as well as reflecting and processing feelings, all of which may increase the client's sense of safety and trustfulness in the therapist.

Spiritual Rigidity as Resistance

Another form of resistance involves rigidity. For example, a therapist may assess a client's spiritual rigidity as maladaptive to the point that it warrants intervention, even though the client may not view it as a problem. Here is a strategy for beginning to deal with such rigidity. Begin by carefully and respectfully exploring the clients' spiritual perspective, particularly how they conceptualize their beliefs. Rather than attempting to modify such dysfunctional beliefs, focus instead on expanding them. Endeavor to offer new conceptualizations from within the clients' spiritual or religious perspective. This might involve religious language, scripture, or stories. This may require consultation with someone with expertise. Utilize the same strategies for expanding rigid psychological beliefs, assumptions, and schemas, when working with spiritually based cognitive distortions. Moreover, focus change efforts at or slightly above the clients' cognitive levels of complexity (Young et al., 2009).

Spiritual Beliefs as Resistance

Sometimes specific religious or spiritual beliefs can significantly interfere with a client's functioning and well-being. This can be thought of as a delimiting belief and a source of resistance. Deconstructing the belief can resolve the resistance and restore well-being. Deconstruction is a systematic inquiry which aims to explicate the interpretive assumptions from which a particular belief arises. This inquiry seeks to both identify assumptions and delineate their cultural origins and context. The purpose is not to destroy a belief but rather to enrich its understanding of the role of the belief in one's life. In this process, the meaning and influence of a belief can be transformed as the individual understands its historical and social context (Griffin & Griffin, 2002).

A case example illustrates this process. In an early session, the client, Sandy, reported that she used to be close to God but now could no longer attend religious services. In response to the therapist query to amplify that remark, Sandy, a graduate student, said she had gotten a call from her friend Emma that had deeply upset her. The friend indicated that Sandy was sinning and displeasing God by having sex with her boyfriend. The therapist asked if it was her belief that she was displeasing God. Sandy answered that it probably was but that she was confused. Utilizing deconstruction, the therapist asked her how she imagined God was responding to her confusion, i.e., her desperation in wanting to return to religious services, and the bad feelings that were keeping her away. Sandy said she believed God was accepting and not displeased and punishing as Emma described. Nevertheless, Sandy had been so upset by Emma's comments that she could not bring herself to return to religious services.

The therapeutic focus shifted to whether a fear that one was displeasing should keep one from drawing close to God. Sandy was asked how she came to her belief in an accepting God in contrast to Emma's belief in a punishing God. Sandy noted that as a little girl her mother taught her to rely on God and not fear him. Not only had she trusted her mother's understanding of God, but Sandy also had experienced God this way, until recently. The therapist then asked how, if she trusted her mother's and her own experience, had Emma become God's spokesperson? Sandy needed time to think about this question. At their next session, Sandy said that she would never choose Emma for that role, and that she would no longer give Emma's words such power over her. She also mentioned that she had found a church in the university community where she might find other like-minded individuals and the possibility of closeness to God (Griffin & Griffin, 2002).

Spiritual Ambivalence and Motivational Interviewing

When it comes to spiritual and religious issues some clients enter therapy "profoundly ambivalent about exploring their spirituality" (Miller & Rollnick, 2002, p. 3). Accordingly, effective therapy addresses that ambivalence in the initial phase of treatment. Motivational interviewing (MI) is a proven strategy to facilitate the process of working with a client's ambivalence and increasing their motivation for change and growth in a person's life, including their spiritual life (Giordano & Cashwell, 2014; Miller & Rollnick, 2023).

MI has four principles that a therapist can utilize to reduce ambivalence and increase motivation to change. They are: express empathy; develop discrepancy; roll with resistance; and support self-efficacy (Miller & Rollnick, 2023). By expressing empathy, the therapist cultivates an atmosphere of acceptance without criticism or judgment and uses reflection of feeling and content to foster understanding and normalize the client's experience of ambivalence.

By developing discrepancy, the therapist points out the disconnects between the client's current behavior and identified values and goals (Miller

& Rollnick, 2023). For instance, a client may describe his efforts to avoid exploring his spirituality and sense of purpose because he feels wary about "this touchy feely stuff." Later, he indicates that he really wants to have more balance in his life, saying "I just want to feel whole for once in my life." The therapist can develop discrepancy by helping the client reflect on this dilemma, where on the one hand he avoids exploring his spiritual life and on the other he longs for integration and a sense of wholeness.

Resistance is viewed as normal, and therapists using MI will respond by reflecting, reframing, refocusing, and confirming the client's control over their change process (Miller & Rollnick, 2023). For the client who states a desire to integrate spirituality into their life but expresses resistance related to incorporating spiritual practices, the therapist can roll with resistance with a double-sided reflection by saying: "The idea of making changes in your spiritual life seems daunting and maybe even a little frightening right now. But, at the same time, there is a part of you that is dissatisfied with your current spiritual life."

Supporting self-efficacy involves increasing a client's belief in their ability to make desired changes (Miller & Rollnick, 2023). For example, the therapist may inquire about past experiences in which the client was successful in efforts to make positive change. The therapist would ask a client who is ambivalent about exploring spirituality to reflect on past experiences in which she had followed through with her decision to investigate an unknown topic or try a new activity. By expanding on those successes, the client may increase her confidence and her willingness to further explore and expand her spiritual life.

Transferences and Countertransferences

The quality of the therapeutic alliance is the foundation upon which all other therapeutic endeavors are based. While there are conditions which facilitate the development and maintenance of an effective therapeutic alliance, there are also conditions which militate against its development and maintenance (Sperry, 2022). This section focuses on one set of these conditions, transference and countertransference, that can and do interfere with the therapeutic relationship as well as therapeutic outcomes. It first describes transference, countertransference, and their enactments, and then describes a strategy for resolving such enactments.

Past experiences with relationships affect subsequent relationships and seldom are individuals consciously aware that they "transfer" feelings and thoughts from past relationships onto current ones. In addition to transferring feelings and thoughts, expectations to act in certain ways are also transferred. Thus, a college student may meet a professor for the first time and react to that professor with the same or similar set of thoughts, feelings, and expectations that she had for her high school biology teacher. She may be surprised and even experience slight confusion when the professor is more friendly but more academically demanding than she expected. This confusion is because transference and countertransference are interpersonal distortions that often do not fit present role expectations (Good & Beitman, 2006).

Just as there are active elements like trust and collaboration in current relationships, there are also active elements of past relationships that both clients and therapists bring to the client–therapist relationship. It is these active elements of past relationships that can negatively impact the treatment process. Transference is such an element. Transference is a phenomenon in which clients inaccurately transfer thoughts, feelings, and expectations about past interpersonal experiences onto their current relationship with the therapist. These distortions tend to be considerably potent and can negatively impact the process of therapy (Good & Beitman, 2006). Transference can be either positive or negative. It is a form of reenactment of the client's old and familiar pattern of relating, a pattern that often involves "unfinished business." In this reenactment clients demonstrate how they felt in the past when they were treated in a particular manner. Transference typically occurs when a therapist—often inadvertently—says or does something that triggers the client's unfinished business (Beitman & Yue, 2004; Sperry, 2022).

Countertransference is a similar phenomenon in which clinicians inadvertently and inaccurately transfer thoughts, feelings, and expectations from past experiences onto clients. Similarly, these distortions can impact the treatment process. Countertransference can be positive or negative. An increasing consensus among clinicians from the various therapeutic orientations is that countertransference can be a useful source of information about the client (Gabbard, 1999).

Spirituality and Countertransference

Countertransference can interfere with the therapeutic relationship. Facilitating the therapeutic alliance requires that clinicians recognize and deal forthrightly with countertransference issues. Issues surrounding prayer may or may not be a countertransference issue, but it can potentially impact the engagement process. Accordingly, countertransference is discussed in the following sections.

Countertransference issues can arise in the course of incorporating the spiritual dimension in therapy. Countertransference can manifest in several ways. These range from actively arguing with clients about spiritual doctrine and regarding it as destructive, to passively avoiding discussion of spiritual topics or labeling them as "resistance" (Lovinger, 1984). Spero (1981) describes several other types of countertransference problems that can arise when religious or spiritual issues are involved. When the client and clinician share the same religious beliefs, there can be idiosyncratic or conflicting differences based on differing needs for religion in the client and clinician. For instance, the client might have expectations and fantasies of magical cure by the clinician, or might even view the clinician as punitive, demanding, and judgmental as a religious figure or parent in their past. The clinician, on the other hand, might experience countertransference reactions to the client that range from rescue fantasies to neurotic projections resulting in contemptuous feelings for the client. The clinician's own spiritual beliefs may result in rejecting or harshly judging clients who engage in an adulterous affair, persist in abusing substances, or refuse to alter lifestyles that are incompatible with spiritual principles.

Spero (1981) provides clinicians with seven strategies for managing countertransference issues that arise in these situations.

1. Develop an understanding of the client's neurotic and non-neurotic needs for religion and spirituality.
2. Identify neurotic forms of religious beliefs, i.e., the ways religion is used as a defense mechanism for aggressive drives, that reflect underlying psychological conflict and must separate these immature forms of belief from mature forms that are adaptive.
3. Perform a self-examination in order to identify one's own neurotic needs for religion and spirituality, and for immature beliefs that arise from those needs. Then recognizing how these are similar to or different from the client's needs and beliefs will help the clinician to avoid or at least be conscious of countertransference reactions during therapy.
4. When experiencing negative feelings toward the client, attempt to recognize if overconcern or overidentification with the client is the cause for such feelings.
5. Avoid special treatment for clients with similar spiritual backgrounds. This should assist in maintaining therapeutic neutrality and objectivity.
6. Recognize the limits placed on therapeutic goals when religious commitments are similar, since this may restrict one's ability to see how such commitments are used as unhealthy defenses by the client.
7. Avoid providing the client with one's own spiritual insights into the client's problems as this can limit one's recognition of how the client's religious beliefs are involved in his or her neurotic conflict.

The Case of Maria

Maria is a 47-year-old, married, Cuban American female who was referred by her gynecologist for evaluation and treatment of depressed moods. The therapist was a psychologist to whom this gynecologist had referred others who had mood issues and were looking for a therapist who was sensitive to spiritual issues. She described sadness, feelings of worthlessness, and worry.

She said she felt so overwhelmed that she took a leave of absence from her job claiming she was unable to handle a class of 5th graders. She stated she could no longer tolerate being around other people and felt that she had failed. She also complained of increased marital discord which stemmed from her husband's complaints that she was neglecting him because she was preoccupied with the unreasonable demands of the parents of two of her students. Three weeks ago, she had been prescribed Celexa (citalopram) but had stopped taking it after two weeks because of side effects. She told her doctor that she was willing to try psychotherapy before trying another antidepressant. Two years ago, she had met with another psychotherapist for six sessions before terminating treatment "because it wasn't helping." When asked if she thought working with the present therapist might be any different, she responded that he just listened and never said anything which she believed could not possibly help her. She also believed that spiritual issues were affecting her life and her mood but that the previous therapist "seemed indifferent to these concerns." However, because of the current therapist's receptivity to the spiritual dimension, she said she was willing to try therapy again. She reported her health to be good, other than taking prescribed medication for mild hypothyroidism. She volunteered that her doctor had said her thyroid problem was mild and unrelated to her depressed mood. She also denied the use of nicotine, alcohol, or recreational drugs, and takes a daily vitamin and calcium.

Therapeutic Relationship

Because therapeutic outcomes depend, in large part, on the client's engagement in the therapeutic process, the therapist elicited Maria's explanation of presenting concerns and expectations for treatment before negotiating mutual agreeable treatment goals and an intervention plan for treatment. Two considerations from her past have the potential for activating negative transference enactments. The first involves emotional withholding, a demanding attitude, and verbal abusiveness from her parents. The second involves the neutrality, perceived withholding, and apparent lack of interest in her spiritual concerns. Accordingly, the current therapist endeavored to foster and maintain a positive therapeutic alliance by displaying emotional connectedness, avoiding demands, even subtle ones, evaluative comments, and interest in her spiritual concern.

Concluding Note

The therapeutic relationship can and does have a profound effect on the treatment process and outcomes in both conventional and spiritually integrated psychotherapy. The chapter described the therapeutic alliance as encompassing therapeutic bond, goals, and tasks. It described both the process of developing and of maintaining the therapeutic alliance. Specific strategies for developing the therapeutic relationship were emphasized, particularly with spiritually sensitive clients. The chapter also described strategies for maintaining the therapeutic relationship and emphasized one for dealing with resistance and countertransference in spiritually integrated psychotherapy.

References

Ackerman, S., & Hillensroth, M. (2003). A review of therapist characteristics and techniques positively impacting the therapeutic alliance. *Clinical Psychology Review*, *23*, 1–33.

Arkowitz, H., Westra, H., Miller, W., & Rollnick, S. (Eds.). (2007). *Motivational interviewing in the treatment of psychological problems*. Guilford.

Beitman, B., & Yue, D. (2004). *Learning psychotherapy: A time-efficient, research-based, and outcome-measured psychotherapy training program* (2nd ed.). Norton.

Bordin, E. (1979). The generalizability of the psychoanalytic concept of the working alliance. *Psychotherapy: Theory. Research and Practice*, *16*, 252–260.

Eames, V., & Roth, A. (2000). Patient attachment orientation and the early working alliance: A study of patient and therapist reports of alliance quality and ruptures. *Journal of Psychotherapy Research*, *10*, 421–434.

Engle, D., & Arkowitz, H. (2006). *Ambivalence in psychotherapy: Facilitating readiness to change*. Guilford.

Friedlander, M. L., Escudero, V., & Heatherington, L. (2006). *Therapeutic alliances with couples and families: An empirically informed guide to practice*. American Psychological Association.

Gabbard, G. (1999). An overview of countertransference: Theory and technique. In G. Gabbard (Ed.), *Countertransference issues in psychiatric treatment* (pp. 1–25). American Psychiatric Press.

Giordano, A. L., & Cashwell, C. S. (2014). Entering the sacred: Using motivational interviewing to address spirituality in counseling. *Counseling and Values*, *59*, 65–79.

Good, G., & Beitman, B. (2006). *Counseling and psychotherapy essentials: Integrating theories, skills, and practices*. Norton.

Griffin, J., & Griffin, M. (2002). *Encountering the scared in psychotherapy: How to talk with people about their spiritual lives*. Guilford Press.

Horvath, A., & Symonds, B. (1991). Relationship between working alliance and outcome in psychotherapy: A meta-analysis. *Journal of Counseling Psychology*, *38*, 139–149.

Horvath, A. O., Del Re, A., Flückiger, C., & Symonds, D. (2011). Alliance in individual psychotherapy. In J. Norcross (Ed.), *Psychotherapy relationships that work* (2nd ed.). Oxford University Press.

Kelly, E. (1995). *Spirituality and religion in counseling and psychotherapy: Diversity in theory and practice*. American Counseling Association.

Ledley, D., Marx, B., & Heimberg, R. (2006). *Making cognitive-behavioral therapy work: Clinical process for new practitioners*. Guilford.
Levenson, H. (1995). *Time-limited dynamic psychotherapy: A guide to clinical practice*. Basic Books.
Lovinger, R. J. (1984). *Working with religious issues in therapy*. Jason Aronson.
Miller, W., & Rollnick, S. (2002). *Motivational interviewing: Preparing people for change* (2nd ed.). Guilford.
Miller, W. R., & Rollnick, S. (2023). *Motivational interviewing: Helping people change and grow* (4th ed.). Guilford Publications.
Morrison, M., & Borgen, W. (2010). How Christian spiritual and religious beliefs help and hinder counselors' empathy toward clients. *Counseling & Values*, *55*, 25–45.
Norcross, J. (2002). Empirically supported therapy relationship. In J. Norcross (Ed.), *Psychotherapy relationships that work: Therapist contributions and responsiveness to patients* (pp. 3–16). Oxford University Press.
Orlinsky, D., Grawe, K., & Parks, B. (1994). Process and outcome in psychotherapy. In A. Bergin & S. Garfield (Eds.), *Handbook of psychotherapy and behavior change* (4th ed., pp. 270–376). Wiley.
Orlinsky, D., Ronnestad, M., & Willutzi, U. (2004). Fifty years of psychotherapy process-outcome research: Continuity and change. In M. Lambert (Ed.), *Bergin and Garfield's handbook of psychotherapy and behavior change* (5th ed., pp. 307–389). Wiley.
Pargament, K. (2007). *Spiritually integrated psychotherapy: Understanding and addressing the sacred*. Guilford.
Pargament, K. I., & Exline, J. J. (2021). *Working with spiritual struggles in psychotherapy: From research to practice*. Guilford Publications.
Rogers, C. (1961). *On becoming a person*. Houghton-Mifflin.
Spero, M. H. (1981). Countertransference in religious therapists of religious patients. *American Journal of Psychotherapy*, *35*(4), 565–575.
Sperry, L. (2022). *Highly effective therapy: Developing essential clinical competencies in counseling and psychotherapy*. Routledge.
Sperry, L., Brill, P., Howard, K., & Grissom, G. (1996). *Treatment outcomes in psychotherapy and psychiatric interventions*. Brunner/Mazel.
Sperry, L., Carlson, J., & Kjos, D. (2003). *Becoming an effective therapist*. Allyn & Bacon.
Sperry, L., & Sperry, J. (2023). *Core clinical competencies in counseling and psychotherapy* (2nd ed.). Routledge.
Young, J., Dowdle, S., & Flowers, L. (2009). How spirituality can affect the therapeutic alliance. In J. Aten & M. Leach (Eds.), *Spirituality and the therapeutic process: A comprehensive resource from intake to termination* (pp. 167–192). American Psychological Association.

Chapter 7

Assessment and Case Conceptualization

Assessment and case conceptualization are critical processes in spiritually integrated psychotherapy. This chapter describes a comprehensive and integrative assessment strategy that includes assessment of personality dynamics, family dynamics, cultural dynamics, and spiritual dynamics. An integrative assessment is an ongoing process that begins with an initial evaluation and continues through termination (Sperry, 2022). As in conventional psychotherapy, case conceptualization is the link between assessment and treatment planning. The chapter also discusses and illustrates how spiritual factors and issues can be incorporated in developing an integrative case conceptualization. Today, the expectation is that therapists will not only be aware of and assess a client's spiritual values and concerns, but will also incorporate them in the therapeutic process, specifically in the case conceptualization. In the past, this was not always an expectation. Accordingly, when therapists were not sufficiently aware of the client's spiritual needs and issues, the result was often "a skewed and narrow case conceptualization of the presenting problem and may have led to inadequate treatment planning, as powerful sources of gains were largely overlooked" (Aten & Leach, 2009, p. 17).

The chapter begins with a description of the common reasons or indications that individuals seek spiritually integrated psychotherapy. This is followed by a brief description of the reasons for performing a spiritual assessment and how to perform a brief and an extended spiritual assessment. Next are sections on the integrative assessment and the integrative case conceptualization. The final section includes a case example that illustrates both an integrative assessment and case conceptualization.

Three Clinical Indications of Spiritually Integrated Psychotherapy

There are three common clinical indications for spiritually integrated psychotherapy. They are: (1) as a spiritual resource for coping with a health

DOI: 10.4324/9781003425991-8

problem, personal, interpersonal, or professional loss or conflict; (2) in situations involving a death or other loss resulting in symptoms reflecting a crisis of faith or meaning in life; or (3) for increased well-being and spiritual growth (Shafranske & Sperry, 2005; Sperry, 2012). There is increasing recognition that spiritual and religious issues are common in and outside of therapy. APA has responded to this recognition in the DSM with the diagnostic code "Religious or Spiritual Problems" (Z65.8). It is a diagnostic category for religious or spiritual problems which includes distressing experiences involving the loss or questioning of one's faith, problems associated with conversion to a new faith, or of questioning one's spiritual values (American Psychiatric Association, 2022). This designation primarily reflects the second of the three clinical indications of spiritually integrated psychotherapy.

Coping with a Serious Stressor

Perhaps the most common of the three clinical indications of spiritually integrated psychotherapy involves the use of spiritual resources in coping with a serious stressors and tragedies (Sperry, 2012). The range of stressors is quite broad and includes serious health problem, significant personal losses, or professional losses, as well as difficult interpersonal and family conflicts. Common religious and spiritual resources for coping with such stressors include prayer, attendance at religious services, emotional support of a faith community, etc. (Pargament & Exline, 2021). Therapists can assist such distressed clients in identifying and utilizing spiritual resources for coping more effectively.

Case Example

Patricia is a 34-year-old, single, African American female who sought therapy following the death of her mother. During the brief spiritual assessment of the initial evaluation, Patricia revealed that while she considered herself a deeply spiritual person, she had stopped attending church as an adolescent against her mother's wishes. Because of a recent job transfer out of town she had no support from either a faith community nor from her extended family. In the weeks following her mother's death she had become increasingly depressed, anxious, tearful, and guilt-ridden. Her constant thought was that her deeply religious mother "begged me not to take that job transfer and look what happened. I should have listened to her." At some level she knows this thought is "ridiculous but my guilt is crushing me and maybe God is punishing me for leaving my mother." Her expectation is that therapy will help her cope better, reduce symptoms, and clarify her issues.

Crises of Faith and Meaning

Any number of tragedies and stressors can provoke a crisis of faith or meaning. These can include betrayals, the death of a child, or other losses resulting in a crisis of faith or meaning in life. Such crises are also called spiritual struggles. "Spiritual struggles are signs of spiritual disorientation, tension, and strains. Old roads to the sacred and old understandings of the sacred itself are no longer compelling. In their place, people struggle to reorient themselves and find a new way to the sacred or a new understanding of the sacred" (Pargament, 2007, p. 112). Pargament identifies three types of spiritual struggles: interpersonal, intrapersonal, and divine. Interpersonal struggles involve family, friends, or congregations about matters such as gossiping, cliquishness, hypocrisy, or disagreement with doctrine. Intrapersonal struggles typically involve uncertainly or doubt about spiritual matters or serious doubts about one's religious tradition. A third form of struggle involves tensions between an individual and the divine often in the face of critical life events when an individual comes to question or doubt God's existence or the belief that God is caring and benevolent in the face of adversity. Such questions and doubts are referred to as crises of faith. These struggles can be temporary expressions of spiritual pain that quickly resolve, or they may be protracted experiences that result in anxiety or depressive conditions with lowered physical and relational functioning and quality of life (Exline & Rose, 2005; Pargament & Exline, 2021).

Case Example

Leila is a 47-year-old, married female who complains of worsening anger, confusion, insomnia, and "down moods" of four months duration. It appears that her symptoms began soon after a priest in her parish was indicted for sexual misconduct with an adolescent. It appears that while Leila had no such history, her younger brother had been abused by a priest from age 13 to 15. After the indictment Leila reports that she stopped all church involvement and began questioning her faith in "a God that would let such terrible things happen to kids."

Spiritual Growth

Spiritual growth refers to the development and formation of the whole person by an intentional focus on increasing one's self-aware consciousness, self-transcendence, and transformation (Sperry, 2012). It involves developing one's spiritual and interior life with spiritual practices and disciplines such as prayer, fasting, simplicity, solitude, and worship

(Walsh, 1999). Such spiritual formation can also include the more intimate and in-depth process of spiritual direction (May, 1992).

Case Example

Martin is a 43-year-old, married executive and had just made an appointment with a psychologist who practiced spiritually integrated psychotherapy. He had been referred by a friend who was involved in "growth counseling" with the psychologist. Martin sought help in "toning down my obsession with work" and "getting more balance in my professional, family, personal, and spiritual life." While Martin regularly worked 60 hours a week, the same or less than his fellow executives, he did not find his work satisfying or as meaningful as it had been in the past. He attributed this to a midlife crisis in which he felt increasingly disconnected from his family and friends and "spiritually impoverished."

It is presumed that an unbiased, systematic spiritual assessment of clients' spiritual life requires that clinicians be sufficiently aware of their own spiritual belief orientations. Furthermore, it is helpful, if not essential, to know something of the basic tenets of a given client's religious tradition. For example, in some clients it may be difficult to differentiate between delusions and compulsions and the basic beliefs and rituals of a different spiritual tradition. If a clinician is unaware of these basic beliefs and rituals, it may be necessary for them to request that clients briefly describe their interpretation of these beliefs or rituals.

The Spiritual Assessment

There are several reasons for performing such an assessment (Richards & Bergin, 2005). Five such reasons are: (1) to understand clients' spiritual orientations and communicating to clients that their entire life experience is of interest and value to the clinician; (2) to determine the degree of health of clients' spiritual orientations and its impact on presenting problems and disturbance; (3) to determine whether clients' spiritual beliefs and communities can be used as healing and coping resources; (4) to determine whether clients' spiritual needs and concerns should be addressed in treatment; and (5) to determine which spiritual interventions may be useful and effective.

Performing a Brief Spiritual Assessment

It is a basic contention of this book that a brief spiritual assessment should be performed on all clients. An increasing number of researchers and clinicians insist that, at a minimum, a brief spiritual assessment should be performed on all clients because of demonstrated health consequences of religiosity and spirituality (Gorsuch & Miller, 1999; Matthews, 1998). Routine screening questions about religion and spirituality can easily be incorporated into the initial evaluation and assessment process.

A brief spiritual assessment can and should be performed in all initial encounters with clients (Sperry, 2012). A focused inquiry about an individual's spiritual status takes less than two minutes using the following screening questions.

1. "Is religion or spirituality important to you?"
2. "Do your religious or spiritual beliefs influence the way you look at your problems and the way you think about your health?"
3. "Would you like me to address your religious or spiritual beliefs and practices with you?"

(Matthews, 1998, p. 274)

If clients answer "no" to the first question the clinician would ask if religion or spirituality were *ever* important to them. Matthews reasons that since research indicates that rejection of religion is associated with higher rates of substance-related disorders and a decline in self-satisfaction and happiness, this information may be a useful prognostic indicator. A positive answer to the third question is followed up to ascertain the client's preferences and expectations. Matthews has added another question: "Are you part of a religious or spiritual community?"(Koenig & Pritchett, 1998, p. 327). This question is added between the second and third previously noted questions. Usually such a screening assessment can be completed in three minutes or less.

Performing an Extended Spiritual Assessment

As already noted, it is assumed that every client in all counseling and psychotherapy settings will be accorded a brief or screening spiritual assessment. For some clients, a more extensive spiritual assessment is indicated. These are the most common indications:

1. The client indicates that religious or spiritual issues are important in his or her life.
2. A spiritual issue or concern is evident in the presenting complaint.
3. The clinical issue involves morality or guilt.
4. A persistent concern regarding meaning or purpose in life is noted.

(Sperry, 2012)

There is some consensus on what constitutes an extended spiritual assessment (Bullis, 1996; Gorsuch & Miller, 1999; Josephson et al., 2000; Pargament & Exline, 2021). At a minimum, the following information is elicited: a spiritual history; the client's God representation; spiritual beliefs; spiritual practices; spiritual identity; and involvement in a spiritual and religious community.

Spiritual History

A detailed spiritual history is the foundational element of the spiritual assessment. In most cases, the spiritual history follows from a review of the presenting complaint. In others, the clinician will need to initiate more specific inquiry. The detailed spiritual history is an assessment tool designed to collect relevant information about the influences and determinants of the client's spiritual life and well-being. Since there are significant differences among members of the same religion or denomination, knowing a client's religious affiliations is of limited value. More useful information is gleaned by examining how the client is spiritual, rather than the religious label attached to that spiritual system (Sperry, 2012). Additional information can be gleaned when clients can describe how their spirituality affects their lives today; what ideas, books, persons, etc., have influenced their current spiritual attitudes; how they have changed from their spiritual orientations as children or young adults; and what spiritual conflicts they now address (Bullis, 1996).

The following are some basic questions useful in conducting a detailed spiritual history.

- What was the spiritual tradition of your parents? Were they strict or lenient in their beliefs? What effect does it have on you today?
- What were their most important spiritual beliefs? Did they pass these on to you? How?
- What is their main religious or spiritual identity? In which spiritual tradition were they raised? Have they remained with this orientation? Why or why not?
- What religious or spiritual issues, if any, have caused problems in your relationship? If resolved, how did you resolve them? If not resolved, how do they affect your relationship?
- If you have children, do you and your significant other agree or disagree on the spiritual orientation with which they are being raised?

God Representation

God representation, also called God image, refers to the way in which an individual views or represents God. The image can vary from positive, e.g., loving and caring, to negative, e.g., stern and wrathful. There are various explanations for how God images develop, the most common being that a child's image of God is linked to the child's perception of their parents or that the child projects characteristics of their father onto their image of God (Hood et al., 1996). Transformational experiences and psychotherapy have been shown to modify the God image. For example, researchers report that an adult client's God image changes as a result of successful psychotherapy even when the therapy did not address spiritual matters. God images changed from a harsh, negative view of God at the outset to images of God as loving and caring at the completion of treatment (Cheston et al., 2003).

Eliciting an individual's God representation is relatively easy. Begin with the question: "What is your image of God?" For most clients, this question and follow-up inquiries provide invaluable information. Clients are encouraged to describe this image, i.e., "judge," "a force," "friend," "policeman," etc., and how they define their relationship to this entity. The God Image Inventory (Lawrence, 1997) is a psychometric instrument for assessing God representations in clinical and pastoral contexts based on Rizzuto's theory (1979).

Spiritual Beliefs

Next, ask about the client's basic values and beliefs. Such traditions have views on the meaning of illness and suffering, the moral and virtuous life, the healthy family, and sources of spiritual authority (e.g., scriptures, religious teachings, and tenets) which may all be relevant to assess. Such core beliefs can powerfully determine an individual's behavior and if the clinician does not inquire about them, an entire treatment process may be undermined (Sperry, 2012).

Here are some questions for eliciting such values and beliefs:

- What are the basic spiritual values that you both wish to impart to your children?
- In what religious or spiritual tradition were you raised? Was your instruction strict or lenient?
- What values and ideas have stayed with you?
- How has your spiritual orientation changed since your upbringing? Why has it changed? What events or experiences helped to change you?
- What is your current religious or spiritual affiliation? What are its major beliefs and values?

Spiritual Practices

An assessment of the role of prayer and meditation, or attempts to communicate with the transcendent, can be included in this line of questioning

(Pargament & Exline, 2021). Inquire about other spiritual practices. These include spiritual reading, mindful walking and eating, fasting, almsgiving, and seeking spiritual direction. Which ones do they practice? How often and for how long? What impact or effect have these practices had?

Spiritual Identity and Involvement in a Spiritual Community

Ask clients if they do or did identify themselves with a spiritual tradition. Then, inquire about any involvement in a religious or spiritual community now or in the past. If they are involved in such a community, relevant questioning examines their level of involvement, the extent of influence of this group or its leaders, as well as the degree of perceived support they have received from the community. Finally, inquire about whether there have been changes in their relationship with the community.

Josephson et al. (2000) and Matthews (1998) provide a more extensive description and rationale for these, and other questions related to an extended spiritual assessment. Here are some questions derived from these two sources that can be useful in performing a brief as well as extended spiritual assessment.

Brief Spiritual Assessment

Is religion or spirituality an important part of your life?

If "yes" ---> "how?"
If "no" ---> "was it ever?" ---> "how?"

Do religious or spiritual beliefs influence your life? (i.e., the way you look at your problems and the way you think about yourself and health?)

If "yes" ---> "how?"
If "no" ---> "why not?"

Are you part of a religious or spiritual community?

If "yes" ---> "how are you involved?"
If "no" ---> "why not?"

Are there spiritual needs or concerns you'd like to discuss?

If "yes" ---> "which ones?" ---> [follow up on preferences and expectations]
If "no" ---> "why is that?"

Extended Spiritual Assessment

"When you were growing up how did you learn about spiritual/religious matters?" ---> [follow up]
"What's your concept of God or a higher power"? ---> [follow up]
"What religious/spiritual beliefs and values are important to you?" ---> [follow up]
"What's the role of prayer or meditation in your life?" ---> [follow up]
"What religious rituals or spiritual practices are important to you?" ---> [follow up]
"How do you identify yourself spiritually (or denominationally)?" "What is your involvement?" ---> [follow up]

Two additional questions can be useful in eliciting

> the spiritual and religious beliefs and practices that support the client's well-being, recovery, and mental health. They include: (1) How do your spiritual and religious beliefs and practices support your well-being and mental health?; and (2) Are there certain spiritual and religious beliefs and practices that you find particularly helpful in dealing with difficulties?
>
> (Vieten & Lukoff, 2022, p. 34)

Initial, Implicit, and Explicit Assessment

Pargament (2007) distinguishes among initial, implicit, and explicit assessment. Initial spiritual assessment involves the use of simple questions to elicit the client's spirituality, religion, problem or struggles, and solution. Implicit spiritual assessment involves listening for implied spiritual content in the client's description and asking questions that suggest the possibility of spiritual experiences. It is appropriate for clients who may be hesitant in discussing spirituality. Explicit assessment delves deeper into the client's resources, pathways, destinations, struggles, and transformations (Pargament, 2007).

The Assessment Process and Integrative Assessment

The spiritual assessment is one component of the larger assessment process. A basic premise of this book is that effective spiritually integrated psychotherapy requires much more than a spiritual assessment; it requires an integrative assessment. An integrative assessment includes an assessment of all relevant personality dynamics, family dynamics, cultural dynamics, and spiritual dynamics that influence the client, and it situates these dynamics within the client's pattern of functioning. This section describes such an integrative assessment. It begins with a brief description of the assessment process and the most common strategies.

Assessment Process

Assessment is a prerequisite for developing a case conceptualization, and a comprehensive assessment is essential in developing a competent and clinically useful case conceptualization (Sperry & Sperry, 2022). Assessment organizes the content of the case conceptualization, focuses treatment goals, clarifies expectations about what can and what needs to change, and then defines the client's and the clinician's roles in the change process (Sim et al., 2005). The irony is that while assessment influences the case conceptualization, at the same time the case conceptualization influences and guides the assessment process.

A comprehensive assessment serves as the basis for identifying a diagnosis and developing a case conceptualization and treatment targets (Sperry & Sperry, 2020). Three approaches of such an assessment are: a diagnostic assessment, a theory-based assessment, and a pattern-based assessment. An assessment is likely to be more complete or comprehensive if it includes at least two of these approaches (Sperry, 2012).

Diagnostic Assessment

A diagnostic assessment is a focused assessment of the client and the current and developmental context influencing the client. The purpose of this assessment is to discover the answer to the question: what accounts for the client's concerns, distress, and/or diminished functioning for which the client seeks therapeutic assistance? A relatively complete diagnostic assessment interview can often be accomplished within the first 30 to 40 minutes of the initial session between client and therapist. However, the time frame necessary to complete such an evaluation may take considerably longer depending on the client's previous history and treatment, sense of ease and trust of the clinician, language, and other psychological and cultural factors.

The focus of the diagnostic assessment is to gather information about the client that is clinically relevant to the treatment process and outcomes. This includes data on the client's current problems, current functioning and mental status, social, cultural, developmental, and medical history, health behaviors, and, particularly, the expectations and resources the client brings to therapy. Since cultural factors such as cultural identity, level of acculturation, and illness perceptions can influence the treatment process, it is imperative that these factors be identified. Similarly, this assessment includes client resources, such as the client's coping skills and support system, previous success in making changes, readiness and motivation for change and treatment expectations (Sperry, 2012).

Theory-Based Assessment

The second assessment approach is theory-based assessment. While diagnostic assessment can be useful in establishing a diagnosis based on grouping a client's symptoms into an ordered pattern which matches DSM-5-TR criteria (American Psychiatric Association, 2022), a diagnosis does not provide an understanding of the client. Neither will the results of such an assessment reveal the personality dynamics nor relational dynamics that activated that particular set of symptoms. Nor can a diagnosis indicate why or how these symptoms began when they did or what maintains them. On the other hand, a theory-based assessment can provide such an understanding, and it is for this reason that theory-based assessment is a valuable component of a comprehensive assessment strategy (Sperry, 2012).

The type of information gathered in a theory-based assessment differs depending on the given theoretical orientations. For instance, CBT-based assessment is likely to focus on questions such as: "What particular dysfunctional thoughts lead to the client's specific emotional and behavioral problems? How, then, does problematic emotion and behavior feedback into the maintenance of dysfunctional cognition?" Assessing such theory-based information is essential in developing a CBT-based case conceptualization (Ledley et al., 2005).

In psychodynamically oriented approaches, such as Time-Limited Dynamic Psychotherapy, the focus of inquiry is more likely to be on eliciting a story or narrative of recurrent maladaptive interpersonal patterns that reflect dysfunctional mental working models and their reenactment in the therapeutic alliance (Strupp & Binder, 1984). Accordingly, identifying the cyclical maladaptive pattern is essential to the dynamic case conceptualization as well as providing a treatment focus (Levenson, 1995).

In contrast to the assessment strategies in CBT and the psychodynamic approaches, the systemic approaches, such as Solution Focused Therapy and Strategic Therapy, focus assessment primarily on solutions and attempted solutions. Accordingly, they pose questions such as: "What have you tried? How did you do that? Exactly what did you say? Did it work?"

Pattern-Based Assessment

Unlike these two types of assessment, a pattern-based assessment is based on pattern identification. It involves querying clients about their underlying pattern. Pattern refers to the characteristic way of perceiving thinking, and responding which is reflected in four dimensions of the client's pattern: presentation, precipitants, predispositions, and perpetuants (Sperry & Sperry, 2020, 2022; Sperry et al., 1992). By identifying the sequence of the client's presenting symptoms or concern, precipitants or triggers, predisposing factors that when activated result in the client's presentation, and identifying the perpetuants or maintaining factors, the client's basic pattern is revealed.

Presentation: Presenting problem and characteristic response to Precipitants.
Precipitant: Triggers that activate the pattern resulting in the Presentation.
Predisposition: Biological, psychological, and social factors that foster adaptive or maladaptive Pattern functioning.
Perpetuants: Factors that maintain the Pattern.
Pattern: Predictable, self-perpetuating way of thinking, feeling, acting, and coping that inform Presentation and are adaptive, flexible, and effective or maladaptive, inflexible and ineffective.

Although pattern-based assessment shares some features with the cognitive behavioral formulation model (Tarrier & Calam, 2002) and the cyclic maladaptive pattern model (Levenson, 1995; Strupp & Binder, 1984), there are differences. The primary difference is that unlike the others, pattern-based assessment is not theory-based nor theory-bound. Another difference, and a primary advantage of this assessment approach, is that it provides an *inclusive model* or map for developing a case conceptualization. As an inclusive model, it provides a framework in which any theoretical orientation can be incorporated, specifically in providing a theoretically based "explanation" for the client's symptoms and situation (as the Predisposing factor). In other words, all three of the other factors (Presentation, Precipitant, and Perpetuants) are the same, only the Predisposing factor differs, irrespective of the theoretical orientation. The advantage of this general model is that trainees and experienced clinicians can relatively easily develop a coherent case conceptualization and pick a best "fit" explanation from the various theoretical approaches in specifying the predisposing factor.

Integrative Assessment

An integrative assessment includes an assessment of relevant personality dynamics, family dynamics, cultural dynamics, and spiritual dynamics that influence the client. Dynamics refers to causes and effects which influence thoughts, feelings, and behaviors, inside and outside the therapy process. Furthermore, it situates these dynamics within the client's Pattern in terms of Presentation, Precipitants, Predisposition, and Perpetuants which are the basis for developing a treatment plan. An integrative assessment often includes a diagnostic assessment which informs the Presentation dimension, and a theory-based assessment which informs the Presentation and Perpetuants dimensions.

However, the central component of the integrative spiritual assessment is reflected in the Predisposition. Note that the Predisposition dimension of an integrative assessment includes personality, family, cultural, and spiritual dynamics. Under the designation spiritual dynamics are spiritual history, God representation, spiritual beliefs, spiritual practices, spiritual identity, and involvement in a religious or spiritual community, spiritual influence on presentation (i.e., struggles, conflict, symptoms), and spiritual influence on therapeutic relationship and interventions.

Predisposition

Predisposing factors include all personality, family, cultural, and spiritual dynamics underlying the client's maladaptive Pattern and influencing the Presentation

- **Personality Dynamics:** Personality style: self-view and worldview, coping skills, strengths and deficits, motivation, and readiness for change
- **Cultural Dynamics:** Cultural identity and acculturation (birthplace, social class, work orientation, etc.) which influence the Presentation, the therapeutic relationship, and the Plan
- **Family Dynamics:** Family narrative; family functioning and style; family identity, acculturation, and support
- **Spiritual Dynamics:**
    - Spiritual history
    - God representation or image
    - Spiritual beliefs and spiritual practices
    - Spiritual identity and involvement in a religious or spiritual community
    - Spiritual influence on Presentation (i.e., struggles, conflict, symptoms)
    - Spiritual influence on therapeutic relationship, Plan, and interventions

In short, an integrative assessment is much broader than a conventional diagnostic assessment in that it is derived from not only personality dynamics, but also family, cultural, and spiritual dynamics.

Case Conceptualization and Integrative Case Conceptualization

Increasingly case conceptualizations are expected or required to inform the practice of psychotherapy. Interestingly, a quick review of nearly all books on spiritually integrated psychotherapy suggests that case conceptualization is not considered necessary or important since the topic is rarely covered. However, one basic premise of this book is that highly effective forms of spiritually integrated psychotherapy are based on integrative case conceptualizations. This section begins by defining case conceptualization, and goes on to describe integrative case conceptualization.

Case Conceptualization

Case conceptualization is "a method and clinical strategy for obtaining and organizing information about a client, understanding and explaining the client's situation and maladaptive patterns, guiding and focusing treatment, anticipating challenges and roadblocks, and preparing for successful termination" (Sperry & Sperry, 2020, p. 4). A case conceptualization consists of four components: a diagnostic formulation, a clinical formulation, a cultural formulation, and a treatment formulation (Sperry, 2022; Sperry et al., 1992). This section briefly describes each of these components.

Diagnostic Formulation

The diagnostic formulation provides a description of the client's presenting situation and its perpetuants or triggering factors. It is a phenomenological description as well as a cross-sectional assessment of the client. It answers the "what" question, i.e., "What happened?" This formulation usually includes a DSM-5-TR diagnosis.

Clinical Formulation

A clinical formulation provides an explanation of the client's presentation. It offers a rationale for the client's symptoms, concerns, functioning, and maladaptive personal and/or relational patterns. It answer the "why" question, i.e., "Why did it happen?" It incorporates relevant individual, cultural, religious/spiritual, and family dynamics. The clinical formulation is the central component in a case conceptualization and serves to link the diagnostic and treatment formulations.

Cultural Formulation

A cultural formulation is a systematic review of cultural factors and dynamics. It answers the "what role does culture play" question. More specifically, the cultural formulation statement describes the client's cultural identity and level of acculturation. It may provide a cultural explanation of the client's condition as well as the impact of cultural factors on the client's personality and level of functioning. It also identifies cultural elements that may impact the relationship between the client and the therapist and whether cultural or culturally sensitive interventions are indicated (Committee on Cultural Psychiatry, 2002). Further discussion of the cultural formulation and culturally sensitive interventions are found in Chapter 10.

Treatment Formulation

Treatment formulation provides an explicit blueprint for intervention planning. It is the logical extension of the diagnostic and clinical formulations, and answers the "how" question, i.e., "How can it be changed?" It contains treatment goals, the treatment focus, and specific interventions, and anticipates challenges and obstacles in achieving those goals.

In the typical practice of psychotherapy the clinical formulation component, as described here, is what most therapists consider to be a case conceptualization. A review of a dozen or so clinical reports and case files is likely to support this contention. In contrast, a well-developed case conceptualization that includes all four formulation components is more likely to foster more positive psychotherapy outcomes.

So how will a case conceptualization for spiritually integrated psychotherapy differ from the four component case conceptualization described here? The answer is that the case conceptualization will be integrative. This section describes such an integrative case conceptualization, and the next section illustrates it with an extended case example.

Before describing the integrative case conceptualization, a single component formulation will be briefly described. It is based on a focused spiritual assessment.

The therapist can choose either a brief or an extended form of the integrative case conceptualization depending on the level of severity and complexity of the case. Cases which are less severe and straightforward are usually better suited to a Brief Case Conceptualization, while those that are more severe and complex tend to be better suited to an Extended Case Conceptualization. The Brief form consists of six dimensions: Presentation, Precipitant, Pattern, Predisposition, Perpetuants, and Plan. The extended form consists of eight dimensions: Presentation, Precipitant, Pattern, Predisposition, Perpetuants, Plan, Protective Factors, and Predictive Factors. The addition of Protective Factors and Predictive Factors is central to the extended case conceptualization because they are essential in focusing and configuring the treatment process and interventions to severity and complexity issues. *Case Conceptualization: Mastering this*

Competency with Ease and Confidence, Second Edition (Sperry & Sperry, 2020) and *The 15-Minute Case Conceptualization: Mastering the Pattern-Focused Approach* (Sperry & Sperry, 2022) provide further information on the indications and utilization of both types.

The first six dimensions are central to the brief form of case conceptualization while all eight dimensions are central to the extended form of case conceptualization (Sperry & Sperry, 2020, 2022).

Presentation: The client's characteristic response to Precipitants; type and severity of symptoms, history, course of illness, diagnosis, and relational behaviors.

Precipitant: The triggers or stressors that activates the pattern resulting in the Presentation.

Predisposition: All personality, family, cultural, and spiritual dynamics underlying the client's maladaptive Pattern and influencing the Presentation.

Perpetuants: Processes by which a client's pattern is reinforced and confirmed by both the client and the client's environment; also called maintaining factors.

Pattern: Predictable, self-perpetuating way of thinking, feeling, acting, and coping that informs Presentation and is adaptive, flexible, and effective, or maladaptive, inflexible, and ineffective.

Plan: Goals (first and second order); therapeutic strategy for reducing symptoms or relational issues and shifting from a maladaptive to a more adaptive pattern; and the specific interventions to accomplish these goals.

Protective Factors: Personal strengths and positive external factors that foster well-being and resilience, and decrease the likelihood of negative outcomes.

Predictive Factors: Anticipated challenges and obstacles based on the Pattern that are useful in developing or modifying the Plan to foster positive clinical outcomes.

Case Conceptualization Based on a Spiritual Assessment

This case conceptualization model can reasonably support spiritually integrated psychotherapy. It is based on an extended but focused spiritual assessment (described earlier in this chapter). It also includes four elements: religious/spiritual identity, religious/spiritual influences, religious/spiritual explanation, and religious/spiritual factors affecting the therapeutic relationship and treatment process (Sperry, 2011). Here are some assessment questions that can be useful in developing a spiritually oriented case conceptualization:

1. *Religious/Spiritual Identity.* "How do religious/spiritual beliefs and practices affect your choices about psychotherapy or medical care?"
2. *Religious/Spiritual Influences.* "Do you consider your religious/spiritual faith and community as a source of strength, or a source of stress?"
3. *Religious/Spiritual Explanation of Presentation.* "Do you believe that there is a religious/spiritual cause to your distress? Will it affect treatment?"
4. *Religious/Spiritual Factors Affecting the Clinician–Client Relationship and Treatment.* "Is the religious/spiritual background of a clinician important in your decision whether or not to get into and remain in psychotherapy?"

(Sperry, 2012)

Case Illustration

Jack N. is a 41-year-old, single, Caucasian male who is a second generation German American Catholic who was referred for counseling at a Catholic Charities Counseling Center by his parish priest. He presents for treatment complaining of relationship problems, inability to control guilt feelings about pornography, and confusion about preferring masturbating with pornography to sexual relations with his girlfriend of three years. Jack's father died when he Jack was 15, and he subsequently functioned as a parentified parent to his two younger sisters. Jack reports that he began masturbating when his teenage sisters would walk around the house in their underwear. Although he considers himself an alcoholic, Jack has maintained sobriety for the past year. After completing an initial diagnostic evaluation, James' assigned therapist developed an integrative case conceptualization which included the cultural formulation statement below. The therapist, Dr. Fernandez, is a 56-year-old, married, highly acculturated, Hispanic American male. He is an elder in the Anglican Church who had been a commercial pilot before he retired. Three years ago, he completed a doctorate in counseling psychology and completed an internship at the Center after which he was hired there as a staff psychologist.

Brief Case Conceptualization of Jack N

Jack's spiritual identity is that of a practicing Catholic. He is a member of the same parish in which he was baptized as a young boy. He grew up with strict Catholic upbringing, his religious beliefs are essentially the same, and he maintains many of the same religious practices from his youth. He believes that his sexual guilt is the result of his family and religious upbringing and has negatively influenced his intimate relationship with women.

He regularly meets with a parish priest who provides spiritual guidance as his confessor and believes that the priest has helped him. Jack considers his parish to be a source of strength, i.e., with his priest's urging and support he has been somewhat successful in reducing his drinking, although not pornography. But the parish life is also a stressor in that he is continually exposed to revelations of sexual misconduct in his diocese by priest pedophiles. Needless to say, this has reinforced his ambivalence toward the Church. In terms of coping strategies, Jack's involvement with AA meetings and his sponsor, along with the encouragement of his priest, seems to account for his current sobriety; at the same time his image of God is negative, and he perceives negative life events as God's punishment. Jack considered that working with an older married male clinician who was not Roman Catholic would be important to him. "There'd be less spiritual baggage since we come from different faith traditions." He believes he can talk freely about his various concerns with the clinician as he has done with the parish priest. Although Jack experienced his alcoholic father as abusive, demanding, and emotionally unavailable while he was alive, it appears that he could easily identify the therapist as a competent and concerned father figure; perhaps similar to the way Jack has identified with the parish priest and his AA sponsor, who are both approximately the same age as the therapist. Countertransference reactions such as judgmental statements and impatience at slow or limited progress will likely strain the therapeutic alliance. Jack is likely to respond to relationally oriented dynamic therapy that is sensitive to his God / biological father conflicts.

Case Commentary

This case conceptualization is clinically useful in that it informs and guides the therapist in considering various therapeutic alliance and intervention implementation considerations, including predictions of likely obstacles to treatment progress. However, the case conceptualization is limited in the extent to which other personality, family, and cultural dynamics are included and incorporated.

Integrative Case Conceptualization

In contrast to a case conceptualization based primarily on a focused spiritual assessment, the integrative case conceptualization advocated here is based on an integrative assessment that accounts for more personality, family, and cultural dynamics as well as spiritual dynamics. Such an integrative case conceptualization involves a diagnostic formulation, an expanded clinical formulation, and a treatment formulation. The expanded clinical formulation accounts for all relevant personality, family, cultural, and spiritual dynamics necessary to explain the client's presentation, i.e., the reason why the client is experiencing the particular religious or spiritual struggle or conflict and the distress and impairment associated with it.

The following case example illustrates both an integrative assessment and a brief integrative case conceptualization. Note that the assessment section highlights the relevant personality, family, cultural, and spiritual dynamics of the case, and then integrates them into a case conceptualization in terms of diagnostic, clinical, and treatment formulations.

Continuing Case of Maria

Background information for this case was provided in Chapter 6. Briefly, Maria is a 47-year-old, married, Cuban American female who presented for the treatment of depressed moods. She was looking for psychotherapy that was sensitive to her spiritual concerns. This section illustrates the results of an integrative assessment and integrative case conceptualization of this client.

Integrative Assessment

A detailed initial evaluation was completed. It included a full assessment of personality, family, cultural, and spiritual dynamics. In the first session, it was noted that Maria exhibited sadness, constricted affect, and some obsessive and narcissistic features.

Personality Dynamics

Psychological assessment included the Millon Clinical Multiaxial Inventory (MCMI–III), the Beck Depression Inventory (BDI), and the Thematic Apperception Test (TAT). The MCMI–III suggested the diagnosis of dysthymic disorder and as well as obsessive-compulsive personality disorder with narcissistic and paranoid features. The BDI score was 18 suggestive of a moderate degree of depression. TAT themes included fathers as demanding individuals whose expectations were impossible to meet, as well as daughters not noticed by fathers. There were also themes of mothers who were ungiving, incompetent, and wanting to be taken care of by daughters.

Maria's self-view was that she was inadequate, driven, and fearful of displeasing others. Her view of the world was that life is unfair and that others are demanding, uncaring, and can be hurtful. Her coping capacity ranges from the ability to focus and work diligently for extended periods of time when she feels understood, confident, and cared for, but very limited when her efforts to please others are unrecognized or rebuffed, or when increased demands foil her efforts to achieve and do things perfectly. Areas of strength that may have potential therapeutic value are six years of employment as a school teacher, perseverance in spiritual practices, and maintaining a long-term relationship with her husband despite conflicts. Her readiness for treatment appeared to be at the action stage (Prochaska et al., 1992).

Family Dynamics

Maria is the oldest of three siblings. Her brother and sister are both alive with professional jobs and families. Maria's parents, highly acculturated Cuban Americans, are alive, retired, and reasonably healthy. Maria denied any family history of psychiatric or substance abuse treatment. She did indicate that a maternal uncle's mood swings were probably related to his suicide. Her health is reported as good. She admits to taking medication for mild hypothyroidism which her doctor says is unrelated to her depressed mood; she denies the use of nicotine, alcohol, or recreational drugs.

Cultural Dynamics

Maria is a third generation Cuban American who identifies herself as an "upper middle class American whose parents happen to be Cuban." The Brief Acculturation Scale suggests that she is highly acculturated (Paniagua, 2013). Maria has been married to Michael for 24 years; they have no children. Michael is a fourth generation Irish who is highly acculturated. Maria is currently a special education teacher while Michael is a partner in an accounting firm.

Spiritual Dynamics

Maria describes herself as a "cradle Catholic" who attended Catholic elementary school, high school, and college. She reports being reasonably active in her local parish. The formal practice of her religion has diminished considerably since her son Alex graduated from a nearby Catholic high school. She indicated that she only kept up church attendance and traditional spiritual practice "to set a good example for my son." For the past several years her spiritual practices have included daily formula prayer, occasional scripture reading, and Sunday worship services. In the past, she had tried to meditate but had given up because she overly distracted and worried. At the outset of treatment, she described her image of God as "judge and taskmaster." Upon further inquiry, God was described as an elderly male who "made hard demands, who checked up on you and wasn't easily pleased." He was also emotionally withholding, unsupportive, and critical. Not surprisingly, her image of God appears to be a composite description of both her parents. For her, faith was the belief that there was a God, but that her salvation was totally up to her. As a result, she worked hard and tried to be perfect. Unfortunately, her perfectionistic beliefs that she was "never good enough" were ego-syntonic with her religious beliefs, i.e., "God helps those..." and "God is always watching and seeing your sins." It shouldn't be surprising that her image of God was that of judge and taskmaster. Not surprisingly, she feared she would be judged as worthless and inadequate by God and the priests in her parish; and she felt uncomfortable there. For several years she held a leadership position in two parish committees. However, for the past three years she has not been active in her parish. She explains that she reduced her involvement because she felt increasingly uncomfortable. This attitude toward her church congregation persisted until it was processed during the course of therapy. Parenthetically, it can be noted that both her parents are active members in another Catholic parish.

Brief Integrative Case Conceptualization

Diagnostic Formulation

Maria did not meet sufficient DSM-5-TR criteria to merit the diagnosis of Major Depressive Disorder, Single Episode, and so was given the diagnosis of Unspecified Depressive Disorder (F32.A). She also met criteria for Obsessive-Compulsive Personality Disorder (F60.5) and was coded for Religious or Spiritual Problems (Z65.8) (American Psychiatric Association, 2022). Because she denied suicidal ideation and did not meet other criteria for inpatient or intensive outpatient treatment, it was determined that outpatient treatment was a reasonable disposition. While there was some genetic loading for depression, personality, family, and spiritual dynamics appear to be more causative of Maria's symptoms and impaired functioning.

Clinical Formulation

The following dynamics appear to be operative: her depressive symptoms, increased marital discord, and subsequent social isolation were precipitated by increasing pressure and demands associated with her job. Personality dynamics are prominent, particularly perfectionism and the need to please others which appear to have fuelled her depressive symptoms and sense of inadequacy. Other predisposing factors involve family dynamics including an avoidant-anxious attachment style reflecting a self-preoccupied and emotionally withholding mother, and a strict, demanding, and abusive father. Furthermore, her maladaptive self-view of being driven and fearful of displeasing others and a worldview that life and others are demanding and uncaring seemed to lead to depression and self-deprecation, particularly when she experienced unrealistic personal and professional demands. These maladaptive beliefs, along with increasing social isolation, seem to be perpetuating this maladaptive pattern. High levels of acculturation for Maria and her parents and no reported experiences of prejudice or even cultural microaggression suggest that cultural dynamics are not operative, at least now. Spiritually, she images God as demanding, critical, and withholding, and she reacts to others with anger and suspiciousness when distressed. Her discomfort with and limited contact with community support, particularly her church, seems related to feelings of unworthiness and perceived non-acceptance by others. The spiritual practices she described—limited to formula prayer and church attendance—were consistent with her religious tradition and seemed to be both fear- and duty-based. It is noteworthy that her religious beliefs about "earning" salvation appear to reinforce her own perfectionistic beliefs and behaviors. She exhibits a high readiness for treatment and strengths which include six years of employment and a long-term marital relationship.

Treatment Formulation

The mutually agreed upon treatment goals were first to reduce depressive symptoms and relational conflict, and then to modify her obsessive-compulsive style. Given that Maria's drivenness, perfectionism, and need to please appear to be directly related to her parents and reflected in her God-image, a psychospiritual treatment focus was reasonable. One potential barrier and therapeutic challenge in working with Maria would be to avoid transference enactments which might result in premature termination. These included being overly neutral or subtle demands or evaluative comments.

Case Commentary

This case illustrates how an integrative assessment was undertaken and how it was reported. It also illustrates how a brief integrative case conceptualization is based on the integrative assessment and includes a diagnostic, clinical, and treatment formulation. The value of such a case conceptualization is that it integrates spiritual dynamics with personality, family, and cultural dynamics for a full and complete view of the client's reality. It also specifies how treatment might effectively proceed to address all the various concerns and dynamics, including spiritual concerns and dynamics. The case of Maria will be continued in subsequent chapters as an illustration of other aspects of the therapeutic process.

Concluding Note

Assessment and case conceptualization are essential to effective spiritually integrated psychotherapy. Accordingly, this chapter has described and illustrated an integrative assessment approach and an integrative case conceptualization approach. Both identify and incorporate relevant personality dynamics, family dynamics, cultural dynamics, as well as spiritual dynamics.

The next chapter describes both psychotherapeutic and psychospiritual interventions that are useful in the practice of spiritually integrated psychotherapy. Some of these interventions will be illustrated in a continuation of the case of Maria.

Appendix: Assessing the Spiritual Dimension with Inventories

A number of instruments have been designed to measure various aspects of the religious and spiritual dimension. However, only a few of these appear to have clinical utility for spiritual assessment. These instruments are not meant to replace the spiritual assessment interview, but rather to supplement it. Five of these instruments are briefly reviewed here.

Spiritual Well-Being Scale

Spiritual well-being is conceptualized as a personal experience related to spiritual health and spiritual maturity. That is, spiritual health and spiritual maturity appear to be enduring underlying states that are expressed in the experiences of spiritual well-being. The Spiritual Well-Being Scale (Ellison, 1994) is a 20-item instrument which can be quickly completed and scored. Its three subscales, i.e., overall spiritual well-being, existential well-being, and religious well-being, can be used as a starting point for exploring of the client's spiritual dimension. The instrument's non-sectarian content makes it appropriate for clients with diverse spiritual beliefs. Individual test items, e.g., "I don't find much satisfaction in private prayer with God," can be used to explore spiritual attitudes pertinent to the client's presenting and emerging spiritual issues and concerns. Chapter 9 contains additional information about this measure, including its use in ongoing monitoring of treatment progress.

Spiritual Health Inventory

The Spiritual Health Inventory was developed by Veach and Chappel (1992). This 18-item instrument purportedly measures four domains, i.e., personal spiritual experience, spiritual well-being, sense of harmony, and personal helplessness. Items include: "It is my experience that developing and maintaining spiritual health requires work and effort" and "I have had a spiritual experience or a sense of spiritual awakening." While only preliminary psychometric data has been reported on this instrument, it may have some value in the spiritual assessment process.

Index of Core Spiritual Experience

The Index of Core Spiritual Experience, also called INSPIRIT, was developed by Kass et al. (1991). It purports to assess two core elements of spirituality: a personal conviction of the existence of God and one's perception of an internalized relationship with God. It consists of seven items, including an item about involvement with spiritual practices. Although more limited in scope than the Spiritual Well-Being Scale, initial results with the Index of Core Spiritual Experience suggest that it may provide a quick and helpful method for assessing the spiritual dimension, particularly as a take-off point for discussing their experience of God.

God Image Inventory

The God Image Inventory is an 8-scale, 156-item instrument that measures image of God, developed by Lawrence (1997) for clinical and pastoral use with individuals. A 6-scale, 72-item and a 3-scale, 36-item version called the God Image Scales are briefer research versions of the God Image Inventory. The God Image Inventory and God Image Scales are based on Rizzuto's (1979) distinction between the God concept and the God image. Both instruments assess belonging (Presence and Challenge scales), goodness (Acceptance and Benevolence scales), and control (Influence and Providence scales). The scales of the God Image Inventory have demonstrated adequate internal reliability and validity. Standards have been developed on a sample of 1580 US adults but appear to be applicable only for Christians. A computerized version is reportedly available.

The Spiritual Experience Index

The Spiritual Experience Index consists of 38 questions and is answered on six-point Likert scales. It was developed to assess spiritual maturity from an object relations, developmental perspective (Genia, 1991). The Spiritual Experience Index is intended to correlate with a five-stage model of spiritual maturity or faith. The stages are: (1) egocentric faith, dominated by splitting; (2) dogmatic faith, characterized by rules of fairness and clearly defined obligations, defensive and utilitarian use of doctrine; (3) transitional faith, religious searching and doubting; (4) reconstructed internalized faith, characterized as a more internal, differentiated and personally integrating religious system; and (5) transcendent faith, for which Genia lists ten criteria. Both of these instruments are helpful to begin to conceptualize the functional, interactive nature of the God–family relationship.

A convenient reference guide for the selection of these and several other measures of spirituality is available in Kapuscinski and Masters (2010).

References

American Psychiatric Association. (2022). *Diagnostic and statistical manual of mental disorders*, 5th edition, Text revision. American Psychiatric Association.

Aten, J. D., & Leach, M. M. (2009). *Spirituality and the therapeutic process: A comprehensive resource from intake to termination*. American Psychological Association.

Bullis, R. (1996). *Spirituality in social work practice*. Taylor & Francis.

Cheston, S., Piedmont, R., Eanes, B., & Lavin, L. (2003). Changes in clients' images of God over the course of outpatient therapy. *Counseling and Values*, *47*, 96–108.

Committee on Cultural Psychiatry of the Group for the Advancement of Psychiatry. (2002). *Cultural assessment in clinical psychiatry*. American Psychiatric Press.

Ellison, C. (1994). *Spiritual well-being scale*. Life Advance.

Exline, J., & Rose, E. (2005). Religious and spiritual struggles. In R. Paloutzian & C. Park (Eds.), *Handbook of the psychology of religion and spirituality* (pp. 315–330). Guilford Press.

Genia, V. (1991). The Spiritual Experience Index: A measure of spiritual maturity. *Journal of Religion and Health*, *30*, 337–347.

Gorsuch, R., & Miller, W. (1999). Assessing spirituality. In W. Miller (Ed.), *Integrating spirituality into treatment: Resources for practitioners* (pp. 47–64). American Psychological Association.

Hood, R. W., Jr., Spilka, B., Hunsberger, B., & Gorsuch, R. (1996). *The psychology of religion: An empirical approach* (2nd ed.). Guilford Press.

Josephson, A., Larson, D., & Juthani, N. (2000). What's happening in psychiatry regarding spirituality? *Psychiatric Annals*, *5*, 533–541.

Kapuscinski, A. N., & Masters, K. S. (2010). The current status of measures of spirituality: A critical review of scale development. *Psychology of Religion and Spirituality*, *2*(4), 191–205.

Kass, J., Friedman, R., Leserman, J., Zuttermeister, P., & Benson, H. (1991). Health outcomes and a new index of spiritual experience. *Journal for the Scientific Study of Religion*, *30*, 203–211.

Koenig, H., & Pritchett, J. (1998). Religion and psychotherapy. In H. Koenig, (Ed.), *Handbook of religion and mental health* (pp. 323–336). Academic Press.

Lawrence, R. T. (1997). Measuring the image of God: The God image inventory and the God image scales. *Journal of Psychology & Theology*, *25*(2), 214–226.

Ledley, D., Marx, B., & Heimberg, R. (2005). *Making cognitive-behavioral therapy work*. Guilford.

Levenson, H. (1995). *Time-limited dynamic psychotherapy*. Basic Books.

Matthews, D. (1998). *The faith factor: Proof of the healing power of prayer.* Viking.

May, G. (1992). *Care of mind, care of soul.* HarperCollins.

Paniagua, F. A. (2013). *Assessing and treating culturally diverse clients: A practical guide.* Sage Publications.

Pargament, K. I. (2007). *Spiritually integrated psychotherapy: Understanding and addressing the sacred.* Guilford.

Pargament, K. I., & Exline, J. J. (2021). *Working with spiritual struggles in psychotherapy: From research to practice.* Guilford.

Prochaska, J. O., DiClemente, C. C., & Norcross, J. C. (1992). In search of how people change: Applications to addictive behaviors. *American Psychologist, 47*(9), 1102–1114.

Richards, P. S., & Bergin, A. E. (2005). *A spiritual strategy for counseling and psychotherapy* (2nd ed.). American Psychological Association.

Rizzuto, A. (1979). *The birth of the living God: A psychoanalytic study.* University of Chicago Press.

Shafranske, E., & Sperry, L. (2005). Addressing the spiritual dimension in psychotherapy: Introduction and overview. In L. Sperry & E. Shafranske (Eds.), *Spiritually integrated psychotherapy* (pp. 11–29). American Psychological Association.

Sim, K., Gwee, K., & Bateman, A. (2005). Case formulation in psychotherapy: Revitalizing its usefulness as a clinical tool. *Academic Psychiatry, 29*, 289–292.

Sperry, L. (2011). From spiritual assessment to spiritually focused cultural formulation. In J. Peteet, F. Lu., & W. Narrow (Eds.), *Religious and spiritual considerations in psychiatric diagnosis: A research agenda for DSM V* (pp. 221–224). American Psychiatric Press.

Sperry, L. (2012). *Spirituality in clinical practice: Theory and practice of spiritually oriented psychotherapy* (2nd ed.). Routledge.

Sperry, L. (2022). *Highly effective therapy: Effecting deep change in counseling and psychotherapy* (2nd ed.). Routledge.

Sperry, L., & Sperry, J. (2020). *Case conceptualization: Mastering this competency with ease and confidence* (2nd ed.). Routledge.

Sperry, L., & Sperry, J. (2022). *The 15-minute case conceptualization: Mastering the pattern-focused approach.* Oxford University Press.

Sperry, L., Gudeman, J., Blackwell, B., & Faulkner, L. (1992). *Psychiatric case formulations.* American Psychiatric Press.

Strupp, H., & Binder, J. (1984). *Psychotherapy in a new key: A guide to time-limited dynamic psychotherapy.* Basic Books.

Tarrier, N., & Calam, R. (2002). New developments in cognitive-behavioral case formulation. Epidemiological, systemic and social context: An integrative approach. *Cognitive and Behavioral Psychotherapy, 30*, 311–328.

Veach, T., & Chappel, J. (1992). Measuring spiritual health: A preliminary study. *Substance Abuse, 13*, 139–147.

Vieten, C., & Lukoff, D. (2022). Spiritual and religious competencies in psychology. *American Psychologist, 77*(1), 26–38.

Walsh, R. (1999). *Essential spirituality: The seven central practices to awaken heart and mind.* Wiley.

Chapter 8

Interventions

Derived from an integrative assessment, an integrative case conceptualization specifies treatment goals and a treatment focus as well as a treatment strategy which specifies various interventions which when implemented achieve the goals of treatment (Sperry, 2022). When the treatment goals include the resolution of spiritual struggles or spiritual growth, various psychological and spiritual interventions can be specified. This chapter describes various interventions that can be clinically useful in addressing spiritual struggles and fostering spiritual growth, and it illustrates how these psychotherapeutic interventions are utilized in spiritually integrated psychotherapy. Such interventions include cognitive restructuring, interpretation, and experiential focusing. The chapter also describes various spiritual interventions for achieving specific treatment goals and treatment targets. Examples of such spiritual interventions include prayer, meditation, mindfulness, and forgiveness. In addition to spiritual interventions are spiritual practices. These practices are focused activities which foster spiritual qualities that can foster a balanced and disciplined lifestyle. Examples of such practices include recognizing the sacred in all, living ethically, fasting, and service to others. When utilized as an adjunctive to the treatment process, spiritual practices can powerfully facilitate the change process and growth.

This chapter begins with a brief discussion of the indications and contraindications for the use of such interventions. Then it describes psychotherapeutic interventions, followed by spiritual interventions, and then spiritual practices and strategies. Finally, the continuing case of Maria illustrates the utilization of these various treatment strategies.

Indications and Contraindications

The use of spiritually integrated interventions can be effective in certain situations and circumstances rather than in others. These interventions include both psychotherapeutic interventions, spiritual interventions, and

DOI: 10.4324/9781003425991-9

spiritual practices. This section lists common indications and contraindications for such interventions.

Indications

An indication refers to a situation or circumstance in which an intervention is likely to be appropriate and warranted. Spiritually integrated interventions appear to be warranted in the following situations and circumstances:

- The client specifically asks for or consents to discussing spiritual issues and/or incorporating spiritual interventions.
- The client has the capacity to consent and to collaborate in the treatment involving a spiritual intervention.
- The spiritual issue or concern is related to the client's presenting problem.

(derived from Koenig & Pritchett, 1998)

Contraindications

A contraindication refers to a situation or circumstance in which an intervention is considered likely to be inappropriate and unwarranted. The following are some useful guidelines for evaluating the appropriateness of including spiritually integrated oriented interventions in the course of treatment. Absolute contraindications refers to situations in which the intervention is not warranted and may prove harmful, whereas relative contraindications refers to situations in which the use of an intervention would be too risky, unlikely to be effective, or otherwise inadvisable (Richards & Bergin, 1997, 2005).

Absolute Contraindications

- Client is unwilling to participate in such interventions.
- Client is delusional or otherwise psychotic.
- Client's presenting problems are clearly unrelated to the spiritual dimension.
- Client is underage and does not have parental permission to discuss religious issues or use spiritual interventions.

Relative Contraindications

- Client is severely psychologically disturbed.
- Client is anti-religious or non-religious.

- Client is spiritually immature.
- Client perceives God as distant and condemning.
- Client has a deferring or passive religious problem-solving style.
- Client is a child or adolescent.

It is speculated that "therapist-initiated, denominationally specific, religiously explicit, and in-session spiritual interventions are probably more risky than client-initiated, ecumenical, religiously implicit, and out of-session interventions" (Richards & Bergin, 1997, p. 253). Furthermore, spiritually integrated interventions may be more risky in the following circumstances: government-supported settings; the therapeutic alliance is weak; there is low therapist–client religious value similarity; therapists lack cultural competence and spiritual sensitivity; or therapists have limited denominational expertise or are spiritually immature.

Psychological Interventions

This section describes and illustrates four different psychotherapeutic approaches and related interventions for incorporating the spiritual dimensions when working with individuals and couples. These include variants of the cognitive-behavioral therapy approach, the dynamic psychotherapy approach, the focused-experiential approach, and a couples or relationship dynamics approach. These represent four different ways of conceptualizing and incorporating the spiritual dimension in psychotherapy.

Cognitive Behavioral Approaches

Cognitive-behavioral therapy appears to offer a treatment approach that is well suited to the assessment and modification of all forms of belief, including religious beliefs, as they affect the psychological and spiritual health and well-being of individuals (Propst, 1988, 1996; Tan & Johnson, 2005). That is because the theoretical perspective of cognitive therapy is a flexible therapeutic framework which can include the spiritual dimension as an active part of the therapeutic process. Although certain intervention strategies and techniques characterize the approach, the content of the therapy can vary greatly based on client need, the creativity of the clinician, and what research indicates to be efficacious for the symptom or concern in question. Propst (1988) describes four intervention strategies in what she calls religious cognitive therapy. They are: understanding the influence of cognition on emotion and behavior; monitoring cognitions, including thoughts, beliefs, and assumptions; challenging cognitions; and cognitive restructuring and behavior modification. Each will be briefly described and then illustrated with a case example.

Understanding the Influence of Cognition on Emotion and Behavior

Since a basic tenet of cognitive therapy is that clients understand and believe that their thoughts and assumptions strongly influence their emotions and psychological well-being, it follows that religious clients and spiritual seekers probably should be given a spiritual rationale for this framework as well as a spiritual rationale for assessing their thoughts and assumptions. Accordingly, Propst suggests that theological reflections could be considered a strategy or tool of cognitive therapy.

Monitoring Cognitions, Including Thoughts, Beliefs, and Assumptions

Spiritual themes are, then, useful therapeutic tools that provide a motivational language to encourage clients to actively monitor cognitions, including their thoughts, beliefs, and assumptions. This should help to overcome any initial resistance to therapy. With such a motivating language, many of the therapeutic tools originated by Beck such as the three column technique (Beck et al., 1979) can be made effective for spiritually oriented clients.

Challenging Cognitions

After clients accept the value of monitoring cognitions and can apply this skill, the next process in cognitive therapy is challenging and subsequent changing of thoughts and assumptions. Themes from most spiritual belief systems can play an important role in this process. Propst (1988) contends that these religious ideas can actually become cognitive restructuring techniques. For example, it is not uncommon for clients to have a cognitive schema in which any error, mistake, or a less than perfect solution to a problem can be catastrophic. Thus, they are more likely to have perfectionistic strivings rather than a basic problem-solving orientation toward life. This attitude may be intensified in some spiritual individuals because of the assumption that God expects perfection, which results in minimal risk taking and increased levels of anxiety and depression. Problem solving, on the other hand, means adopting the general orientation toward life that problems are a natural part of life and that coping with those problems is only a natural part of living.

Since assumptions of perfectionism can be rooted in an individual's religious beliefs, Propst (1988, 1996) reasons that therapeutically challenging such perfectionistic schemas can be most effective when such schemas are linked to a client's religious beliefs. She notes that influential thinkers in most spiritual traditions emphasize that life is not perfect, and that life has a tragic element, and that believers will rarely be problem-free or even find a perfect solution to all their problems.

Cognitive Restructuring and Behavior Change

The use of religious imagery is an additional cognitive restructuring technique that is helpful within a spiritual context. Propst (1996) understands images as an individual's responses rather than stimuli to which individuals respond. Furthermore, images can have a greater capacity than thoughts for intensifying traumatic memories and, thus, may allow clients to focus more fully on emotionally laden ideas. Accordingly, she has found that using images of Jesus in calling forth problematic, stressful scenes such as those resulting from post-traumatic stress responses has been useful for many Christian clients (Propst, 1988). For example, Christian female clients with abuse histories are often able to experience the image of the abuse when they imagine Jesus with them in the image. The meaning of the image begins to change at the point they can visualize Jesus present in that image (Propst, 1988, pp. 130–138).

Such an ameliorating of the negative intensity of the image may permit the client to work through the terrifying aspects of the images and their meanings. Techniques of thought stopping, cognitive rehearsal, and confrontation of dysfunctional forms of thinking complement the use of biblical and theological reflection in the examination of core beliefs and assumptions. Finally, behavior modification methods have also been found useful.

The effectiveness of cognitive-behavioral therapy appears to be enhanced if aspects of the client's religious belief system are used to provide not only a motivation for self-examination, but also a challenge to some of the client's dysfunctional schemas. Usually, clients are asked to view their religious and spiritual beliefs somewhat differently. Other times, they are asked to pay attention to aspects of their religious beliefs that have previously been ignored, i.e., the notion of a triune God, the Trinity, can be an appropriate model for respect and mutuality in interpersonal relationships such as marriage.

Finally, Propst (1988) indicates that the disconfirmation of clients' dysfunctional beliefs is usually supported by the religious or spiritual authorities when queried by clients. She notes this is especially when clinicians have been careful to stay within the clients' religious tradition. However, when clients may find themselves in a conflict between the clinician and their religious community, Propst (1988) notes that such clients find other congregations within the same faith that offer them more support. A few clients will drop out of therapy. However, this is rare if the clinician has been careful to attempt to stay within the bounds of the individual's spiritual tradition when suggesting reinterpretations. The following case example is inspired by Propst (1993).

Case Example

Jennifer is a 32-year-old, single, female, Christian client presenting with loneliness and sadness for several weeks. Her only reported social outlet was involvement in church activities. Yet, she was extremely fearful of social contacts, and devastated by even mild social criticism. She met DSM-5-TR criteria for persistent depressive disorder and avoidant personality disorder (American Psychiatric Association, 2022).

The assessment identified her core maladaptive schema that any type of negative emotions, social criticism, or uncomfortable circumstances were unbearable. Furthermore, Jesus was portrayed in therapy as one who chose suffering to accomplish a purpose: he was not a passive victim but a courageous person who laid down his life and experienced pain for a purpose. It was emphasized that he put himself in difficult situations with possible negative consequences. Biblical illustrations provided valuable sources of inspiration and aided in the cognitive restructuring for this client. They were not imposed on the client but, rather, were used to reflect her predominant faith orientation as a believer who viewed Jesus as the model for human perfection.

When she admitted believing that it was always easier to avoid pain, including the pain of possible rejection, she was asked whether Jesus held that belief. Jennifer responded "No." The therapist underscored that Jesus had made the choice to go to the cross, and that facing that pain resulted in a transformation, his Resurrection. The client responded that this was new understanding for her since she had always believed that the Christian ideal was to avoid all pain.

Consistent with the spiritual beliefs of individuals with avoidant personality disorder, she firmly believed that negative feelings were bad and that, since she experienced such feelings, she must be unhealthy. Applying Beck's three-column technique (Beck et al., 1979), she was asked to rate her belief in the notion that Jesus was vulnerable and in pain, but still a healthy human person. She rated it as 100%. Then Jennifer was asked to rate the belief that if she was vulnerable and in pain, she could also be a healthy person. Initially, she rated it as only 10%. Soon there was a recognition response, then she smiled and said she was expecting more of herself than she did of Jesus.

By means of this strategy Jennifer was also able to confront her highly critical, overbearing, and possessive parents. In addition, she also undertook the challenge of forming social relationships. Prior to the completion of treatment, she had established a romantic relationship. Although initially finding the relationship rather threatening, she approached it with the thought that being a Christian means risking the pain of rejection.

Dynamic Approaches

There are several dynamic approaches to psychotherapy. Of these, a small number are sensitive to the spiritual dimension. These include a contemporary Jungian approach to spiritually integrated psychotherapy (Corbett & Stein, 2005), and a psychoanalytic approach to spiritually integrated psychotherapy (Shafranske, 2005).

This section focuses on the object relations approach which emphasizes the client's God representation (Rizzuto, 1979, 1991, 1996, 2005). The reader is referred to Chapter 2 of this book for an extended discussion of the object relations perspective and God representations. A brief sketch of the formation of this representation is given followed by its therapeutic implications and application. A case example then illustrates this approach.

God representations are transitional phenomena which serves the same function in relation to God that they serve with other objects. Representations permit the mind to know existing realities. Without the representation of the breast or of the mother, the infant has no means to know the mother. However, neither the mother nor the breast she provides is the representation. Similarly, the God sought for by the spiritual seeker should not be confused with the representation of God. Representations belong to different layers of reality. The God representation is the psychic means the mind has to seek God and its developmental and dynamic sources are unconscious and not accessible without psychic exploration. God, however, appears to the spiritual seeker as the object of conscious belief as an existing being beyond the limits of the mind (Rizzuto, 2005).

Spiritual practices and religious elements such as prayers, scriptures, and ritual are also part of the dialectic processes of attachment and separation from parents. Each carries deep emotions and the potential for integration or rejection. With psychotherapeutic exploration their unconscious motivational and dynamic sources can be revealed.

The affective component of spiritual experience is its main source of personal meaning and is rooted in all relational exchanges extending from the beginning of life to the moment when it occurs. Thus:

> all encounters with God, as with any other person, are preceded and conditioned by the psychic structure and by the momentary psychic reality of the person who is having the experience... The final shape of the experience of God is always the result of complex psychic compromises between available representations, accepted and rejected feelings and wishes, superego pressures, and the effort at self-integration aided by defensive maneuvering.
>
> (Rizzuto, 1996, p. 419)

This formulation of the formation of God representations suggests that every child who has grown up in a religious culture will come to treatment with some conscious representation of God. Even though religion may be irrelevant to the person coming for psychotherapy, the clinician must not forget that in most children the God representation has played a psychic role during development and that when it emerges it may be fruitfully explored.

Rizzuto (1996) notes that three types of clients can be encountered in therapy: (1) seekers and believers for whom their belief is not a problem; (2) non-believers who are at peace with their religious situation and accept the treatment without any religious considerations; and (3) seekers who are concerned about their religion and fear that therapy may change their faith or their moral commitments.

Therapeutic Strategies

How does an analytically oriented psychotherapy proceed? It begins with a detailed spiritual assessment. Rizzuto (1996, 2005) advocates the taking of a comprehensive spiritual assessment, which she refers to as a "religious history." This assessment should include the religious affiliation of each parent, the family's religious practices and attitudes, as well as its degree of integration within the spiritual community. It is also important to elicit the individual's major spiritual landmarks, i.e., baptism, circumcision, bar mitzvah, confirmation, etc., including their private and public meaning. Finally, the client's current involvement in and attitudes toward religious institutions, beliefs, and spiritual practices is elicited. In short, this type of spiritual assessment reveals the client's perceptions of the significant other and self in the spiritual development process.

The clinical significance of such a spiritual assessment is enormous. For instance, in eliciting a social-developmental history a client reports that her father was a good provider for the family, but moments later in the spiritual assessment indicates that God never answers her prayers. Noting this object discrepancy, the astute clinician might speculate that the client needs to maintain the idealization of her father whereas God can tolerate her angry complaints.

Rizzuto (1996) contends that clinicians should not reveal their religious affiliation, beliefs, or any other personal information. Withholding such information maximizes the potential for the development of a transference based on the client's psychic processes, unrestricted by factual data. Nevertheless, the clinician must show respect for the clients' spiritual experiences, spiritual concerns, doubts, moral quivering, and commitments.

Does the God representation change in the course of this type of analytic treatment? Rizzuto (1989) would say that it most likely will change since it is a process of self-transformation. It is a "transformation of the ways of receiving one's own experiences and self-representations, questioning them, examining them, attending to them, being amazed that they can be looked at from another angle. As you do that you have a new self-representation" (Rizzuto, 1989, p. 3). She also speculates that the God representation is transformed even if God is not discussed in the course of treatment. She bases this on the basic assumption of object relations theory that one cannot change oneself without changing one's view of others. Even though the individual may not be consciously aware of the transformation of their God representation, "it may remain quietly in the background and at the moment when you may have the need for a God it may reappear… a conscious transformation of the God representation" (Rizzuto, 1989, pp. 3–4).

A number of other therapeutic strategies are useful in this approach which some call the "transitional figure method." These include the traditional psychoanalytic method of processing: clarification, confrontation, interpretation, and working through, as well as guided imagery and dream analysis.

Case Example

Jason is a 46-year-old, single, white male who presented for psychotherapy with insomnia and difficulty concentrating. While he did not meet criteria for a clinical depression, he appeared to be experiencing a delayed grief reaction. His father had died of inoperable cancer 14 months ago, and it appears Jason did not begin the mourning and grieving process until the first anniversary of his death some two months ago.

Jason's developmental and spiritual history was instructive. He was baptized and reared by fairly strict and devout Catholic parents who had high expectations for their only child. Their expectation was that Jason would become a priest, and if not, would work for and assume leadership of the family printing business when his father retired. However, Jason's only desire was to become a high school science teacher. During elementary school, Jason found himself striving to please his teachers and to be almost obsessed with the idea of "saving his soul" through achievement and by being a good boy. He recalled that his father was emotionally unavailable and never seemed satisfied with his achievements. And he was embarrassed to add that he was, then and now, as critical as or more critical than his father. During these years Jason's view of God was that of taskmaster and judge.

There was considerable tension between father and son throughout Jason's teen years. While he continued to complain to his mother that he felt unloved by his father, his mother's only response was "your father does care about you." But since he didn't feel it, Jason couldn't believe his mother. When Jason was in college it became clear that he would not fulfill his father's dream. As a result, several years of near silence ensued between father and son. Nevertheless, Jason became a well-respected teacher at the same high school he himself had attended. He also volunteered as a teacher in his church's Sunday morning religious education program. Curiously, in this capacity he wrote, illustrated, and published a small book entitled *God Loves All the Little Children*. While somewhat interested in women, he never married, although he was never sure why he believed he was meant to remain a bachelor.

Over the course of 34 sessions Jason was able to sufficiently work through his grief and gain a greater perspective on and appreciation of his father. The brief course of psychotherapy helped him deal with the overpowering effect of his relationship with his father. He came to understand his grief as a call to deal with the unmet needs in his early life. Rather early in therapy, Jason began to realize that his failure to get his father's love and approval did not mean that he was unloved or unlovable. He discovered that not only had his paternal grandfather deeply cared about him, but so did his father, who also bragged about him to the grandfather. He had identified with his father and judged himself as sternly as he always did. Somewhat later, he began to see that remaining a bachelor was his solution for obeying his father, at least in part, i.e., priests don't marry, while at the same time pursuing the career he wanted. Furthermore, he discovered his unconscious belief that the God of his feelings was as harsh as him and impossible to please, while the God of his conscious belief was quite different. He came to believe in a God who loved him. And, in the process, a gradual change in his God representation occurred.

A transforming experience involved spending a long afternoon alone with his 87-year-old paternal grandfather. Whereas he had previously felt unwelcome by his grandfather, this day was different. During this afternoon, his grandfather brought out a family photo album and reminisced about pictures of Jason's birth and baptismal ceremony. He pointed out how proud Jason's father was of his son, and casually mentioned that it had always been like that. When Jason queried his grandfather about his statement, he learned that his father regularly told the grandfather, with pride, about his son's life and achievements, especially his many academic and teaching awards. When Jason sadly said he had no idea his father felt this way, his grandfather began to tear and said: "Son, the men in this family never learned how to show their love and appreciation to those they really cared about." For the first time Jason came to understand that his father really cared for him but could not show it directly.

Later, as therapy focused on his criticalness, Jason recalled an incident that occurred two months before his father died. While driving his father to a chemotherapy appointment, Jason became impatient at a slowly moving car that he could not get around. He repeatedly honked the car horn and began the kind of name-calling that he had learned from his father. Rather gently his father pointed out that there were elderly occupants in the other car and that he, the father, was in no hurry. After relaying this experience in therapy, he began to cry when it was interpreted that perhaps Jason's father was growing and changing even as he was dying. As this was further clarified and interpreted, Jason came to understand and accept that the angry, critical image he had of his father was also changing. As treatment terminated, Jason's grief work was well under way and his representation of God had been transformed to that of a proud father.

Experiential Focusing Approach

The Experiential Focusing Method, developed by Eugene Gendlin (1969, 1981), is a useful psychospiritual intervention strategy for working with issues related to the spiritual dimension. Gendlin's theory of experiencing (1969) and his Experiential Focusing Method (Gendlin, 1969, 1981), hereafter called "focusing," have been applied to the process of spiritual growth in psychotherapy and counseling by Hinterkopf (1994, 1998, 2005).

Hinterkopf (2005) suggests a number of indications for utilizing focusing in helping clients integrate their spiritual experiences. For example, focusing can help clients with difficulty getting in touch with the spiritual dimension because of negative experiences with religious practices during childhood. Focusing can be used to work through such blocks and to integrate the positive aspects of their past religious experiences. It can also deepen and develop spiritual experiences that already exist. Furthermore, it can foster new spiritual experiences.

Focusing is a process of paying attention to something unclear in one's experience, and letting it unfold into new, explicit meanings. When the process has been carried forward, it involves psychospiritual growth. Although focusing is a natural, flowing process, it is frequently taught in six steps (Gendlin, 1981). This process can be guided by the clinician within the session prescribed as a spiritual technique to be practiced between sessions.

Step 1. Here, the client takes an inventory of presently felt problems or issues and notes the inner experience of each issue. As each issue is identified, the client imagines setting each problem outside to perceive it more clearly and to feel better physically in order to work on it. Then one issue is chosen as a point of focus. It is usually the problem that is felt most strongly. Within the treatment setting, clients typically begin by discussing a chosen issue, and thus, the clinician may omit Step 1 and begin with Step 2 at the appropriate time.

Step 2. Now, the client is instructed to attend to the "felt sense" of the issue. The felt sense is multifaceted involving emotional tones and qualities, bodily sensations, and felt meanings; it can also involve images, movements, sounds, and smells. Initially, it is unclear and vague, i.e., the uncomfortable feeling individuals experience leaving home and realizing they forgot something but are uncertain as to what it might be.

Step 3. Here, the client finds words or images to describe the emotional qualities of the felt sense, i.e., "empty," "tense," or "expanding."

Step 4. At this step the client determines whether the words describing the felt sense are the best words to describe the felt sense at the present time. It may be changed, or other words added to more accurately describe the felt sense. At times, resonating may simply involve being with the felt sense.

Step 5. The clinician may suggest that the client ask the felt sense an open-ended question. Usually, asking such an open-ended question brings new meanings for the client, e.g., "What leaves you feeling this way?" The client directs the question to the felt sense and continues to attend to it, waiting for an answer. Hinterkopf (1998) notes that an answer tends to emerge in a minute or less. A new felt meaning, called a "felt shift," is a physiological change in the client which brings a sense of relief or a release of life energy. It can be likened to the relief experienced when remembering the forgotten item. A felt shift indicates that psychospiritual growth has occurred.

Step 6. Finally, this step involves integrating the answer that elicits the felt shift. To help the client receive an answer, the clinician affirms a client's felt shift. This can be accomplished by suggesting that the client take time to notice the felt shift and the answer that came with it, by body language such as sitting more upright or looking more interested, or by adding a note of excitement to voice tone.

As noted earlier, the focusing process can be used inside or outside the treatment setting. Outside the treatment setting Steps 2 through 5 are usually recycled until a felt shift occurs. In the treatment setting a selected few of the six steps can be utilized. Whatever the context, the client is taught the importance of keeping a number of attitudes while attending to feelings. A receptive attitude involves allowing feelings and symbols to enter into awareness rather than trying to control or force them to happen. Other attitudes include being friendly, kind, patient, and self-accepting. Focusing, which results in physiological release and increased life energy, is contrasted with a critical self-attitude, which results in increased tension and dullness. Furthermore, clients are taught to maintain some distance from their problems, i.e., remaining close enough to achieve a felt sense but sufficiently removed to appreciate that one's life is greater than one's problems. Maintaining such a distance fosters the development of an "observer self."

Case Example

Hinterkopf (1998, pp. 56–57) illustrates the focusing process with a professional athlete who consulted her about increasing levels of anxiety. He reported that he had always been healthy and successful in life. He also prided himself on maintaining tight control of his emotions during the course of his athletic career. However, six weeks before the consultation, he was diagnosed with hypertension and soon thereafter noted anxiety and worry that quickly increased. He could not really explain the source of his anxiety except that he was a little concerned about his hypertension. In answer to a query about recent stressors, he mentioned a fire in his home and the arrest of his adolescent son, both occurring in the past year. But he insisted that neither incident had really fazed him. He repeatedly told himself that there was nothing to worry about; nevertheless, his anxiety and worry continued. He was agreeable to engage in the focusing process during the consultation.

In Step 1 the client was instructed to quiet his mind, become relaxed, and to focus on his breathing. Then he was asked "What stands in the way of you feeling fine?" As he named each issue, the therapist asked, "How does this whole thing feel in your body now?" As he noticed how the house fire felt in his body, he realized that there was some remaining fear and sadness about the losses involved. He imagined setting aside this issue, along with the fear and sadness. As he thought about his son, he noticed his sadness and anger about the arrest. He imagined putting this issue, along with his sadness and anger, into a place where his son was staying. He then named the news from the doctor about his slightly high blood pressure. He said that it felt like a large, prickly ball with anxiety in it. As he imagined setting this issue, along with the anxiety, outside of himself, he breathed a sigh of relief. He then chose this issue for focusing.

In Step 2 he was asked to notice how the news from the doctor felt in his body. In Step 3, he reported that it still felt like a ball and that it could grow larger than himself. In Step 4, it was suggested that he stay with the thing and notice if he had the right words to describe it. He replied that he had the right words, and that he also noticed darkness. In Step 5, he was asked "What was it about the news from the doctor that leaves you with a large, prickly, dark ball with anxiety in it?" He directed this question to the felt sense and waited a few moments. With a big sigh of relief he said, "the straw that broke the camel's back." Then, he realized he had repressed his feelings about the fire in his house and his son's arrest. He noted that his blood pressure was really not as important as the fire and his son's arrest. He reported feeling relieved and more relaxed, and no anxiety. In Step 6, it was suggested that he stay with and notice the feelings of relief and relaxation that came with the words "the straw that broke the camel's back."

After he had experienced the felt shift and the focusing segment of the session was completed, he indicated that he was able to take his emotions more seriously. This client was able to transcend his former frame of reference and to reach out to more parts of himself; specifically, his emotional self. Later, he reported an increasing acceptance of the emotions of others in his life. This example illustrates how focusing often leads clients to experience their spirituality and, consequently, to undergo psychospiritual growth.

Focusing offers a non-judgmental approach to the spiritual and religious dimensions in psychotherapy and counseling because it is process oriented. This means that, when using focusing, the clinician follows a client's feelings and how they unfold into new meanings, rather than focusing entirely on the contents of what the client is saying. Since words have special meanings or connotations for each person, the clinician follows the client's experiencing process rather than being concerned with the vocabulary that the client is using. After the focusing segment of the session has been completed, the clinician assists the client to examine the contents and clarify the vocabulary. In focusing, whatever is said or done is checked with the client's feelings to monitor changes in life energy associated with transcending one's former frame of reference (Hinterkopf, 1994).

Relational Dynamics Approach

Clients who seek out spiritually integrated psychotherapy are presumed to be relationally unattached individuals searching for spiritual change or growth in personal therapy. The reality is that many spiritual seekers are married or in committed relationships and have embarked on the spiritual journey together. Whether they present for individual or conjoint therapy these individuals or couples come with a system of spiritual beliefs and values that affect their relational thoughts, attitudes, and behaviors. Their spiritual orientation and religiosity influence various aspects of their lives together from ideals about marriage to power, sexuality and intimacy, gender roles, and perhaps the raising and disciplining of children. As such, religion and spirituality can either serve as an important resource or a significant source of resistance for therapy. Accordingly, it is incumbent for psychotherapists to understand the dynamics of the spiritual beliefs and spiritual practices of the couples.

Sperry and Giblin (1996) have described an eclectic approach to working with relational issues. Unlike the first three approaches described in this chapter, their approach easily accommodates spiritual practices. This section briefly overviews some of the spiritual beliefs impacting therapy and assessment strategies, as well as intervention strategies described by Sperry and Giblin (1996) as useful in working with such relationship issues. Two brief cases illustrate these strategies.

Couples experiencing problems can derive significant benefits from spiritual beliefs and practices. Clinicians can assist couples in utilizing their spiritual beliefs and practices as vehicles for growth. For instance, clinicians can encourage the development of spiritual practices that support family cohesion such as family rituals and customs associated with religious holidays. Furthermore, clinicians can encourage the replacement of religious practices that negatively impact growth and functioning with more positive religious behaviors and practices. For example, parents can be counseled to substitute limit setting and forgiveness for threats and guilt when talking to adolescents about attendance at religious services.

But which religious beliefs and practices are helpful to families and facilitate the therapeutic process, and which do not? A survey of family-life professionals' (Brigman, 1984) perceptions of religious beliefs and practices helpful to families identified the following: beliefs such as love, faith, hope, forgiveness, grace, reconciliation, parenthood of God, and divine worth of persons were reported as helpful. Similarly, these professionals identified loving, caring, sharing, giving to others, taking responsibility, and shared religious observances as lifestyles or behaviors that helped strengthen families. Furthermore, these professionals perceived that the social support and networking that religious groups and organizations provide can greatly strengthen families. Brigman (1992) believes that such affiliations not only reduce loneliness and isolation with a feeling of belonging and acceptance, but also ease the burden of guilt and contribute to a sense of hope.

Several studies have demonstrated a positive relationship between marital satisfaction and spiritual well-being and/or religious maturity. Giblin (1993) proposed that in the therapeutic context the affective, cognitive, and behavioral shifts from marital conflict to marital satisfaction are potentially mediated by the couple's spiritual resources, and that there is a sense in which the dynamics accompanying marital conflict are the direct inverse of a marital spirituality.

On the other hand, some religious attitudes can be detrimental to families (Pruyser, 1977). Religious beliefs and practices that could be harmful to families were also identified by family life professionals in Brigman's (1984) study. These included rigid doctrine that is insensitive to human need, negativity regarding issues like family planning, sexuality, divorce and remarriage, and an overemphasis on concepts such as sin, a judgment leading to guilt feelings and low self-esteem. Other harmful beliefs and practices identified were the promotion of traditional, patriarchal sex roles, a bias toward the indissolubility of marriage on any grounds, and an emphasis on the individual to the exclusion of emphasis on the family, particularly by activities that separate family members (Brigman, 1984).

Just as it is important for the clinician working with couples to evaluate whether spiritual beliefs and practice contribute to integration and growth or disintegration, so too must the clinician ascertain the couple's or family's expectations and perceptions of therapy. Generally speaking, the more orthodox or conservative their religious beliefs, the more sensitized and concerned they are about clinicians attacking their beliefs or encouraging them to go against their religious beliefs or the standards of the religious group to which they belong (Brigman, 1992; Koltko, 1990). Such perceptions and expectations are less likely to be present among those with less conservative beliefs, irrespective of creed.

Respect for and incorporation of the spiritual dimension in couples or relationship therapy does not necessitate an arsenal of specific strategies and techniques. Quite the opposite. More harm is likely to be done to clients by clinicians equipped with ready scriptural reference for each presenting problem, by untimely or overused prayer, and by simplistic rendering of the mysterious and paradoxical sides of life. Instead, clinicians need a range of flexible approaches including: (1) therapeutic use of self; (2) a sense of how explicitly or implicitly the spiritual dimension can be used; and (3) consideration of the appropriateness and timing of interventions such as prayer with or for clients, sacred readings such as scripture, spiritual bibliotherapy, forgiveness, and other spiritual practices and resources.

When clients are both aware of and able to articulate their relationships with the transcendent, the clinician can more directly and explicitly incorporate the spiritual dimension in therapy. For example: "Where do you think God is in your decision making?" or "What do you think God wants for each of you and for your relationship?" However, when clients lack such awareness or articulation, clinicians do well to incorporate the spiritual dimension in a more indirect fashion, never speaking directly about God, but always keeping an ear open for understanding clients' value, belief, and meaning systems.

More important than any other single factor is the clinician's own spiritual journey and his/her awareness of and ability to articulate that process. Couples need to know they have found a "spiritual friend." Spiritual friends are familiar with the religious resources, scriptures, rituals, traditions, and spiritual reading materials that the client mentions. And, if not directly familiar with these resources, will become familiar. Even more important, they have firsthand experience with clients' struggles with finding meaning, with experiences of loss—in all its psychological and spiritual dimensions—as well as with hope and resurrection. Couples also need to know their values and beliefs will be respected and that they will not be shamed, ridiculed, or evangelized.

How do a couple's values and the decisions they make embody the spiritual? One's deepest desire is for self-transcendence (Conn, 1998). The pulls of denial and addiction (May, 1988), materialism, careerism, and egoism (Watchell, 1983) are strongly opposed to the recognition of this desire. The more open clients are to evaluate decisions in trusted relationships the more likely they will overcome blind spots in their decision making.

What are the dynamics of change and growth? Is it a cognitive, affective, or behavioral shift that initiates and maintains lasting change? From a spiritual perspective, growth or change takes time, and typically involves waiting and letting go. Hendrix (1988) notes that what one partner needs the most is what the other partner is least able to give, as well as being the precise area where that partner needs to grow.

Change and growth involves differentiation in relation to spiritual dimension as well. It is painful but all too easy to go along with the cultural and religious expectations for marital and family life while failing to listen to the deeper desires and stirring of self, partner, and family members. For example, one may believe that from a spiritual point of view anger should be repressed and that self-sacrifice is always valued over self-awareness and one's own needs.

As Rizzuto (1979) notes, God representations are an admixture of parental, developmental, imaginative, and familial and religious influences. How a client images God, whether as distant, demanding, and critical and/or warm and nurturing, can influence the process and outcome of therapy. For example, in a client whose image of God is punitive, demanding, and unforgiving it might be a therapeutic error to initially focus treatment on forgiveness. Asking such a client to begin to forgive herself and accept her behaviors when she hears criticism, judgment, and non-acceptance from her spouse and her parents and also imagines God to be saying similar things could present an insurmountable obstacle to therapy.

The clinician also needs to determine how directly or indirectly the spiritual dimension is to be used. Experience suggests that clinicians move slowly and indirectly toward the spiritual dimension and only after a relationship has developed with the couple. Then comments that are semi-direct are likely to be acceptable and useful. For instance, "I wonder how God can accept you when you find it so difficult to accept yourself?" or "I wonder what God would think about this decision?" The goal is to plant seeds, to suggest alternative ways of looking at and experiencing relationships, to create an openness to the spiritual dimension.

Case Examples

Two cases are presented which illustrate various interventions with client presenting relationship issues. Jack is a 38-year-old, highly verbal, minimally insightful, married man. He has two children and added a third during therapy. He is Roman Catholic, a graduate of a parochial high school and college, a weekly participant in a men's prayer and scripture study group, and a daily churchgoer. Jack is dissatisfied with his professional work and envisions himself called to be an evangelizer, minister, or perhaps a missionary. He is about to "give it all up" to follow his "call," and he declared bankruptcy to pay off debts. He reports marital satisfaction but appears minimally committed to either marriage or parenting. In terms of spiritual assessment Jack's spirituality is fueled by perfectionist images and is self-centered. It differs markedly from a spirituality that asks, "What is God doing in my life?" and is God-centered.

Jack is articulate about his Christian belief system, but it appears to function in a largely defensive fashion: (1) calling him out of responsible partnering, parenting, and economic providing; (2) bolstering an otherwise weak sense of self and providing a sense of specialness and entitlement; and (3) having little to do with any altruistic sense of service. In terms of Pruyser's categories, Jack presented as follows. (1) Awareness of the holy: Jack strongly identified with the church and its rituals. He was an active church participant on the daily level. He spoke of a strong sense of God, a God who was primarily otherworldly. (2) Providence: he had little sense of trust in himself and placed all his trust in God and God's representatives, the clergy. (3) Faith: he struggled with an appropriate locus for his commitments. It was surprising how little impact a pregnancy and birth in the family had on him during therapy. (4) Grace, gratefulness: Jack had little sense of thanksgiving for his life and relationships; he had a strong sense of existential guilt for not being more successful with his life. (5) Repentance: he had a legal, rule-governed sense of morality and would not take work that would apparently compromise his values. (6) Communion: he had little sense of connectedness. (7) Vocation: this was a critical question for him. What would he choose to do with his life that would provide him a sense of meaning and purpose? There was a strong sense that Jack was operating less based on his heart's desires than an external sense of validation. Overall, Jack presented with what seemed to be a fairly rigid belief system, a strong sense of connectedness to the institutional church, and with much less of a sense of personal spirituality.

Betty is a 47-year-old, divorced woman who presented for therapy to deal with her ex-husband. She is the mother of six grown children, one of whom was diagnosed with cancer only months after Betty separated from her husband. She was seeking a separation rather than divorce; however, she was soon served with divorce papers. Her son died two years later for which she was blamed by her ex-husband and her elderly parents. Both pointed to her separation as the catalyst for the son's illness. Betty's grief and rage were palpable; her spiritual seeking was passionate but filled with doubt and questioning. Her upbringing allowed for little anger or vulnerability, much independence, and dogmatic religious practice. Not surprisingly, Betty's image of God at the outset of treatment was punitive, demanding, and unforgiving.

Spiritual Interventions

Spiritual interventions are increasingly being utilized in psychotherapy (Aten et al., 2011). This section will describe eight spiritual interventions that have the potential to foster spiritual and psychological development based on Walsh's seven spiritual interventions (Walsh, 2000). They are: prayer, meditation, mindfulness, forgiveness, fasting, written spiritual resources, moral instruction, and service.

Prayer

Prayer is probably the most distinctive and characteristically spiritual of all activities associated with the spiritual dimension. It is a spiritual phenomenon that is central to most seekers on the spiritual journey. Most clients pray at least occasionally and many use it frequently for coping with life's difficulties. Prayer can serve as a journey marker for clients demarcating important struggles and events in their lives. Clinicians can view their clients' prayer lives as a measure of their spiritual and psychosocial functioning. It can also be utilized as a vehicle for fostering cognitive and behavioral change. McCullough and Larson (1999) note that many clients are favorably disposed to an assessment and discussion of their prayer lives in the treatment context.

Types of Prayer

Various typologies of prayer have been proposed. Meadow and Kahoe (1984) described six types: petitionary, meditation, thanksgiving, adoration, confession, and intercessory. Paloma and Pendleton (1989) describe four types: adoration, thanksgiving, petition, and intercession. Intercessory prayer is also known as healing prayer. It was once "one of the chief therapeutic tools of the nineteenth century physician, but more recently prayer has been squeezed out of the therapeutic setting by chemicals, machines, and heroic surgical procedures" (Lipp, 1986, p. 314). Today, intercessory prayer has been reintroduced in the clinical context.

There are four variants of intercessory prayer utilized by clinicians in psychotherapy practice. The first, and most controversial, involves the clinician praying directly with a client. The second involves praying for the healing of the client outside the treatment context. The third involves praying for guidance on diagnostic or treatment matters. Finally, the fourth involves the clinician allowing the client to pray within the session while the clinician remains silent. Prayer may be the most common spiritual practice in psychotherapy and counseling, second only to spiritual assessment (Sperry et al., 2007).

The use of intercessory prayer by mental health professionals is widespread but controversial. For example, among social workers 28% report engaging in verbal prayer with clients, while 57% report praying privately. An extensive systematic review—including a meta-analysis—of the use of intercessory prayer with clients found small but significant effect sizes (Hodge, 2007). The use of intercessory prayer in clinical settings is controversial because some contend that prayer is not a psychotherapeutic intervention but rather a spiritual practice. Adding to the doubt about its use in treatment is that intercessory prayer is classified as an "experimental" rather than as an "empirically supported" intervention. This conclusion is based on criteria developed by Division 12 of the American Psychological Association for empirically supported interventions. This leads the study's author to conclude that the study's "findings are unlikely to satisfy either proponents or opponents of intercessory prayer" (Hodge, 2007, p. 185).

Prayer in the Treatment Context

Prayer can have a significant impact, positively or negatively, on the therapeutic relationship and the treatment process. It is essential for the therapist to carefully consider if and when prayers can foster a positive impact. There are at least four different ways prayer can become a part of the treatment process: (1) the clinician may pray *for* the client's healing and well-being outside treatment sessions; (2) the clinician may pray silently *for* guidance about diagnostic and treatment issues as they come up in a session; (3) the clinician may allow or encourage the client to pray silently or aloud in the session; or (4) the clinician may pray with the client during the treatment session.

Clients with religious backgrounds and/or spiritual needs may expect that clinicians will pray with them in treatment sessions. Some clinicians believe that it is appropriate and useful to respond to such requests or even to offer to pray with clients. Praying with clients in the context of psychotherapy and counseling is a controversial intervention, particularly for clients with severe emotional issues (Koenig & Pritchett, 1998). Incorporating this form of the spiritual dimension may have unpredictable consequences on the therapeutic relationship. Some clinicians may recoil at any mention of prayer in psychotherapy and view it as a clear violation of clinician-client boundaries. Unfortunately, at this time there are no research studies nor professional standards nor a consensus among experts on guidelines to guide clinical practice. Prayer remains a delicate issue with psychotherapy clients because of the matter of boundary issues. Praying with clients can produce an intimacy that is threatening to both patient and therapist. Some experts express deep reservations about clinicians praying with clients in treatment sessions (Richards & Bergin, 2005).

In specific circumstances, a clinician may choose to pray *with* certain clients. But what are the benefits and risks of praying with clients? There are at least four benefits: (1) prayer can effect comfort and hope that can extend beyond the treatment session; (2) it can convey a sense of the clinician's caring and commitment for the client; (3) it can combat the client's sense of isolation and loneliness; and (4) it can enhance trust in the client–clinician relationship. At least four risks are possible in praying with clients during a treatment session: (1) prayer could be dangerous in some circumstances, i.e., fragile clients with poor ego boundaries and a history of intimacy issues that prayer could activate; (2) it could threaten the therapeutic alliance; (3) it could adversely affect the client's psychological stability; and (4) it could disrupt the clinician's neutrality and objectivity, i.e., in some psychoanalytically oriented psychotherapies (Koenig & Pritchett, 1998). In short, routinely praying with all clients is probably unwise and contraindicated. If the client insists on it and the clinician feels uncomfortable with the request, referral to a religious professional is a reasonable option.

Indications for Praying with Clients

Koenig and Pritchett (1998) list five *general indications* for determining the advisability of utilizing prayer as a treatment intervention. The five are: (1) the client clearly indicates that religion is an important way for them to cope with problems; (2) the client and clinician are from the same religious background; (3) the client either asks for prayer or shows no hesitation when the clinician asks for permission to pray; (4) the client has sufficient ego strength and stability, and disturbance of boundaries is not an issue; and most important, (5) the situation indicates that prayer would help advance the goals of treatment.

What are appropriate *specific indications* for praying with client? These include (1) acute situational stressors such as the death or serious injury of a loved one; (2) deep personal disappointment such as marital separation or job loss; and (3) life-threatening medical illness such as a diagnosis of cancer or need for major surgery.

Prayer can also be helpful to clients struggling with chronic behavioral problems that seem impossible to overcome such as a chronic substance use or compulsive gambling. It might also be helpful in counteracting the feeling of hopelessness that might otherwise paralyze further efforts to overcome the problem.

Protocol for Praying with Clients

Koenig and Pritchett (1998) offer a protocol that they suggest is non-intrusive, non-offensive, and minimizes risks of adverse consequences. The protocol is:

1. Assess whether prayer is congruent with the client's worldview. If so, the clinician might say: "Some clients find comfort in prayer while others do not. Would my praying with you over this situation be helpful to you, or do you feel that it would not be particularly helpful?" The client must be given clear and explicit permission to reject the offer for prayer without feeling uncomfortable or that they have disappointed the clinician. Even if the clinician has prayed with the client before, the same cautious approach should be taken each time a new occasion for prayer arises.
2. If the patient agrees and shows sincere interest in proceeding, then prayer might be conducted in the following manner. The prayer should be brief, lasting less than one minute, particularly if the clinician does the praying. It is preferable for the client to do the praying, in which case the clinician can listen attentively and answer "Amen" at the end of the prayer. By carefully listening to the client's prayer, the clinician might learn things about the client's motivation and priorities that may otherwise not be revealed.
3. If the client asks the clinician to pray, then the prayer should be general, supportive, affirming, and hopeful.
4. Finally, during a subsequent session, explore the client's reaction to the prayer, encouraging both negative and positive experiences.

Meditation

Meditation has been described in many ways. It has been described as a means of relaxing the body-mind, as a way of training and strengthening awareness, as a method for centering and focusing the self, as well as a means of reducing high blood pressure and other cardiovascular conditions, relieving stress, bolstering self-esteem, and reducing the symptoms of anxiety and depression (Carrington, 1998). But it is first and foremost a spiritual practice.

There are two general types of meditation described in both the spiritual and research literatures. They are concentrative meditation and external awareness meditation. Concentrative meditation seeks to restrict awareness by focusing attention on a specific object of attention such as the breath, a candle flame, a mandala, or a mantra, i.e., a repeated word or sound. Transcendental Meditation or TM is probably the most common form of concentrative meditation practiced in the US. Unfortunately, TM and some other forms of Eastern meditation practice may be viewed negatively by some Christian clients (McLemore, 1982).

External awareness meditation, on the other hand, focuses on developing or "opening up" one's awareness of the external environment. This form of meditation focuses one's awareness on a sacred word, image, or feeling as they consciously occur on a moment-to-moment basis. This form of meditation is also referred to as insight or mindfulness meditation. Centering prayer is one of the more commonly practiced forms of mindfulness meditation and is acceptable to most Christians.

There is an extensive and evolving literature on the use of meditation as an adjunct to psychotherapy. Marlatt and Kristeller (1999) and Cortright (1997) ably review this literature and discuss the various benefits and limitations of prescribing meditation to clients or actually incorporating meditation techniques within therapy sessions. Marlatt and Kristeller (1999) offer a number of guidelines for incorporating meditation techniques in clinical practice, including indications and contraindications. The interested reader is referred to these references.

Because of its acceptability to a wide variety of clients, centering prayer will be highlighted in the remainder of this section. Clinicians looking for resources and references about other forms of meditation, including the concentrative form, might consult Lawrence LeShan's (1974/1999) classic book *How to Meditate* or Patricia Carrington's compendium (1998).

Centering prayer is a passive form of meditation in which a sacred word or an image is silently introduced when one becomes aware of thoughts (Keating, 1992, 1995). It is a method for centering or focusing on one's intention of consenting to God's presence. Since it is not a concentrative form of meditation, it is not an exercise in *attention* which cultivates the faculty of the mind. Rather, it is an exercise of *intention* which cultivates the faculty of the will. In short, it is a spiritual practice for developing habits conducive to responding to the inspirations of the Spirit.

Centering prayer has been described as an initial form of contemplative prayer. Contemplative prayer is a process of interior transformation, a relationship initiated by God and leading to divine union. One's way of perceiving reality changes in this process. A restructuring of consciousness takes place that empowers one to perceive, relate to, and respond with increasing sensitivity to the divine presence and action in, through, and beyond everything that exists.

Centering prayer is not an end in itself but a beginning. It is not done to produce spiritual consolation but rather to increase the experience and expression of charity, joy, peace, self-knowledge, compassion, inner freedom, and humility. To achieve this end, centering prayer must be done regularly, preferably for a minimum of 20 minutes twice a day. To maximize the process, additional spiritual practices are recommended throughout the day. These might include: repetition of a prayer sentence, unconditional acceptance of others, and releasing upsetting emotions as soon as they arise.

Centering prayer is a method designed to facilitate the development of other forms of meditation, particularly contemplative prayer. Centering prayer is an attempt to present the ancient teaching of this method in an updated form and to put a certain order and regularity into it. It is not meant to replace other kinds of prayer; it simply puts other kinds of prayer into a new and fuller perspective. During the time of prayer, the individual consents to God's presence and action within.

How is centering prayer practiced? The following method is described and outlined by Keating. It is recommended that centering prayer be practiced daily, preferably for a minimum of 20–30 minutes twice a day.

1. A sacred word is chosen as a symbol of one's intention to open and yield to God's presence and action within. It could be one of the names of God or a comforting word, i.e., presence, silence, peace, stillness, oneness.
2. Sit comfortably and with eyes closed, relax. Then silently introduce the sacred word as the symbol of one's consent to God's presence and action within.
3. When one becomes aware of any thought, feelings, memories, reflections, or images, return ever so gently to the sacred word. This is the only activity one needs to initiate after centering prayer has begun.
4. During the prayer time, avoid analyzing the experience or harboring expectations. Also avoid attempting to achieve any specific goal, i.e., having no thoughts, making the mind blank, feeling peaceful or consoled, repeating the sacred word continuously, or achieving a spiritual experience.
5. At the end of the prayer time, remain in silence with eyes closed for a short time. This allows the psyche a brief space to readjust to the external senses and a transfer of the atmosphere of interior silence into subsequent activities (Keating, 1992, 1995).

Mindfulness

Mindfulness, as noted in the section on "Meditation" was described as a basic of formal meditation practice, i.e., insight or mindfulness meditation.

Mindfulness meditation appears to have a number of positive health effects including increasing brain and immune function (Davidson et al., 2003). In this section, mindfulness will be described as spiritual intervention separate from the formal practice of meditation. As such it has considerably wider applicability since this form of mindfulness focuses on recognizing the sacred in all dimensions of creation in everyday life situations and circumstances. This form of mindfulness is about being fully mindful in the present moment. It is about being fully aware and attentive to the full range of experiences that exist here and now, moment to moment. Mindfulness permits an individual to experience things directly and immediately, seeing for themselves that which is present and true. It brings to bear one's whole personhood, one's entire, heart, mind, and attention to each moment.

Mindful awareness is based on an attitude of acceptance. Rather than judging one's experiences as good or bad, healthy or sick, worthy or unworthy, mindfulness accepts all thoughts, feelings, persons, objects, and events as exactly as they are in the present moment. Mindful acceptance of difficult thoughts or emotional states can transcend their negativity and defuse aggression. Rather than suppressing emotions or indulging them, a mindful attitude allows one to view them with acceptance (Marlatt & Kristeller, 1999).

A valuable clinical application of mindfulness is the capacity to adopt what Deikman (1982) called an "observing self," which carefully monitors one's thoughts and feelings as they occur in the present moment. The observing self is a "bridge" between meditation and cognitively oriented psychotherapy techniques such as self-monitoring and cognitive restructuring strategies. While these approaches have some clinical utility, it comes with a price. The price is that these strategies conceptualize the individual's thought patterns as "themselves." Instead of conceptualizing an individual's identity as a reflection of their thoughts, feelings, and actions, mindfulness views an individual's thoughts as "simply thinking" rather than as personal directives that must be yielded to or followed.

The clinical value of mindfulness is that the process of momentarily stepping back and objectively viewing one's compulsive behaviors and patterns permits individuals to dis-identify themselves from these patterns. That is, "we begin to see that those thoughts and feelings are not us. They come along accidentally. They are neither an organic part of us nor are we obliged to follow them" (Snelling, 1991, p. 55).

How can clients be advised to practice mindfulness in daily life activities? Four steps are involved in the practice of daily mindfulness. First, assist the client to pick a given daily activity, such as eating, walking, watching, or listening, and a given time frame. Second, practice being totally present to the activity for that time frame.

Third, observe and reflect on one's thoughts and feelings of this experience. Fourth, take these thoughts and feelings into the next activity. For example, a client wants to be totally present and mindful during a 20 minute walk in the park. The client is advised to gently look around and find something of beauty such as a child playing, a tree swaying in the wind, or a squirrel eating an acorn. Whatever it is, full attention and sensitivity is directed at it. If it is a tree, the different colors are noticed as is the swaying of branches, and the movements of individual leaves. At the same time, thoughts and feelings, such as appreciation of the pleasure that beauty brings, should be noted. Finally, these pleasant thoughts and feelings are extended to other activities. More specific instructions and guidelines for utilizing the spiritual practice of mindfulness with clients can be found in two books by Jon Kabat-Zinn (1990, 1994).

Forgiveness

Next to prayer, forgiveness may be the most commonly practiced spiritual practice. Forgiveness can be defined as "a motivational transformation that inclines people to inhibit relationship destructive responses and to behave constructively toward someone who has behaved destructively toward them" (McCullough et al., 1997, p. 321). Forgiveness is a capacity and a skill that must be practiced. It is also more than a change in feeling; it is a change in cognition as well as in action. Like many other spiritual practices, it should not be surprising that all spiritual traditions recognize their value and offer similar instructions for its practice (Worthington et al., 2005).

How does forgiveness occur? Among the various spiritual traditions there is agreement that five steps are required. First, personal responsibility must be acknowledged. Second, sincere regret must be expressed. Third, suitable reparation must be made, if at all possible. Fourth, a promise to stop the offending behavior must be made. And fifth, forgiveness must be requested. An apology that lacks personal, sincere, or suitable qualities, or one that is followed by repeated offenses, is considered inadequate and unacceptable (Sanderson & Linehan, 1999).

Interestingly, there has been an unprecedented interest in forgiveness among researchers and clinicians in the past five years. Besides numerous articles and research studies a national institute to promote research on forgiveness has been founded. Known as "A Campaign for Forgiveness Research," it has received extensive funding from the John Templeton Foundation and the Fetzer Institute, among other philanthropic organizations.

Coming out of these research endeavors have been a number of protocols and guidelines. Enright (1996), McCullough and Worthington (1995), and Worthington (1998) have developed forgiveness protocols. A few of these are reviewed here.

Protocol for Forgiveness

Worthington (1998) describes the Pyramid Model of Forgiveness. It is more comprehensive than the empathy-based model of McCullough and Worthington (1995). The steps of the protocol spell the word REACH. (1) R is for "recalling the hurt" as objectively as possible. (2) E stands for "empathize" which means attempting to feel the offender's feeling and identifying with the pressures on the offender. (3) A is for "altruistic gifts of forgiveness" and refers to the induction of a state of humility in the forgiver through the experience of guilt, gratitude, and gift. Although empathy is what mediates forgiveness, it is insufficient unless forgiveness is actually given. This step facilitates that process. (4) C stands for "commit to forgive." Being covert, forgiveness is subject to later doubts. To reduce the likelihood of a later denial, the individual should make a public commitment of the forgiveness beyond the offender. This usually takes the form of telling someone else, i.e., a therapist or friend, and writing a letter about the forgiveness, and not necessarily sending it but saving it for later reference. (5) H stands for "holding on to forgiveness" which refers to efforts to maintaining the act of forgiveness (Worthington et al., 2005). Worthington offers six strategies for maintenance that are similar to relapse prevention strategies.

Guidelines for Letting Go of Anger and Giving Forgiveness

1. Consider the pros and cons of forgiving the person vs. not forgiving the person, including the effects of anger on one's psychological and physical health.
2. Use cognitive refraining to understand the offending person's behavior.
3. If the offending person is sincerely sorry, practice validation of his or her distress.
4. Act opposite to angry feelings by engaging in conciliatory behavior.

(Sanderson & Linehan, 1999, p. 213)

Guidelines for Requesting Forgiveness

1. Give a sincere and validating apology.
2. If possible, repair the hurt.
3. Commit to not engaging in the injurious behavior again.
4. Follow through on the commitment by changing that behavior.
5. Engage in conciliatory acts.

(Sanderson & Linehan, 1999, p. 210)

Finally, what about reconciliation? Although related to forgiveness, reconciliation "is a restoration of a violated trust (which) is earned through mutually trustworthy behavior" (Worthington, 1998, p. 129). Whereas forgiveness occurs within an individual, reconciliation occurs within relationships. Reconciliation can and does occur without forgiveness as when the offender has died, moved or it is not safe to reconcile, i.e., the offender is a sexual abuser. Furthermore, forgiveness can occur without reconciliation, such as when individuals are forced to forgive, or the offense is considered insignificant or even too hurtful. Nevertheless, forgiveness can facilitate reconciliation (Worthington, 1998).

Written Spiritual Resources

Each of the major spiritual traditions in the East and the West view their sacred writings as a source of spiritual wisdom. There are few who discount the importance and value of sacred writings in individuals' lives. Throughout history, including the present time, the bible remains the all-time bestselling book in America. Albert Ellis (1993) acknowledges that the bible has been the single most significant self-help book in human history.

The purpose for reading sacred writings can differ by traditions and individual clients' needs. Some will study their tradition's sacred writings for intellectual reasons such as to increase their doctrinal understanding of their tradition's theology or philosophy, while others will read them to find comfort or insight about particular concerns. However, a major reason spiritual seekers read and reflect on sacred writings is to put themselves into the presence of the divine.

Sacred writings can be used for a variety of purposes in spiritually integrated psychotherapy. These include: (1) challenging and modifying dysfunctional beliefs; (2) reframing and understanding life and problems from a spiritual perspective; (3) clarifying and enriching understanding of the religious doctrines; and (4) seeking enlightenment, comfort, and guidance (Richards & Bergin, 2005).

Before implementing a spiritual intervention that uses sacred writings in some way, the clinician should carefully assess their clients' beliefs and attitudes about sacred writings, and only utilize such an intervention if it is compatible with clients' spiritual beliefs. Many spiritual seekers believe that sacred writings are a means for helping them communicate with God and know of his will for them. With clients with such beliefs, it would not be unreasonable for clinicians to encourage them to read and reflect on spiritual writings with the purpose of seeking divine insight into their problems and concerns. However, it should also be noted that such an intervention can be misused, as when clients have been advised by ministers or other spiritual leaders that engaging in prayer or sacred reading will be a magical cure for their problems. If clients do read the sacred writings seeking enlightenment about coping and overcoming their problems and do not realize those outcomes, clinicians "need to be prepared to process such 'failures' with their clients" (Richards & Bergin, 1997, p. 211).

When a clinician believes that a client's understanding of a specific sacred writing is erroneous, referral to an appropriate religious leader for doctrinal discussions and clarification is preferable to discussing the matter in therapy. When client and clinician share the same belief system, it may be appropriate for clinicians to invite clients to explore specific writings that would help clarify their misunderstandings, being careful not to assume the mantle of spiritual authority.

Lectio divina is a time-tested method of praying with Christian sacred writings, particularly scriptural texts. It has been practiced in many forms by monks and other spiritual seekers for over a thousand years. *Lectio divina* has been described as the "art of letting God speak to us through his inspired and inspiring Word" (Pennington, 1998, p. xi) and then responding, since it is a two-way communication. The method for practicing *lectio divina* is a relatively straightforward and simple three-step process. The first is to take the sacred text and call upon the Holy Spirit. The second is to listen—read or hear—to the Lord speaking through the text for about ten minutes. Then reflect on it and respond. Third, choose a word or phrase from the text and take it to reflect on for the rest of the day.

A related spiritual intervention is spiritual bibliotherapy (Pargament, 2007) which is the use of literature and films to foster spiritual growth. To utilize this intervention, it is necessary to first assess the impact of literature, movies, and videos on clients and the therapeutic process. Where client readings serve to maintain rigid defensiveness, prescribed reading may economically expand perspectives, correct misinformation, challenge misperceptions, and contribute to a sense of belonging and understanding. Clinicians need to have read the material they assign, follow up on their assignments, and process client understanding and/or interpretation of the material.

Spiritual Practices

Spiritual practices are rituals and other intentional activities that, with ongoing practice, can foster spiritual development (Plante, 2009). Indirectly, they can also foster psychological development. Psychotherapists who are sensitive to the spiritual dimension often utilize spiritual practices in their work with clients. Just as spiritual interventions can be utilized as homework or intersession activities, spiritual practices are often utilized as intersession activities. While some spiritual interventions may be similar or the same as spiritual practices, e.g., prayer and forgiveness, the main difference between practices and interventions is that specific spiritual practices may already be a part of the client's religious or spiritual tradition and even part of his or her daily repertoire.

The fact that psychotherapists are increasingly utilizing spiritual practices with clients is reflected in the growing number of articles, book chapters, and books on the subject. For example, APA Books has recently published a professional book on spiritual practices in psychotherapy (Plante, 2009). It describes the use of 13 such spiritual practices which include meditation, charitable works, ethical values, and approaching others with compassion. There are seven spiritual practices that are common across all the religious traditions (Walsh, 2000). In the Foreword to Walsh's book, the Dalai Lama notes that all seven spiritual practices are essential to developing and practicing the virtue of compassion. It should be pointed out that Walsh distinguishes spiritual practices from spiritual techniques and exercises. He uses the term "practice" to refer to the disciplines of developing crucial capacities of the heart and mind, while the terms "technique" and "exercise" refer to specific methods for achieving a spiritual practice.

For instance, the techniques of meditation and centering prayer are highly effective in achieving the practice of developing a peaceful mind. Some techniques can be useful in achieving two or more spiritual practices, i.e., meditation is also a useful method for cultivating wisdom and spiritual intelligence. Furthermore, these various practices are interrelated and follow a developmental sequence. For example, developing a peaceful mind, spiritual practice four, is facilitated by cultivating the first three spiritual practices. Each of these seven spiritual practices is described here. Two others, fasting and service to others, are also described.

Purifying Motivation

The purpose of this spiritual practice is to reduce one's cravings and redirect one's desires For most individuals, this means relinquishing attachments to beliefs, feelings, possessions, and the desire for possessions or experiences or vices that impede them in their quest for true happiness. In so doing persons become better able to transform their motivations by reducing cravings and find their soul's basic desire or higher motives, which Walsh indicates is a central goal of all spiritual practices. He notes that at the peak of higher motives is the pull to self-transcendence which is defined as "the desire to transcend our usual false, constricted identity, to awaken to the fulness or our being, and to recognize our true nature and our three relationship with the sacred" (Walsh, 2000, p. 53).

Walsh (2000) recommends two complementary exercises that are effective in reducing cravings and attachments. Craving is usually a word associated with the abnormal longing or desire to ingest a specific substance such as food, snacks, drugs, liquids, smoke, or solvents, i.e., glue sniffing. Cravings involve strong physiological and psychological longings for the object of desire. Attachment refers to abnormal longing or desire for certain objects, activities, relationships, belongings, etc. Generally speaking, attachment involves only psychological longings. The purpose of these exercises is twofold: (1) to reduce and eliminate that compelling and uncontrollable desire and its associated craving or attachment for things that do not bring true happiness, but instead enslave individuals to difficult-to-control and habit-forming activities or even harmful addictions; and (2) set the stage to redirect one's desires to those things which bring true happiness. Walsh notes that both of these exercises are recommended in nearly all the spiritual traditions.

Reducing Cravings

There are three simple and straightforward instructions for this spiritual practice. First, have the client choose a specific attachment and a specific date; throughout that entire designated day, they are to indulge and enjoy that attachment and its craving as fully as possible. For example, if a client craves candy, have them buy a few bags or boxes of their favorite kind and prescribe that they eat as many as possible. The second instruction is for the client to mindfully experience while indulging that craving. As with other spiritual practices, the greater the degree of awareness, the more likely the benefit. Mindfully indulging the particular attachment or craving in this manner should clearly illuminate its limitations. Have the client compare how the tenth piece tasted compared to the first. By the law of satiation, the taste and pleasure should be considerably lessened. Third, process this experience in the next therapy session.

Reducing Attachments

This exercise nicely complements "indulging an attachment." The directions are straightforward. First, have the client choose a specific craving or attachment and a designated time frame, i.e., 24 hours, during which the individual contracts to forgo the attachment. Establishing a realistic time frame for this practice is important, i.e., the decision to frustrate the addiction of cigarette smoking for one a low stress work day is more likely to lead to a positive outcome than a global decision to stop cold turkey forever. Second, have the client carefully attend to all sensations, thoughts, and feelings experienced during this period of frustrating the attachment.

Writing down these experiences during the course of the exercise is preferred. Third, encourage the client to reflect on the experience immediately after the exercise, and then in your next session. Many individuals expect to feel anxious and fearful about the deprivation of their attachment only to find that they were able to cope rather well (Walsh, 2000).

Cultivating Emotional Wisdom

Since emotions tend to rule a seeker's life, transforming one's emotions is an essential spiritual practice. The great religious and spiritual traditions indicate three ways in which this occurs: (1) by mastering and reducing toxic and painful affects such as fear and anger; (2) by fostering positive attitudes such as gratitude and generosity; and (3) by cultivating such positive emotions as love and compassion. The goal is neither indulgence nor repression of emotions, but rather appropriateness, balance, and equanimity, i.e., the capacity to experience the inevitability of the ups and downs of life without becoming victim to mood lability. Learning how to release, transform, and appropriately use emotions is the basis of emotional wisdom.

Living Ethically

Walsh contends that "ethical living is one of the most powerful yet misunderstood of all religious practices" (Walsh, 2000, p. 117). However, when it is correctly understood and practiced it is an essential means for spiritual growth, and without it progress is difficult. Unethical acts "create deep deposits of fear and guilt, paranoia and defensiveness... agitate and cloud our minds, making it difficult to achieve calm and clarity" (Walsh, 2000, p. 121). Unethical living is destructive to both self and others, and has immediate and long-term consequences, i.e., we become what we do and how we act. To live ethically involves practicing right speech and right action. It also involves dealing with the emotional residue remaining from past unethical behavior, i.e., making restitution and dealing with guilt feelings.

Developing a Peaceful Mind

As individuals are less compelled by craving and compulsive need, less troubled by painful affects, and less disturbed by ethical lapses, they become better disposed to concentrate and focus their attention resulting in a sense of calm and inner peace. "This peace is the doorway to the sacred, when the mind is focused and unperturbed, it opens effortlessly to its Source" (Walsh, 2000, p. 168). The challenge of mastering this sense of attention and inner peace is a slow process aided by such methods as meditation, contemplation, yoga, and continuous prayer. It also involves transforming the busyness of everyday life and, as much as possible, transforming daily activities into sacred rituals and moments of awareness. Needless to say, it requires the regular and habitual use of various meditative and focusing methods.

Recognizing the Sacred in All

Awakening sacred vision is another term for discerning or seeing the sacred in all persons, things, and situations. It is also referred to as underscoring the sacredness of all (Plante, 2024a). This is a principle focus of spiritual direction in the Christian tradition as it is in other religious systems that advocate formal spiritual direction or spiritual guidance. "What we perceive is selected by our desires, colored by our emotions, and fragmented by our wandering attention. What we see outside us reflects what is inside us. The result: we do not see ourselves or the world clearly or accurately" (Walsh, 2000, p. 175). Living mindlessly, like this, exacts a significant toll physically, emotionally, and spiritually, and unhealthy cravings, motives, and emotions are most likely to surface during these moments of mindlessness. The corrective is mindfulness. "To love mindfully is to bring greater awareness to each activity, to be more present in each moment, and to catch subtle experiences that all too often go unnoticed (Walsh, 2000, p. 177). Mindfulness not only enhances our awareness of relationships and the world within and around us, but also frees us from automaticity, the sense of being locked on mental autopilot. With regular practice of mindfulness, these "initial glimpses gradually become a recurrent vision, peak experiences extend into plateau experiences, altered states of consciousness became altered traits of consciousness..." (Walsh, 2000, p. 206).

Cultivating Wisdom and Spiritual Intelligence

Walsh defines wisdom as "deep understanding and practical skill in the central issues of life, especially existential and spiritual issues" (Walsh, 2000, p. 216). The crux of wisdom includes finding meaning and purpose in life, managing relationships and aloneness, living in the face of mystery, coping with illness, suffering, and death, and knowing and truly accepting oneself. The wise person is one who has developed deep insight into these issues and skills for dealing with them. Wisdom is a liberating spiritual capacity. It can dissolve one's delusions about self, just as it can reduce one's suffering and speed the awakening of one's heart and mind. Finally, by "loosening the bonds of egoism, wisdom also fosters concern and compassion for others" (Walsh, 2000, p. 248).

Engaging in the Services of Others

Altruism or helping others is viewed by the great religions as a central human desire, and recent psychological research seems to confirm that individuals are altruistic by nature. "So esteemed are generosity and service that some traditions regard them as the essence of spiritual life, the practice upon which all other practices converge... the supreme goal of enlightenment is sought, not for oneself alone, but to better serve and enlighten others" (Walsh, 2000, p. 256). Thus, as spiritual seekers become increasingly enlightened it is to be expected they will become sages, sages who dedicate themselves to the welfare of others and of life. Walsh notes that the first six spiritual practices lay the groundwork for generosity. Nevertheless, he describes several specific methods and techniques for cultivating generosity directly. This spiritual practice has the advantage of transforming all of one's daily activities into spiritual practices.

> With its help we need not change what we are doing so much as how and why we are doing it... With this approach, work and family, far from being distractions from spiritual life, become central to spiritual life, and each project or family activity can be transformed into a sacred act.
>
> (Walsh, 2000, p. 266)

Fasting

Fasting means abstaining from food or eating sparingly. There are various reasons for fasting: as a means of weight loss, detoxification of the body for medical purposes, or as a spiritual practice. Done as a spiritual practice, fasting is abstention from food for the purpose of purification of one's motivation. All the great spiritual traditions recognize its merits.

More than any of the other spiritual practices, fasting can surface and uncover not only the obvious but also the more subtle cravings and desires that control one's life. Food and other substances permit individuals to camouflage aspects of their inner life, which fasting quickly surfaces. Foster notes:

> If pride controls us, it will be revealed almost immediately. Anger, bitterness, jealousy, strife, fear—if they are within us, they will surface during fasting. At first we will rationalize that our anger is due to our hunger; then we will realize that we are angry because the spirit of anger is within us.
>
> (Foster, 1988, p. 55)

There are other benefits as well. Fasting can foster balance in life. In addition to revealing cravings, it uncovers how non-essentials have taken precedence in one's life. This is important self-knowledge that might not otherwise come to awareness. Fasting also helps increase awareness of the plight of others. In commenting on the social dimension of fasting, Walsh says: "I try to use each feeling of hunger to remind me of the many hungry people around the world. That way each hunger pang not only reduces the craving but also elicits concerns and compassion for the hungry" (Walsh, 2000, p. 50).

What instructions should clinicians give clients about fasting? The first is that, as with all the spiritual practices, a steady progression and moderation should be observed. That means beginning with a partial fast with a duration of no more than 24 hours. Fasting from lunch of one day to lunch of the next is the initial recommendation. This means that two meals are skipped, i.e., dinner and breakfast. Only water and fruit juices are taken during this period of fasting. This initial fast is recommended once a week for several weeks. The client should monitor both the physical and spiritual experience during each period of fasting. Keeping a journal or log can be valuable. Particular attention should be directed at the inner attitude of the heart. As individuals go about their regular duties during this time of fasting, they are advised to inwardly pray and to be aware of thoughts and spiritual promptings, and cultivate a "gentle receptiveness to divine breathings" (Foster, 1988, p. 57). This initial form of fasting is broken with a light meal of fresh fruits and vegetables.

After two or three weeks of this form, the client may be ready for a fast in which only water is consumed. After completing several fasts with a degree of spiritual success, move on to a 36-hour fast: three meals. Fasts lasting longer than this probably should be medically supervised.

Service

Service is another type of spiritual practice. Whether called "altruistic service" (Richards & Bergin, 2005), "true service" (Foster, 1988), or "awakened service" (Walsh, 2000), service involves doing something for others. Foster's distinction between "self-righteous service" and "true service" is worth noting. Self-righteous service is concerned with making impressive gains and achieving results; it usually requires the reward of recognition by others, picks and chooses whom to serve, and may be affected by moods and whims. True service, on the other hand, makes no distinction between big and small service, is contented with hiddenness, i.e., no recognition, and fosters such virtues as humility and gratitude (Foster, 1988).

Service can take numerous forms, such as providing food to the hungry or clothes and money to the poor, providing emotional support to those who are discouraged or grieving, visiting the sick, or volunteering in one's religious or spiritual community. The expected type and the frequency of service may vary in different spiritual traditions, nevertheless service is an extension of the Golden Rule, i.e., "Do unto others as you would have them do to you," or Silver Rule of Confucianism, i.e., "Do not do unto others what you would not have them do to you," and is central to all spiritual traditions (Walsh, 2000). It can be formal and planned or informal and spontaneous. In the later instance it might involve slowing down long enough to practice the service of listening in a context that one might rush on past while preoccupied with needs, obligations, or time constraints (Foster & Yanni, 1992). The results of a national survey of volunteers across the US found that individuals who helped others consistently reported better health than non-volunteers and that many believed that their health improved after beginning their volunteer service. Furthermore, the vast majority reported that service provided them with a sense of euphoria, greater calm and relaxation (Luks, 1993).

Not every client will benefit from the prescription for service involvement. Some clients may actually be overcommitted to service in their religious communities, perhaps even to the point of burnout. Instead, they may need help in reducing their service to the community so they can attend to their own needs and growth (Richards & Bergin, 2005).

How can service be prescribed as a spiritual practice? Advise clients to select an hour, a morning, or a day for the spiritual practice of service. Five steps are suggested: Begin by dedicating the time and what you will be doing during it. Second, look for ways to serve wherever you are, whoever you are with, and whatever you are doing. Third, try to accomplish the activity in a spirit of service. Fourth, be mindful of the intention to serve in such a way that you learn from each activity while releasing any attachments or bias you may have about those being served. And, finally, reflect on how this experience affects your spiritual journey (Foster & Yanni, 1992; Walsh, 2000).

Ignatian Spiritual Strategies

For centuries various religious and spiritual traditions have offered strategies for better living. While initially practiced by believers and spiritual seekers, these strategies have more recently been introduced into psychotherapy practice, for example from the Buddhist tradition. Mindfulness is a common therapeutic intervention that has been incorporated into both spiritually integrated psychotherapy and secular psychotherapy practice. Other strategies and practices such as yoga from the Hindu tradition have also found their way into psychotherapy practice. Others are also emerging.

One set of strategies is based on the Spiritual Exercises (Mottola, 1964) which was developed by Ignatius of Loyola from the Catholic tradition. The Spiritual Exercises are a compilation of meditations, prayers, and spiritual practices to assist individuals in deepening their relationship with God and increasing personal well-being and flourishing. From the Exercises, Plante has modified six Ignatian strategies for use in spiritually integrated psychotherapy and secular psychotherapy practice. These include seeing God or the sacred in all things; caring for the whole person; practicing discernment; using the Examen as an end-of-day review and reflection; managing conflict with accommodation, humility, and the expectation of goodness; and acting with civility, hospitality, solidarity, and mutuality. Extensive case material demonstrates the use of these strategies (Plante, 2024a). A companion workbook for clients is also available (Plante, 2024b).

Continuation of the Case of Maria

As noted earlier, the initial goal of psychotherapy would be reducing Maria's depressive symptoms, along with reducing stressors that triggered depression and fostered relational conflict at her job and with her husband. The first ten therapy sessions addressed this goal and involved three joint sessions with her husband.

The longer-term goal was to modify her obsessive-compulsive style first from the disordered range to the adequate range, and then to a more optimal level. The focus of this goal would be on processing psychological and spiritual aspects of her drivenness and perfectionism as they related to her parents and her God-image. Specifically, this meant attempting to transform her basic perfectionistic pattern so that she might become more comfortable with affects, less reliant on her thinking function, and thereby become more spontaneous and playful. Her core beliefs or schemas about being hardworking, good, and avoiding mistakes in order to feel accepted and worthwhile were examined and processed as well as her need to be in control and overly responsible. Interpretation and cognitive restructuring were the main therapeutic strategies employed to modify the affective, cognitive, and relational aspects of her obsessive style. The specific goal was to increase her capacity for emotional involvement. This is represented as "average" level of functioning on the obsessive developmental line. Whereas the ultimate goal of conventional psychotherapy with someone like Maria would be more adaptive functioning, the goal of this therapy focused also on personal and spiritual growth and well-being.

The general therapeutic strategy for fostering Maria's movement from the adequate to the optimal range involved both reconstructive strategies and developmental strategies. With regard to reconstructive strategies, an initial treatment focus is to help the client specify those limited number of situations where it is reasonable or necessary to be especially goal-directed and conscientious. For Maria this would mean 8:00 am to 3:00 pm Monday to Friday nine months a year for her teaching job, and perhaps another ten hours a week on household duties and volunteer activities in her church. It would also mean that she would practice becoming more spontaneous and less rigid in important and meaningful relationships in which she feels reasonably safe, such as with her husband, her boss, and her pastor.

With regard to the obsessive-compulsive personality style that characterized Maria, three ranges of functioning can be noted. In the disordered range, the individual is characterized by: perfectionism and feeling avoidance that interferes with task completion and relationships. The individual's thinking and attitudes are overly rigid, and they tend to be pessimistic and feeling avoidant. In the adequate range of functioning, individuals are less perfectionist but there is rigidity in tasks and relationships with some degree of emotional involvement and responsiveness. In the optimal range, individuals are conscientious, but not driven, and are more spontaneous. They are individuals who display a balance of personal integrity with generosity, hopefulness, and kindness.

A number of specific strategies were utilized in working toward this goal of psychological transformation. These included focusing on the theme of perfectionism in a fine-grained and focused manner. For example, Maria's self-view or self-schema was that "I am responsible if something goes wrong," while her underlying view of the world was that "Life is always unpredictable and expects too much. So, I must always work hard, be in control, right, and not make mistakes." Characteristic of the disordered range is the absolute conviction that they must be responsible in all situations and that life is always unpredictable and demanding, and she must do her best in all situations. At the average range, however, her schemas would be less absolute, which means that there are a limited number of circumstances and situations in which she could let down her guard with regard to conscientiousness, rigidity, and feeling avoidance. The rest of the time she was likely to be on her guard. In the optimal range, these convictions are still operative but are highly situation specific, meaning that Maria could be more spontaneous and playful in many situations.

Another useful strategy was to help her master some of her subtle and persistent perfectionistic patterns, i.e., those trigger events or thoughts that initiate a sequence of perfectionistic thinking—including self-righteousness—and behaviors and related responses. Maria's more subtle perfectionistic patterns involved safeguarding her money and being overly focused on time. In terms of money, her husband affectionately referred to her as "my little tightwad" because she shopped for bargains, used coupons, and looked for discounts. The transformation of this attitude of stinginess is generosity. In terms of time and deadlines, she reported setting her watch and clocks in her home and car 20 minutes ahead so that she would be "always be early for appointments," which was quite interesting since she was 5–10 minutes late for some therapy sessions. Her packed schedule allowed no time for traffic delays—which were not supposed to happen in a perfect world! Needless to say, Maria was extremely conscientious of time and resented others wasting her time. The transformation of this attitude of time conscientiousness is becoming more spontaneous and playful.

Similarly, being fun loving and carefree was very difficult for her. A common underlying maxim for her had been: "Do it and do it perfectly." The transformation of this attitude of duty-conscientiousness would involve achieving a degree of balance in her life among conscientiousness, spontaneity, and integrity. In addition, she tended to live in the future rather than in the present. Accordingly, the transformation of this pattern involves the prescription to live in the present moment.

Not surprisingly, experiential focusing exercises were initially quite difficult for Maria given her ruminative cognitive style. She was constantly processing new and old concerns, so much so that she became overwhelmed by this mental chatter and background noise which made it all but impossible to focus on the present. Because both centering meditation and focusing require a quieting or derailing of this ruminative style, she learned to utilize a simple breath prayer, saying "Yahweh" as she breathed in and out, to derail this mental chatter.

Characteristically, Maria was very demanding of herself as well as of others. She constantly monitored the actions of others against social norms as well as her own personal norms. Not surprisingly, few people matched up to her standards and she would judge others as being irresponsible. The actions of others triggered her moral indignation. Needless to say, she came across to others as judgmental and sometimes moralistic. In addition, her perfectionistic strivings were often subtle, and, unfortunately, were reinforced by the American culture of achievement and success. Maria began to recognize that they were inhibiting her personal and spiritual development and that changing them would be challenging. For Maria, the transformation of this overall attitude would be hopefulness and kindness.

Such a therapeutic direction with Maria was effective to the extent it focused on these fine-grained dimensions of perfectionism with the goal of becoming a conscientious but spontaneous person who could balance personal integrity with generosity, hopefulness, and kindness. In other words, instead of being compulsively perfectionistic in all matters, she might intentionally strive for a high level of excellence in a few select areas of her life but not in other areas.

For Maria modifying the triggers for her perfectionistic pattern was essential in transforming this dynamic. On closer examination we found that self-righteous thoughts such as: "That's not right" or "That's sloppy work" inevitably triggered her perfectionistic pattern. Subsequently, we worked together to find ways of neutralizing such triggers and replacing them with a non-righteous thought: "This moment is as perfect as it can be." Such a neutralizing thought became like a mantra that Maria repeated whenever she was in "high risk" situations that might possibly trigger her perfectionistic pattern. With a little experimenting Maria also found that if she hummed to herself while going into "high risk" situations she could also derail the perfectionistic pattern.

A few spiritual interventions were also incorporated into the treatment process. These included prayer, particularly centering prayer and meditation, spiritual journaling, and participation in a healthy religious community. This participation provided her social support as well as a corrective emotional experience regarding some of her harsh and perfectionistic religious beliefs and attitudes. Spiritual discussion of her life situation and stressors in light of their spiritual meaning was a part of the therapeutic process. Furthermore, cognitive restructuring of dysfunctional religious beliefs appeared to influence a shift in her image of God.

After about 18 months of therapy, Maria was somewhat less self-critical and driven and more patient and at peace with herself. Supplementing the in-session therapeutic focus, she regularly practiced the focusing strategy she had learned during a retreat. The result was that her moods were more stable and positive.

Concluding Note

The chapter has described several psychotherapeutic interventions, spiritual interventions, and spiritual practices that if appropriately implemented in spiritually integrated psychotherapy can result in positive clinical outcomes, including personal and spiritual growth. If, when, and how such interventions are utilized depends on the adequacy of the case conceptualization. A competent case conceptualization will specify whether such interventions are indicated, which ones to utilize, and how they will be implemented in the treatment process. This process of specifying and implementing interventions may seem somewhat daunting, however it is a competency that can be learned and mastered with supervised experience. The continuing case of Maria illustrates this process of specifying and implementing several psychotherapeutic and spiritual interventions as well as spiritual practices. Finally, it should be noted that there are other spiritually integrated approaches that have not be presented because of space limitations. These include a humanistic approach (Elkins, 2005), an interpersonal psychotherapy approach

(Miller, 2005), a transpersonal-integrative approach (Lukoff & Lu, 2005), a theistic integrative psychotherapy approach (Richards, 2005), and a spiritually integrated psychotherapy approach (Sperry, 2005; Sperry 2013; 2024).

References

American Psychiatric Association. (2022). *Diagnostic and statistical manual of mental disorders*, 5th ed., Text revision. American Psychiatric Association.

Aten, J., McMinn, M., & Worthington, E. (Eds.). (2011). *Spiritually integrated interventions for counseling and psychotherapy*. American Psychological Association.

Beck, A., Sokol, L., Clark, D. et al. (1979). *Cognitive therapy of depression*. Guilford Press.

Brigman, K. (1984). Churches helping families: A study of the effects of religion on families and how churches can help strengthen families. *Family Perspectives*, *18*, 77–84.

Brigman, K. (1992). Religion and family strengths: Implications for mental health professionals. *Topics in Family Psychology and Counseling*, *1*(1), 39–52.

Carrington, P. (1998). *The book of meditation*. Element Books.

Conn, W. (1998). *The desiring self*. Paulist.

Corbett, L., & Stein, M. (2005). Contemporary Jungian approaches spiritually integrated psychotherapy. In L. Sperry & E. Shafranske (Eds.), *Spiritually integrated psychotherapy* (pp. 51–73). American Psychological Association.

Cortright, B. (1997). *Psychotherapy and spirit: Theory and practice in transpersonal psychotherapy*. State University of New York Press.

Davidson, R., Kabat-Zinn, J., Schumacher, J., Rosenkranz, M., Muller, D., Santorelli, S., Urbanowski, F., Harrington, A., Bonus, K., & Sheridan, J. (2003). Alterations in brain and immune function produced by mindfulness meditation. *Psychosomatic Medicine*, *65*, 564–570.

Deikman, A. (1982). *The observing self*. Beacon Press.

Elkins, D. (2005). A humanistic approach to spiritually integrated psychotherapy. In L. Sperry & E. Shafranske (Eds.), *Spiritually integrated psychotherapy* (pp. 131–152). American Psychological Association.

Ellis, A. (1993). The advantages and disadvantages of self-help therapy materials. *Professional Psychology: Research and Practice*, *24*(3), 335–339. https://doi.org/10.1037/0735-7028.24.3.335

Enright, R. D. (1996). Counseling within the forgiveness triad: On forgiving, receiving forgiveness, and self-forgiveness. *Counseling and Values*, *40*(2), 107–126.

Foster, R. (1988). Celebration of discipline: *The path to spiritual growth* (Revised and expanded ed.). Harper San Francisco.

Foster, R., & Yanni, K. (1992). *Celebrating the disciplines: A journal workbook*. Harper San Francisco.

Gendlin, E. (1969). Focusing. *Psychotherapy: Theory, Research and Practice*, *6*, 4–15.

Gendlin, E. (1981). *Focusing*. Bantam.
Giblin, P. (1993). Marital conflict and marital spirituality. In R. Wicks and R. Parsons (Eds.), *Clinical handbook of pastoral counseling (Vol. 2)*. Paulist Press.
Hendrix, H. (1988). *Getting the love you want: A guide for couples*. Harper and Row.
Hinterkopf, E. (1994). Integrating spiritual experiences in counseling. *Counseling and Values*, *38*(3), 165–175.
Hinterkopf, E. (1998). *Integrating spirituality in counseling: A manual for using the experiential focusing method*. American Counseling Association.
Hinterkopf, E. (2005). The experiential focusing approach. In L. Sperry & E. Shafranske (Eds.), *Spiritually integrated psychotherapy* (pp. 207–234). American Psychological Association.
Hodge, R. (2007). A systematic review of the empirical literature on intercessory prayer. *Research on Social Work Practice*, *17*, 174–187.
Kabat-Zinn, J. (1990). *Wherever you go, there you are: Mindfulness meditation in everyday life*. Hypericon.
Kabat-Zinn, J. (1994). *Full catastrophe living: Using the wisdom of your body and mind to face stress, pain and illness*. Delta.
Keating, T. (1992). *Open mind, open heart*. Continuum.
Keating, T. (1995). *Intimacy with God*. Continuum.
Koenig, H. G., & Pritchett, J. (1998). Religion and psychotherapy. In H. G. Koenig (Ed.), *Handbook of religion and mental health* (pp. 323–336). Academic Press.
Koltko, M. E. (1990). How religious beliefs affect psychotherapy: The example of Mormonism. *Psychotherapy*, *27*, 132–141.
Lipp, M. R. (1986). *Respectful treatment: A practical handbook of patient care*. Elsevier.
LeShan, L. (1974/1999). *How to meditate: A guide to self-discovery*. Little, Brown.
Lukoff, D., & Lu, F. (2005). Transpersonal-integrative approach to spiritually integrated psychotherapy. In L. Sperry & E. Shafranske (Eds.), *Spiritually integrated psychotherapy* (pp. 177–206). American Psychological Association.
Luks, A. (1993). *The healing power of doing good*. Ballentine.
Marlatt, A., & Kristeller, J. (1999). Mindfulness and meditation. In W. Miller (Ed.), *Integrating spirituality into treatment: Resources for practitioners* (pp. 67–84). American Psychological Association.
May, G. (1988). *Addiction and grace*. Harper and Row.
McCullough, M., & Larson, D. (1999). Prayer. In W. Miller (Ed.), *Integrating spirituality into treatment: Resources for practitioners* (pp. 85–110). American Psychological Association.
McCullough, M. E., & Worthington, E. L., Jr. (1995). Promoting forgiveness: The comparison of two brief psychoeducational interventions with a waiting-list control. *Counseling and Values*, *40*, 55–68.
McCullough, M. E., Worthington Jr, E. L., & Rachal, K. C. (1997). Interpersonal forgiving in close relationships. *Journal of Personality and Social Psychology*, *73*(2), 321–336.
McLemore, C. (1982). *The scandal of psychotherapy*. Tyndale House.
Meadow, M. J., & Kahoe, R. D. (1984). *Psychology of religion: Religion in individual lives*. Harper & Row.

Miller, L. (2005). Interpersonal psychotherapy from a spiritual perspective. In L. Sperry & E. Shafranske (Eds.), *Spiritually integrated psychotherapy* (pp. 153–176). American Psychological Association.

Mottola, A. (1964). *The spiritual exercises of St. Ignatius: Saint Ignatius' profound precepts of mystical theology*. Doubleday.

Paloma, M. M., & Pendleton, B. F. (1989). Exploring types of prayer and quality of life: A research note. *Review of Religious Research*, *31*, 46–53.

Pargament, K. I. (2007). *Spiritually integrated psychotherapy: Understanding and addressing the sacred*. Guilford Press.

Pennington, B. (1998). *Lectio divina: Renewing the ancient practice of praying the scriptures*. Crossroads.

Plante, T. (2009). *Spiritual practices in psychotherapy: Thirteen tools for enhancing psychological health*. American Psychological Association.

Plante, T. G. (2024a). *Spiritually informed therapy: Wisdom and evidence based strategies that work*. Cognella.

Plante, T. G. (2024b). *Living better with spiritually based strategies that work: Workbook for spiritually informed therapy*. Cognella.

Propst, L. (1988). *Psychotherapy in a religious framework: Spirituality in the emotional healing process*. Human Sciences Press.

Propst, L. (1993). Defusing the powers with Jesus as a model of empowerment: Treating the avoidant personality. *Journal of Pastoral Care*, *47*, 230–238.

Propst, L. (1996). Cognitive-behavioral therapy and the religious person. In E. Shafranske (Ed.), *Religion and the clinical practice of psychology* (pp. 391–408). American Psychological Association.

Propst, L., Ostrom, R., Watkins, P., Dean, T., & Mashburn, D. (1992). Comparative efficacy of religious and non-religious cognitive-behavioral therapy for the treatment of clinical depression in religious individuals. *Journal of Consulting and Clinical Psychology*, *60*, 94–103.

Pruyser, P. (1977). The seamy side of current religious beliefs. *Bulletin of the Messenger Clinic*, *41*, 329–340.

Richards, P. S. (2005). Theistic integrative psychotherapy. In L. Sperry & E. Shafranske (Eds.), *Spiritually integrated psychotherapy* (pp. 259–286). American Psychological Association.

Richards, P. S., & Bergin, A. (1997). *A spiritual strategy for counseling and psychotherapy*. American Psychological Association.

Richards, P. S., & Bergin, A. E. (2005). *A spiritual strategy for counseling and psychotherapy* (2nd ed.). American Psychological Association.

Rizzuto, A. (1979). *The birth of the living God: A psychoanalytic study*. University of Chicago Press.

Rizzuto, A. (1989). Ana-Marie Rizzuto of God representation. *Psychologists Interested in Religious Issues Newsletter*, *14*(2), 1–4.

Rizzuto, A. (1991). Religious development: A psychoanalytic point of view. *New Directions for Child Development*, *52*(Special Issue: Religious Development in Childhood and Adolescence), 47–60.

Rizzuto, A. (1996). Psychoanalytic treatment and the religious person. In E. Shafranske (Ed.), *Religion and the clinical practice of psychology* (pp. 409–432). American Psychological Association.

Rizzuto, A. (2005). Psychoanalytic considerations about spiritually integrated psychotherapy. In L. Sperry & E. Shafranske (Eds.), *Spiritually integrated psychotherapy* (pp. 31–50). American Psychological Association.

Sanderson, C., & Linehan, M. (1999). Acceptance and forgiveness. In W. Miller (Ed.), *Integrating spirituality into treatment: Resources for practitioners* (pp. 199–216). American Psychological Association.

Shafranske, E. (2005). A psychoanalytic approach to spiritually integrated psychotherapy. In L. Sperry & E. Shafranske (Eds.), *Spiritually integrated psychotherapy* (pp. 105–130). American Psychological Association.

Snelling, J. (1991). *The Buddhist handbook*. Inner Traditions.

Sperry, L. (2005). Integrative spiritually integrated psychotherapy. In L. Sperry & E. Shafranske (Eds.), *Spiritually integrated psychotherapy* (pp. 307–330). American Psychological Association.

Sperry, L. (2013). Distinctive approaches to religion and spirituality: Pastoral counseling, spiritual direction, and spiritually integrated psychotherapy. In K. I. Pargament, A. Mahoney, & E. P. Shafranske (Eds.), *APA handbook of psychology, religion, and spirituality (Vol. 2): An applied psychology of religion and spirituality* (pp. 223–238). American Psychological Association. https://doi.org/10.1037/14046-011

Sperry, L. (2024). Spiritually integrative psychotherapy: An impending paradigm shift in theory and practice. In L. Miller (Ed.), *The Oxford handbook of psychology and spirituality* (2nd ed., pp. 314–332). Oxford University Press.

Sperry, L. (2022). *Highly effective therapy: Effecting deep change in counseling and psychotherapy*. (2nd ed.). Routledge.

Sperry, L., & Giblin, P. (1996). Marital and family therapy with religious persons. In E. Shafranske (Ed.), *Religion and the clinical practice of psychology* (pp. 511–532). American Psychological Association.

Sperry, L., Hoffman, L., Cox, R., & Cox, B. (2007). Spirituality in achieving physical and psychological health and well-being. In L. L'Abate (Ed.), *Handbook of low-cost interventions to promote physical and mental health* (pp. 435–452). Springer-Verlag.

Tan, S.-Y., & Johnson, W. B. (2005). Spiritually integrated cognitive-behavioral therapy. In L. Sperry & E. Shafranske (Eds.), *Spiritually integrated psychotherapy* (pp. 77–104). American Psychological Association.

Walsh, R. (2000). *Essential spirituality: The 7 central practices to awaken heart and mind*. Turner Publishing Company.

Watchell, P. (1983). *The poverty of affluence*. Free Press.

Worthington, E. (1998). An empathy-humility-commitment model of forgiveness applied within family dyads. *Journal of Family Therapy*, *20*(1), 59–76.

Worthington, E., Mazzeo, S., & Canter, D. (2005). A forgiveness-promoting approach: Helping clients REACH forgiveness through using a longer model that teaches reconciliation. In L. Sperry & E. Shafranske (Eds.), *Spiritually integrated psychotherapy* (pp. 235–258). American Psychological Association.

Chapter 9

Termination and Evaluation

Termination is often neglected in conventional psychotherapy training. In fact, there is a very limited research and professional literature in this area. There is even less literature on termination in spiritually integrated psychotherapy. This chapter describes the process of termination as well as termination issues that arise when spiritual issues have been a focus of therapy. It also describes the importance of evaluation of treatment outcomes, both overall evaluation of outcomes and session-by-session monitoring of therapeutic progress. The chapter begins with treatment evaluation and then considers the termination process in both conventional and spiritually integrated psychotherapy. Finally, the continuing case of Maria illustrates a number of key points regarding evaluation and termination in spiritually integrated psychotherapy.

Treatment Evaluation

In this age of accountability, the expectation is that therapists will not only provide effective treatment but be able to demonstrate that the treatment is effective. This expectation has given rise to two different perspectives on how to achieve such evidence. One perspective emphasizes "evidence-based practice" which is based on the premise that specific treatment interventions must have been empirically demonstrated to be effective with specific psychological problems. The other perspective emphasizes "practice-based evidence" which is based on the premise that effectiveness is more a function of therapist–client collaboration than of specific treatment interventions (Sperry et al., 1996). This second perspective places a premium on assessing specific treatment processes and outcome measures and requires therapists to monitor treatment processes and outcomes. This chapter emphasizes the second perspective.

Until recently, the focus of research and clinical practice was on the final or overall assessment of treatment outcomes. More recently, the focus has shifted to ongoing assessment, i.e., session-by-session monitoring of

DOI: 10.4324/9781003425991-10

therapeutic progress. Arguably, both forms of assessment are necessary and clinically valuable.

When it comes to evaluating clients' response to treatment, therapists are not particularly good at predicting the effectiveness of their client–therapist relationship nor of treatment outcomes. Rather, research reveals that client ratings of the client–therapist alliance are more accurate and a better predictor of client involvement in treatment than therapist ratings. Research also shows that a client's subjective experience of change early in the treatment process is the best predictor of treatment success compared to all other measures and predictors (Orlinsky et al., 2003). So, how can therapists know and evaluate a client's response to treatment? The answer is simple: monitor treatment outcomes.

The basic premise of treatment outcome research is that therapists need feedback. Research consistently suggests that when therapists receive feedback on their work with clients, their therapeutic relationships and treatment effectiveness increases significantly. When both therapist and client know how the client rates the therapeutic relationship and treatment outcomes, three things can be predicted: (1) an effective therapeutic relationship is more likely to be developed and maintained; (2) the client will stay in treatment; and (3) positive treatment outcomes result. Thus, ongoing monitoring of the treatment process and outcomes appears to be essential for effective therapy (Miller et al., 2006).

Routine Outcome Monitoring

In the past, it was assumed that the use of pre-therapy and post-therapy outcome measures were a valuable clinical strategy. However, recent research has demonstrated serious limitations of this strategy. Essentially, when clients who have been responding poorly are identified only at the end of treatment, it is too late to modify treatment that could result in a more favorable outcome (Lambert, 2017). This is the primary reason for continually monitoring the client treatment response during the course of therapy and for providing therapists with feedback so they can refocus it (Carlier & van Eeden, 2017). This continuous monitoring is called routine outcome monitoring (ROM).

Clients who begin therapy do not inevitably have a positive outcome. Despite evidence that psychotherapy has a positive impact, 30% of clients fail to respond during clinical trials, and upward of 65% of those in routine care leave treatment without a measurable benefit. Without ROM, therapists tend to overestimate client progress and are particularly poor at identifying patients at risk of a negative outcome (Lambert, 2017). For clients who are not progressing in therapy, it is the therapist's utilization of ROM that spells the difference between positive outcomes and limited outcomes or premature termination (Boswell, 2015). ROM can be an important quality tool for measuring the clinical response of clients during the course of therapy and for optimizing clinical decisions based on outcomes. In a large meta-analysis of 24 studies, two-thirds of therapists that used ROM were found to be superior to treatment-as-usual offered by the same therapists. Not surprisingly, ROM usage was found to be particularly effective in the monitoring of clients who were not doing well in therapy (Lambert et al., 2018).

It should be noted that if ROM data is collected but not incorporated in optimizing treatment it is useless. In other words, there is little clinical value in collecting ROM data unless it leads to feedback-informed therapy (van Sonsbeek et al., 2014). Finally, it is becoming increasingly evident that ROM represents a major revolution in the practice of psychotherapy (Miller et al., 2015).

Treatment Outcomes Measures

Several psychometrically sound outcome measures are available. While some are commonly used in conventional psychotherapy they can be used in spiritually integrated psychotherapy practice as well. Other measures are primarily used in spiritually integrated psychotherapy.

OQ-45.2

The OQ-45.2 (Lambert et al., 2004) is the current version of the OQ-45. It is a brief 45-item self-report outcome and tracking instrument that is designed for repeated measurement of client progress through the course of therapy and following termination. It measures client functioning in three domains: symptom distress; interpersonal functioning; and social role. Functional level and change over time can be assessed which allows treatment to be modified based on changes noted. The OQ-45.2 also contains risk assessment items for suicide potential, substance abuse, and potential violence at work. It has been translated into more than ten languages and is based on normative data and has adequate validity and reliability. It can be administered and scored in either electronic or paper format.

Session Rating Scale

The Session Rating Scale (SRS) (Duncan et al., 2003) is a short and easy-to-administer measure of therapeutic alliance which consists of four items. The instructions are simple and straightforward. The client is given a sheet of paper on which four horizontal lines 10 cm long are printed. On the first line the client rates how well understood and respected he or she felt in the just-completed therapy session. On the second line the client rates how much the client and therapist worked on what he or she wanted to talk about. On the third the client rates how good a "fit" the therapy approach was for him or her. On the third line the client rates his or her social and work life. On the fourth the client rates how satisfied he or she felt about the session. The scale is completed by the client immediately after the session has ended. Use of the SRS is free of charge to individual mental health practitioners by a license agreement found at www.talkingcure.com.

Outcomes Rating Scale

The Outcomes Rating Scale (ORS) (Miller & Duncan, 2000) is a short and easy-to-administer outcomes measure consisting of four items. The instructions are simple and straightforward. The client is given a sheet of paper on which four horizontal lines 10 cm long are printed. The client is asked to mark with a pen stroke, somewhere along each horizontal line, how things went in the past week. On the first line the client indicates how he or she had felt. On the second line the client rates his or her relationships. On the third line the client rates his or her social and work life. On the fourth the client rates his or her well-being. The scale is typically completed by the client immediately before the session begins, although it may be administered after the first meeting. Use of the ORS is free of charge to individual mental health practitioners by a license agreement found at www.talkingcure.com.

Clinical Outcomes in Routine Evaluation

Clinical Outcomes in Routine Evaluation (CORE) is an easy-to-use assessment measure for common presentations of psychological distress. It was developed during the late 1990s and early 2000s and psychometric properties were published by Barkham and associates (2013). It is intended to both screen and track treatment progress as a ROM. The CORE-10 is a ten-item measure for assessing anxiety, depression, trauma, physical problems, functioning, and risk to self. It has six high-intensity/severity and four low-intensity/severity items. It has been translated into 21 languages (Zeldovich & Alexandrowicz, 2019). CORE-10 is available to clinicians without cost, as is the manual at: www.corc.uk.net/media/2311/perinatal-roms-manual-a4-final-print-december-2019.pdf.

Spiritual Outcomes Measures

In this era of accountability, clinicians are expected to demonstrate the effectiveness of the treatment they provide. As a result, monitoring treatment progress with clinical outcome measures is increasingly expected, including for those who practice spiritually integrated psychotherapy (Hill & Pargament, 2003). Unfortunately, this expectation is routinely neglected by clinicians, in part because of the perceived lack of empirically valid and clinically useful spiritual outcome measures (Hall et al., 1994; Hill & Pargament, 2003). Actually, there are some measures that are suitable for assessing spiritual outcomes. Fortunately, there are two well-regarded spiritual measures that have value in ROM. They are the Spiritual Well-Being Scale and the Clinically Adaptive Multidimensional Outcome Survey.

Spiritual Well-Being Scale

The Spiritual Well-Being Scale (SWB) is a global measure of an individual's perception of spiritual well-being (Ellison, 1983). It is a 20-item self-report scale that assesses well-being in two subscales: relationship to God and relationship to others and the world. Odd-numbered items assess well-being in relationship to God and comprise the Religious Wellbeing Scale (RWB), while even numbered items assess well-being in relationship to other persons and the world, comprising the Existential Wellbeing Scale (EWB). Responses are reported on a six-point Likert scale from strongly agree to strongly disagree, with no midpoint.

Research indicates that this scale has high levels of internal consistency with alpha coefficients that range from .89 to .94 for the overall SWBS, .82 to .94 for RWB, and .78 to .86 for EWB (Paloutzian & Ellison, 2021) as well as construct validity. It is a good measure of general spiritual changes and correlates positively with the importance of religion, frequency of church attendance, spiritual maturity, and other indicators of spiritual health (Bufford et al., 1991). The scale and the manual are available free as a download. The SWB has been used or highlighted in more than 300 research articles and book chapters and 200 doctoral dissertations and master's theses, and has been translated into 20 languages with versions for use with children and adolescents. It can be administered as a paper-pencil instrument or on a website. While first developed as an initial assessment it is well suited for ongoing monitoring of the treatment process.

Clinically Adaptive Multidimensional Outcome Survey

The Clinically Adaptive Multidimensional Outcome Survey (CAMOS) is a 42-item outcome measure for assessing six dimensions: therapy expectations, relationship distress, psychological distress, physical health distress, spiritual distress, and work/school distress (Sanders et al., 2018). Items are scored on a six-point scale in which 1 = never and 6 = always. CAMOS is designed to be used in the initial intake sessions as a broad, multidimensional assessment. CA-COM is the 25-item short form of CAMOS for use as a ROM in assessing treatment progress. It assesses five dimensions: psychological distress, spiritual distress, relationship distress, physical health distress, and therapy progress (Sanders, 2015). Robust reliability and validity are reported for both versions. CAMOS and CA-COM were integral to the Bridges studies (Sanders et al., 2018).

Subsequent studies have focused on the spiritual distress and psychological distress subscales of the CAMOS (Currier et al., 2024). The Spiritual Distress scale includes four items assessing ways that clients might have struggled with their R/S over the past week (example items include "I felt concerned about my religious or spiritual life," "I felt distant in my relationship with God or Higher Power," "I felt guilt and regrets over mistakes that were inconsistent with my religious beliefs"). The Psychological Distress scale includes seven items assessing emotionally troubling symptoms of depression, anxiety, and posttraumatic stress over the past week (example items include "I felt sad or depressed," "I felt worried, agitated, or tense," "I had images or thoughts I couldn't get out of my head"). Sanders et al. (2018) recommend a cutoff score of 21 or higher on the Psychological Distress scale to identify clients with a probable need for treatment.

Other Spiritual Instruments

Six other instruments may prove to be useful measures of spiritual outcome measures. This includes the Index of Core Spiritual Experiences (ICSE; Kass et al., 1991), the Spiritual Transcendence Scale (STS; Piedmont, 1999), the Spiritual Assessment Inventory (SAI; Hall & Edwards, 1996), and the Spiritual Health Inventory (SHI; Veach & Chappel, 1992). The Religious Commitment Inventory (RCI-10; Worthington et al., 2003) is a ten-item instrument that measures the adherence of a person to his or her spiritual values, beliefs, and practices in daily life. The Theistic Spiritual Outcome Survey (TSOS; Richards et al., 2005) is a 17-item outcome instrument designed for serial (weekly) monitoring of therapy sessions that can be administered weekly in therapy to assess clients' perceptions of their spirituality. Three factors or subscales are noted: love of God, love of others, and love of self. Initial psychometric indicators of reliability and validity are promising, with alphas ranging from. 80 to .93 for the three factors and medium to large positive correlations with religious measures (Kapuscinski & Masters, 2010).

Termination

Termination is the last phase of treatment and represents both an event and a process. As an event, termination means client–therapist contact ends, and as a process it means that the client's level of responsibility increases as the nature of the client–therapist relationship changes. Facilitating the process of terminating and preparing the client for it is the therapist's primary focus in the last phase of treatment. Preparing for termination is a time for clients to express their thoughts and feelings about what the therapeutic process and the therapist has meant to them, as well as an opportunity to review their progress in achieving treatment goals. It is also a time to plan for maintaining treatment gains and to anticipate the inevitable lapses and setbacks that may ensue. Finally, preparing for termination is a time to reflect on what remaining therapeutic tasks clients might work on in the future, and what additional therapeutic contact with the therapist or other treatment might be indicated.

Too often the clinical competency of preparing for termination has been neglected or downplayed in training programs and in textbooks. The situation has not improved appreciably in the past 30 years since this criticism was leveled at training programs: "not only are criteria and techniques for termination not taught and discussed, but termination as a valuable therapeutic opportunity is undoubtedly neglected" (Weddington & Cavenar, 1979, p. 1303). An indicator of this neglect is high dropout rates from psychotherapy. Premature termination rates are approximately 50% (Clarkin & Levy, 2003; Wierzbicki & Perarik, 1993), but appear to be much higher in training programs. A recent study found that the rate of premature termination observed in a training clinic was 77% (Callahan et al., 2009)!

Nevertheless, effective and competent psychotherapy practice assumes the capacity to deal effectively with termination issues. Accordingly, this competency is addressed in this chapter as well as a related competency: maintaining treatment gains. This section begins with a discussion of maintaining treatment gains and relapse prevention before discussing the competency of termination. Then it describes termination considerations in spiritually integrated psychotherapy.

Maintaining Treatment Gains

Making progress in therapy usually consists of some combination of gaining insights, being less symptomatic, feeling better, thinking more positively, or acting in more adaptive ways. There is no guarantee that such progress or treatment gains will be maintained. Progress in therapy can be additive but just as often regressions occur. The client's challenge is to stay on course and continue to practice and apply the skills and strategies learned in the course of therapy. Such ongoing efforts are essential for maintaining gains (therapeutic change). Relapse prevention and self-therapy are important components of the early and middle phases of therapy and are also critical components of the final phase of therapy when preparing the client for termination.

CBT, in particular, has been shown to help clients to make lasting changes: when clients have a plan and the skills to prevent relapse, and are motivated and have a plan for continued growth, the treatment effect is likely to be maintained and even increased (Gloaguen et al., 1998). In other words, relapse prevention is a key factor in maintaining treatment gains.

Preventing Relapse

Relapse prevention is a self-control strategy for assisting clients on how to anticipate and cope with the problem of relapse or recurrence of symptoms or problematic behaviors (Daley, 1989). While it was initially developed as a treatment adjunct with addictive behaviors (Marlatt & Gordon, 1985), it has been applied to smoking cessation, pain control, weight management, sleep disorders, as well as to most psychiatric disorders (Sperry et al., 2003). In short, relapse prevention is a strategy for anticipating and reducing the likelihood of relapse.

Relapse prevention planning (Marlatt & Gordon, 1985) begins with the assessment of a client's likely interpersonal, intrapersonal, environmental, and physiological risks for relapse and specific stressors and situations that may precipitate it. Once these potential triggers and high-risk situations are identified, cognitive and behavioral techniques are implemented that incorporate both specific interventions to prevent or manage them if they do occur. It also involves a discussion of more global strategies to address lifestyle balance, craving, and cognitive distortions that could expose the client to high-risk situations where relapse is most likely. Such a relapse plan is likely to increase the client's sense of self-efficacy and effectiveness in maintaining treatment gains (Carroll, 1996).

Self-Therapy

It is commonly said that the ultimate goal of treatment is to assist clients in becoming their own therapists. But how do clients become their own therapists? Beck (1995) addresses this question and suggests how clients can develop what she calls a "self-therapy" program. In self-therapy clients take responsibility for conducting their own therapy much like their sessions with a cognitive behavior therapist. That is, they set an agenda, review past homework, address a particular problem, process it, decide on new homework, and schedule their next self-therapy session. Becoming one's own therapist begins during the last phase of therapy. Here clients are urged to apply self-therapy as problems or issues arise, and then discuss their efforts with their therapist in the next scheduled session. Thus, after termination a client will already have the experience of doing self-therapy and be able to handle most problems, relapses, or setbacks themselves. "If she is unsuccessful, at least she has had an opportunity to use her skills once more. If she does need another appointment, the therapist can help the patient discover what got in the way of her handling the setback or problem independently, and they can plan what the patient can do differently in the future" (Beck, 1995, p. 278).

Preparing for Termination

While preparing a client for termination is usually considered a key task of the final phase of therapy, some approaches such as Cognitive Therapy consider it a task that begins much earlier (Beck, 1995). As noted previously, the treatment formulation component of the case conceptualization serves as a guide to both specifying treatment outcomes and anticipating obstacles and challenges to achieving those outcomes. More specifically, it assists the therapist in anticipating particular difficulties a specific client may experience with termination. Thus, the therapist will not be surprised when a particular client experiences difficulty with termination because of a history of losses or a pattern of clinging or dependency on others (Cucciare & O'Donohue, 2008).

Indicators of Readiness for Termination

Different therapeutic approaches describe theory-specific criteria for determining when termination is indicated. However, there are also some general indicators common to these various approaches which are useful in assessing a client's readiness for termination from treatment. These include:

1. The client's presenting problem is essentially resolved, or symptoms are reduced or alleviated.
2. The client has developed sufficient insight to understand the problem and patterns that lead to treatment.
3. The client's coping skills are sufficiently improved for dealing with life circumstances.
4. The client has more capacity to plan and work productively.

(Based on Heaton, 1998)

During the course of a planned termination several activities and processes are commonly observed. These include: "a retrospective look at how therapy has proceeded, sharpening of client's future plans for life without the therapist, discussion of possible return appointments, and a statement of appreciation by both client and therapist" (Good & Beitman, 2006).

The therapist does well to begin the process by asking the client to recount the most important changes the client has made in the course of treatment. "Reviewing progress with patients may enable them to more clearly see the significance of their treatment gains, potentially motivating them to continue maintaining gains and building on the progress that they have made during treatment (Dobson & Haubert, 2008, p. 314). A corollary is to discuss the skills they have learned in therapy.

Termination Considerations in Spiritually Integrated Psychotherapy

In short, the objectives of termination in conventional psychotherapy are to provide clients with a healthy ending to therapy and the therapeutic relationship, to review clients' progress and growth, and to prepare clients for future challenges. The same objectives also hold for spiritually integrated psychotherapy. The following sections describe these objectives and challenges which arise in the termination process with spiritually sensitive clients.

Preparing for Termination

When therapy has been sensitive to their spiritual concerns, clients usually want the spiritual dimension included in preparing for termination to experience a sense of closure. Preparing for termination begins with a review of client progress. A useful starting point for this review is to pose the question: what role has spirituality played in the treatment process? Further reflection can be facilitated with related questions (adapted from O'Grady & Richards, 2009) such as:

- What are some of the ways my spirituality has become more personally meaningful?
- How has my image of God changed?
- What role has spirituality played in my relationship with my therapist?
- How has my faith served as a spiritual resource?
- How has including spirituality in therapy affected my healing and growth?
- How has my style of spiritual coping changed?

Discussion of these considerations can provide the client with a sense of peace in ending the therapeutic relationship as well as a measure of confidence in facing future challenges.

Client Difficulty with Termination

The termination phase provides opportunities for spiritually sensitive therapists to address spiritual issues and concerns (Aten et al., 2009). Clients may have difficulty ending relationships because they lack healthy models for interpersonal relations. Their developmental histories may include experiences of unexpected loss, abandonment, or abuse and neglect by parents or caretakers. Similarly, their spiritual history may include feelings of being unloved or abandoned by God. Whatever the case, clients may rely on their spiritual beliefs, practices, and past experiences with spiritual communities to make sense of therapeutic relationships that are ending. Since most spiritual traditions have rituals at the end of spiritual services (e.g., benedictions at worship services, weddings, and funerals), it is not surprising that clients draw on these experiences because of their familiarity. Whether consciously or unconsciously, they may draw on these models of closure. In fact, clients who have such spiritual beliefs and experiences for interpreting and facilitating endings in other situations may expect the same in the termination phase of psychotherapy "even if spirituality has not been explicitly addressed in the earlier stages of treatment" (Aten et al., 2009, p. 220).

Therapist Difficulty with Termination

Termination can also be a concern for therapists, particularly if it brings up unresolved or painful experiences of past losses. Accordingly, termination may result in strong emotions associated with spiritual strain. Such spiritual strain may occur if an individual feels abandoned by God or blames God because of a loss or some other negative event (Exline & Rose, 2005). Or a therapist may experience feelings of apprehension or doubt about their capacity to effectively terminate treatment because of previous negative experiences with the termination process. Whatever the circumstances, therapist self-reflection when approaching termination is recommended (Aten et al., 2009).

Spiritual Community Involvement

Client involvement in a spiritual community can facilitate the termination process. In the termination phase, clients who are deeply spiritual may

> make the transition easier if they become more integrated into a spiritual community. Hence, therapists may consider encouraging clients to continue participation in healthy spiritual communities... Depending on the client's presenting issue and expressed desire for involvement in spiritual communities, such involvement can ease the process of termination.
>
> (Aten et al., 2009, p. 230)

Boundary Issues

Another key strategy for facilitating the termination process is to maintain therapeutic boundaries. Maintaining such boundaries fosters the client's ongoing trust of the therapist and provides the client a firm relational foundation from which to end therapy successfully. This can be somewhat problematic if therapists and former clients later have contact in worship services or other spiritual community events (Aten et al., 2009). Depending on the size of the geographical area such contact is possible or even inevitable. Anticipating such contact, the therapist would do well to initiate a discussion to prepare the client for how such interactions outside of therapy will be handled. This presumes that the therapist is not involved in the same spiritual community as the client in the early stages of treatment. If they are, at least two options are available. One option is to consider referral, assuming other therapists are available (Aten et al., 2009). Another option is to explain the importance of maintaining the therapeutic boundary and then to discuss how to deal with such situations.

Engaging in multiple relationships can create boundary problems for some clients because of their spiritual backgrounds. For example, clergy commonly provide pastoral or spiritual guidance to parishioners as well as officiating at religious services.

> [Such] clients who have received counsel from spiritual leaders may expect much the same tenuous termination from therapists. To avoid these types of potential problems, therapists should establish clear boundaries from the onset of the therapeutic relationship and reiterate expectations as termination is approaching.
>
> (Aten et al., 2009, p. 231)

Continuation of the Case of Maria

Evaluation

After ten sessions Maria was less symptomatic, experienced more energy and hopefulness, and was able return to teaching. Her increasing trust in the treatment process facilitated her willingness to continue in ongoing therapy. Therapy then shifted to a focus on personality and spiritual change with an emphasis on personal growth and spiritual transformation. Maria continued with her teaching position which, in time, included supervising new teachers in the school district. Early the following year, her husband left his job to begin his own accounting firm. For the first several months he had limited income and no benefits, resulting in increased reliance on Maria's salary and benefits. The prospect of taking such responsibility was initially daunting as Maria feared that she might somehow falter and not be the perfect wife and educator. These concerns were processed from both a psychological and spiritual perspective. In time sufficient progress was made that sessions were reduced to monthly and then quarterly. This progress was monitored by the Outcomes Rating Scale which was administered at the beginning of each session, and the Spiritual Well-Being Scale which was administered every fourth session.

The therapeutic focus was adjusted based on feedback from these instruments.

Termination

After a little more than two years, Maria had become much more spiritually and psychologically centered, considerably less driven, and had less of a need to please others in order to feel accepted and worthwhile. As a result, she felt much better about herself, and it was mutually agreed to prepare for termination.

Accordingly, treatment progress was reviewed, and it was agreed that Maria had achieved her stated treatment goals. She felt quite good about her progress and very confident about the future. A relapse plan was mutually established, with a follow-up a session at three months and then phone contact at three month intervals for the first year. It was understood that, if indicated, an emergency session could be arranged. As therapy was winding down her GAF (Global Assessment of Functioning) was now in the low 90s,whereas at the outset of therapy it had been in the mid-60s. About nine months later the therapist received a Christmas card with a note. Maria indicated that she was continuing to do well. She also mentioned that she was now involved in giving women's retreats in her diocese, something she had never imagined herself doing.

Concluding Note

This chapter discussed the importance of evaluation of treatment outcomes in conventional psychotherapy as well as in spiritually integrated psychotherapy. It also described the process of termination in conventional psychotherapy as well as termination considerations that arise when spiritual issues have been a focus of therapy. That termination has been a neglected topic in conventional psychotherapy training and in research, and that there is even less literature on termination in spiritually integrated psychotherapy should now be obvious to the reader. Finally, the continuing case of Maria has illustrated how the processes of evaluation and termination are addressed in spiritually integrated psychotherapy.

References

Aten, J., Mangis, M., Campbell, C., Tucker, B., Kobeisy, A., & Halberda, R. (2009). Spirituality in therapy termination. In J. Aten & M. Leach (Eds.), *Spirituality and the therapeutic process: A comprehensive resource from intake to termination* (pp. 217–239). American Psychological Association.

Beck, J. (1995). *Cognitive therapy: Basics and beyond*. Guilford.

Boswell, J. F. (2015). Psychotherapy: Process, mechanisms, and science–practice integration. *Psychotherapy*, *52*(1), 38–44. https://doi.org/10.1037/a0038579

Bufford, R. K., Paloutzian, R. F., & Ellison, C. W. (1991). Norms for the Spiritual Well Being Scale. *Journal of Psychology and Theology*, *19*(1), 56–70.

Callahan, J., Aubuchon-Endsley, N., Borja, S., & Swift, J. (2009). Pretreatment expectancies and premature termination in a training clinic environment. *Training and Education in Professional Psychology*, 3, 111–119.

Carlier, I. V. E., & van Eeden, W. A. (2017). Routine outcome monitoring in mental health care and particularly in addiction treatment: Evidence-based clinical and research recommendations. *Journal of Addictions Research and Therapy*, *8*, 332. https://doi.org/10.4172/2155-6105.1000332

Carroll, K. (1996). Relapse prevention as a psychosocial treatment: A review of controlled clinical trials. *Experimental and Clinical Psychopharmacology*, *4*, 46–54.

Clarkin, J., & Levy, K. (2003). Influence of client variables on psychotherapy. In M. Lambert (Ed.), *Handbook of psychotherapy and behavior change* (5th ed.). Wiley.

Cucciare, M., & O'Donohue, W. (2008). Clinical case conceptualization and termination of psychotherapy. In M. O'Donohue & W. Cucciare (Eds.), *Terminating psychotherapy: A clinician's guide* (pp. 121–146). Routledge.

Currier, J. M., McDermott, R. C., Sanders, P., Barkham, M., Owen, J., Saxon, D., & Richards, P. S. (2024). Practice-based evidence for spiritually integrated psychotherapies: Examining trajectories of psychological and spiritual distress. *Journal of Counseling Psychology*. https://doi.org/10.1037/cou0000727

Daley, D. C. (1989). *Relapse prevention: Treatment alternatives and counseling aids*. TAB Books.

Dobson, K. S., & Haubert, L. C. (2008). Termination with persons with depressive disorders. In M. O'Donohue & W. Cucciare (Eds.), *Terminating psychotherapy: A clinician's guide* (pp. 303–324). Routledge.

Ellison, C. W. (1983). Spiritual well-being: Conceptualization and measurement. *Journal of Psychology and Theology*, *11*(4), 330–340.

Exline, J., & Rose, E. (2005). Religious and spiritual struggles. In R. Paloutzian & C. Parks (Eds.), *Handbook of the psychology of religion and spirituality* (pp. 315–330). Guilford Press.

Gloaguen, V., Cottraus, J., Cucharet, M., & Blackburn, I. (1998). A meta-analysis of the effects of cognitive therapy in depressed patients. *Journal of Affective Disorders*, *49*, 59–72.

Good, G., & Beitman, B. (2006). *Counseling and psychotherapy essentials: Integrating theories, skills, and practices*. Norton.

Hall, T. W., & Edwards, K. J. (1996). The initial development and factor analysis of the Spiritual Assessment Inventory. *Journal of Psychology and Theology*, *24*, 233–246.
Hall, T. W., Tisdale, T. C., & Brokaw, B. F. (1994). Assessment of religious dimensions in Christian clients: A review of selected instruments for research and clinical use. *Journal of Psychology and Theology*, *22*, 395–421.
Heaton, J. (1998). *Building basic therapeutic skills: A practical guide for current mental health practice*. Jossey-Bass.
Hill, P. C., & Pargament, K. I. (2003). Advances in the conceptualization and measurement of religion and spirituality. *American Psychologist*, *58*, 64–74.
Kapuscinski, A. N., & Masters, K. S. (2010). The current status of measures of spirituality: A critical review of scale development. *Psychology of Religion and Spirituality*, 2(4), 191–205.
Kass, J. D., Friedman, R., Lesserman, J., Zuttermeister, P., & Benson, H. (1991). Health outcomes and a new index of spiritual experience. *Journal for the Scientific Study of Religion*, *30*, 203–211.
Lambert, M. (2017). Maximizing psychotherapy outcome beyond evidence-based medicine. *Psychotherapy and psychosomatics*, *86*(2), 80–89.
Lambert, M., Morton, J., Hatfield, D., Harmon, C., Hamilton, S., & Reid, R. (2004). *Administration and scoring manual for the Outcome Questionnaire-45*. American Professional Credentialing Services.
Lambert, M. J., Whipple, J. L., & Kleinstäuber, M. (2018). Collecting and delivering progress feedback: A meta-analysis of routine outcome monitoring. *Psychotherapy*, *55*(4), 520–537. https://doi.org/10.1037/pst0000167
Marlatt, G., & Gordon, J. (1985). *Relapse prevention: Maintenance and strategies in the treatment of addictive behaviors*. Guilford Press.
Miller, S., & Duncan, B. (2000). *The Outcome Rating Scale*. Author.
Miller, S., Duncan, B., Brown, J., Sorrell, R., & Chalk, M. (2006). Using outcome to inform and improve treatment outcomes: Making ongoing, real-time assessment feasible. *Journal of Brief Therapy*, *5*, 5–23.
Miller, S., Hubble, M. A., Chow, D., & Seidel, J. (2015). Beyond measures and monitoring: Realizing the potential of feedback-informed treatment. *Psychotherapy*, *52*(4), 449–457. https://doi.org/10.1037/pst0000031
O'Grady, K., & Richards, P. S. (2009). Case study showing inclusion of spirituality in the therapeutic process. In J. Aten & M. Leach (Eds.), *Spirituality and the therapeutic process: A comprehensive resource from intake to termination* (pp. 241–265). American Psychological Association.
Orlinsky, D. E., Ronnestad, M. H., & Willutzki, U. (2003). Fifty years of process-outcome research: Continuity and change. In M. Lambert (Ed.), *Bergin and Garfield's handbook of psychotherapy and behaviour change* (5th ed., pp. 307–390). Wiley.
Paloutzian, R., & Ellison, C. (2021). *Manual for the Spiritual Well-Being Scale: Version 2.0*. www.westmont.edu/sites/default/files/users/user401/SWBS%20Manual%202.0_0.pdf
Piedmont, R. L. (1999). Does spirituality represent the sixth factor of personality? Spiritual transcendence and the five-factor model. *Journal of Personality*, *67*, 985–1013.

Richards, P., Smith, T. B., Schowalter, M., Richard, M., Berrett, M. E., & Hardman, R. K. (2005). Development and validation of the Theistic Spiritual Outcome Survey. *Psychotherapy Research*, *15*(4), 457–469.
Sanders, P. W. (2015). *Development of short-form versions of the Clinically Adaptive Client Outcome Measure (CA-COM)*. Unpublished doctoral dissertation, Brigham Young University, Provo, Utah.
Sanders, P. W., Richards, P. S., & McBride, J. A. (2018). Development of the clinically adaptive multidimensional outcome survey. *Psychotherapy Research*, *28*(6), 925–939.
Sperry, L., Brill, P., Howard, K., & Grissom, G. (1996). *Treatment outcomes in psychotherapy and psychiatric interventions*. Brunner/Mazel.
Sperry, L., Lewis, J., Carlson, J., & Englar-Carlson, M. (2003). *Health promotion and health counseling: Effective counseling and psychotherapeutic strategies*. Allyn & Bacon.
van Sonsbeek, M. A., Hutschemaekers, G. G., Veerman, J. W., & Tiemens, B. B. (2014). Effective components of feedback from Routine Outcome Monitoring (ROM) in youth mental health care: Study protocol of a three-arm parallel-group randomized controlled trial. *BMC Psychiatry*, *14*, 1–11.
Veach, T. L., & Chappel, J. N. (1992). Measuring spiritual health: A preliminary study. *Substance Abuse*, *13*, 139–147.
Weddington, W., & Cavenar, J. (1979). Termination initiated by the therapist: A countertransference storm. *American Journal of Psychiatry*, *136*, 1302–1305.
Wierzbicki, M., & Perarik, G. (1993). A meta-analysis of psychotherapy dropout. *Professional Psychology: Research and Practice*, *24*, 190–195.
Worthington Jr., E. L., Wade, N. G., Hight, T. L., Ripley, J. S., McCullough, M. E., & Berry, J. W. (2003). The Religious Commitment Inventory—10: Development, refinement, and validation of a brief scale for research and counseling. *Journal of Counseling Psychology*, *50*, 84–96.
Zeldovich, M., & Alexandrowicz, R. W. (2019). Comparing outcomes: The Clinical Outcome in Routine Evaluation from an international point of view. *International Journal of Methods in Psychiatric Research*, *28*(3), e1774.

Chapter 10

Cultural and Ethical Considerations

Practicing psychotherapy that is sensitive to spirituality and spiritual issues involves recognition of various cultural, ethical, and legal considerations. Just as professional ethical standards require therapists to be sensitive to cultural issues, therapists are also required to be sensitive to spiritual issues influencing their clients. This chapter discusses several cultural, ethical, and legal considerations in the practice of spiritually integrated psychotherapy. It begins with a discussion of some key cultural considerations. These include the complex relationship between spirituality and culture, and the importance of cultural sensitivity and competence in the practice of spiritually integrated psychotherapy. Next, ethical considerations common in spiritually integrated psychotherapy are addressed. These include informed consent, boundaries, and praying with clients. These ethical considerations are described and illustrated. Then, the discussion shifts to legal considerations. Of particular concern for licensed clinicians is the matter of scope of practice, which refers to the type and extent of practice that a licensure board considers acceptable professional practice. It discusses the scope of practice issues involved in the practice of spiritually integrated psychotherapy. To summarize the discussion of the chapter, seven practice guidelines are then highlighted. Finally, key points of this chapter are illustrated with the continuing case of Maria.

Cultural Considerations

This section begins with a discussion of the complex and inextricable relationship between spirituality and culture. Then it reviews the relationship between cultural dynamics and spiritual dynamics. This is followed by definitions of cultural awareness, cultural sensitivity, and cultural competency. Then, the different types of culturally sensitive treatments are described.

DOI: 10.4324/9781003425991-11

Relationship Between Spirituality and Culture

As cultural awareness has increased among the mental health professions, spirituality has recently been recognized as an element of culture, and a domain of cultural assessment and practice. The ADDRESSING framework (Hays, 2016) reflects this recognition. According to this framework, culturally sensitive practice should address the ten domains of Age, Developmental or acquired Disabilities, Religion and spiritual orientation, Ethnicity, Socioeconomic status, Sexual orientation, Indigenous heritage, National origin, and Gender. Despite the comprehensiveness of the domains listed, the relationship among these ten domains is not described. Neither is the relationship between spirituality and culture specified.

Arguably, the relationship between the two is complex as noted by Corkery (2005) and Martsolf (1997). "Spirituality refers to how we live our lives. Culture... is the way we live together" (Corkery, 2005, p. 25). Spirituality is about living life in depth and in a particular way in a given culture. Spirituality exists in all dimensions in which culture does because culture "hosts" it. Likewise, their relationship is inextricable in that spirituality cannot be independent of culture, and culture cannot be devoid of spirituality. "Spiritualities... bear the mark of their cultural context, even if they also challenge those contexts" (p. 26).

Another way of considering the relationship between spirituality and culture is in terms of three points of intersection. The first intersection is that spirituality can be defined completely by one's culture. The second is that spirituality can be individually defined by personal experiences unrelated to the culture. The third is that spirituality can be defined by culture and personal experiences but can be quite different from the cultural norms (Martsolf, 1997).

What are the implications of the relationship of spirituality and culture for spiritually integrated psychotherapy? At a minimum, it means that an integrative spiritual assessment must include an assessment of the client's culture, the client's personal spiritual beliefs and practices, as well as the spiritual beliefs and practices common to that culture. It should also include incorporating the client's expectations and preferences for spiritual interventions and for the providers of spiritual care into the treatment process.

Cultural Dynamics and Spiritual Dynamics

To further clarify the relationship between the spiritual and cultural dimensions one can compare the cultural dynamics and spiritual dynamics that are identified in the integrative assessment and case conceptualization of spiritually integrated psychotherapy (cf. Chapter 7).

Here is a list of the essential spiritual dynamics that are assessed: spiritual history; God representation or image; spiritual beliefs and spiritual practices; spiritual identity and involvement in a religious or spiritual community; spiritual influence on clinical presentation, e.g., struggles, conflict, and symptoms; and spiritual influence on therapeutic relationship and interventions (Gellerman & Lu, 2011). Related but different are the cultural dynamics that are assessed. They are cultural history; cultural identity and acculturation, e.g., birthplace, social class, work orientation, etc.; explanatory model of presentation; cultural influence on clinical presentation, i.e., struggles, conflict, symptoms; and cultural influence on therapeutic relationship and interventions.

Cultural Awareness, Cultural Sensitivity, and Cultural Competency

Terms like cultural knowledge, cultural awareness, cultural sensitivity, and cultural competency are often used synonymously when the reality is that they are quite different (Sperry, 2022). For example, it is possible to possess cultural knowledge without cultural awareness, cultural sensitivity, or cultural competence. Cultural knowledge is a familiarity with selected cultural characteristics, like the history, values, beliefs, and behaviors of another cultural heritage. In contrast, cultural awareness requires cultural knowledge plus some degree of openness to another cultural heritage. Furthermore, cultural sensitivity requires cultural awareness plus the capacity to appropriately respond to the attitudes, feelings, and circumstances of clients and others of a different ethnic, racial, religious, or cultural heritage. The operative phrase is "capacity to appropriately respond," also referred to as "culturally responsive." Finally, cultural competence requires cultural sensitivity and the capacity to translate cultural sensitivity into actions that have positive influence on an individual or individuals from another cultural heritage (Sperry, 2022). In a clinical context, cultural competence is the capacity to translate a therapist's cultural sensitivity into behavior that results in an effective therapeutic relationship and treatment process, as well as positive treatment outcomes (Paniagua, 2005).

Culturally Sensitive Treatments

When cultural dynamics are prominent, it is expected that culturally sensitive treatments will be planned and implemented. Here is a brief description of three types of culturally sensitive treatments: cultural interventions, culturally sensitive therapies, and culturally sensitive interventions (Sperry, 2022; Sperry & Sperry, 2020).

Cultural Intervention

Cultural interventions are healing methods or activities that are consistent with the client's belief system regarding healing and potentially useful in effecting a specified change. Some examples are healing circles, prayer or exorcism, and involvement of traditional healers from that client's culture. Sometimes, the use of cultural interventions necessitates collaboration with or referral to such a healer or other expert (Paniagua, 2005). Still, a clinician can begin the treatment process by focusing on core cultural values, such as *respito* and *personalismo*, in an effort to increase the "clinician's achieved credibility," i.e., the cultural client's perception that the clinician is trustworthy and effective.

Culturally Sensitive Therapy

Culturally sensitive therapies are psychotherapeutic interventions that directly address the cultural characteristics of diverse clients, i.e., beliefs, customs, attitudes, and their socioeconomic and historical context (La Roche & Christopher, 2008). Because they utilize traditional healing methods and pathways, such approaches are appealing to certain clients. For example, Cuento Therapy addresses culturally relevant variables such as *familismo* and *personalismo* through the use of folk tales (*cuentos*) and is used with Puerto Rican children (Costantino et al., 1986). Likewise, Morita therapy originated in Japan and is now used throughout the world for a wide range of disorders ranging from shyness to schizophrenia (Li & He, 2008). These kinds of therapy appear to be particularly effective in clients with lower levels of acculturation.

Culturally Sensitive Intervention

A culturally sensitive intervention is a conventional psychotherapeutic intervention that has been adapted or modified to be responsive to the cultural characteristics of a particular client. Because of their structured and educational focus, cognitive behavior therapy (CBT) interventions are acceptable to many cultures and are the most often modified to be culturally sensitive (Hays & Iwanasa, 2006). For example, particularly in culturally diverse clients with lower levels of acculturation, disputation and cognitive restructuring of a maladaptive belief are seldom the CBT interventions of choice, whereas problem solving, skills training, or cognitive replacement interventions (Sperry, 2022) may be more appropriate.

Ethical Considerations

This section begins with a summary of the key ethical considerations in the practice of conventional psychotherapy. It is followed by a more detailed description of three common ethical considerations in the practice of spiritually integrated psychotherapy.

Ethical Considerations in Psychotherapy

The various ethical issues arising in psychotherapy practice can be subsumed in four core considerations: confidentiality, informed consent, conflict of interests, dual or multiple relationships, and competency (Sperry, 2007). These considerations are summarized in Table 10.1.

Ethically Competent Decision Making in Psychotherapy Practice

Among other considerations, ethical competence requires that clinical decisions are based on whether a therapeutic intervention meets three criteria. The criteria are: (1) is it safe?, (2) is it effective?, and (3) is it appropriate for a given client with a specified concern, diagnosis, or need? (Sperry, 2018). Needless to say, these criteria reflect both ethical competence as well as clinical competence.

Table 10.1 Core Ethical Considerations

Consideration	*Description*
Competence	The professional's capacity to provide a minimum quality of service within the professional's scope of practice, which requires sufficient training, supervision, and experience to provide that service. Makes clinical decision based on whether interventions are effective, safe, and appropriate.
Confidentiality	The professional's obligation to respect the privacy of clients by not revealing to others the information communicated to them by a client during treatment.
Conflict of Interest	The professional's obligation to avoid competing interests that would interfere with faithfully exercising his or her professional judgment and skill in working with a client; the professional's obligation to refrain from assuming one or more roles with a client besides that of therapist. Even if these other relationships seem harmless a conflict of interest exists, and the professional's judgment can be affected by a loss of objectivity.
Informed Consent	The client's right to make a decision about participating in treatment after it has been adequately described and explained in a manner that is understandable to the client.

Based on Sperry, 2007, 2018

A necessary step in making clinical decisions is specifying the indications and contraindications for the use of a particular intervention. The reality is that some therapeutic interventions can be quite effective with specific indications but not with others. Take the commonly utilized intervention of mindfulness. For most clients, many mindfulness interventions are indicated and presumably will be safe, effective, and appropriate. However, with certain depressive conditions some mindfulness interventions can be effective but neither safe nor appropriate. For example, the specific mindfulness intervention called loving-kindness meditation is not considered safe nor appropriate for clients with recurrent depression because of safety concerns (Segal et al., 2013). In short, ethical competence requires knowledge of the clinical and research literature of specific interventions that a therapist considers when making clinical decisions in psychotherapy, including spiritually integrated psychotherapy.

Ethical Considerations in Spiritually Integrated Psychotherapy

Because of the context in which spiritually focused services are provided, role conflicts and multiple relationships can be a complex ethical consideration, as can informed consent. Also, ethical considerations can arise when prayer is utilized as a spiritual intervention. All three are briefly discussed.

Potential Role Conflicts and Multiple Relationships

In contrast to psychotherapists who provide spiritually integrated psychotherapy, ministry personnel such as priests, pastors, rabbis, and others who provide pastoral counseling or spiritual direction often experience potential role conflicts—referred to as dual or multiple relationships—with clients who may also be members of their congregations. While the Ethical Principles of Psychologists and Code of Conduct, also called the APA Ethics Code (American Psychological Association, 2017), exhorts psychologists to avoid such relationships, dual and multiple relationships are often an expected part of the job duties for ministry personnel. For example, a pastor who also functions as a pastoral counselor or spiritual director may preach to his parishioners about religious values, exhort them to virtue, raise money from them, as well as counsel them on marital concerns. As long as reasonable boundaries are maintained, such multiple roles often are not problematic for such ministry personnel.

Informed Consent

Ethical practice requires that client consent be given freely without coercion and without value imposition. Because spiritually integrated psychotherapy is value based it is useful to distinguish value imposition from value exposure (Hathaway & Ripley, 2009). Value exposure involves the disclosure of therapists' values when appropriate and without an agenda, whereas value imposition involves disclosure with an agenda. Typically, value imposition involves therapists imposing their values or religious beliefs on clients, or persuading a client to accept a course of treatment or an intervention. It is unethical because it undermines the client's right to decide about the specifics of treatment (Sperry, 2007). Value imposition can be less a concern for clients seeking spiritual direction or pastoral counseling since these clients have opted for spiritually integrated care. The situation can be considerably different for clients seeking psychotherapy since they may not be seeking spiritually integrated psychotherapy.

Consequently, numerous complaints have been filed by clients, or their guardians, to state licensing boards or professional organizations about spiritually integrated treatment being provided that they had not sought or wanted. Case law contains a number of cases where psychotherapists have been fired for providing unwanted spiritual treatment to clients (Bullis, 1996). Accordingly, therapists would do well to elicit client expectations for treatment and to engage in mutual treatment decision-making so that adequate informed consent is achieved.

Prayer as an Intervention

One of the more sensitive and complex ethical issues that therapists face are requests from clients to pray with them. The advisability of utilizing prayer as a treatment intervention is an important professional and ethical consideration, and fortunately, the matter of indications and contraindications has been addressed (see Chapter 8). Even though therapists may not be fully conversant in these matters, it is expected that they have access to such information through references or consultation, and therapists utilizing prayer must be cognizant of the ethical considerations of this intervention. Two forms of prayer are addressed here: the first is praying *with* clients during sessions, while the second is praying *for* clients outside of sessions. With regard to praying for clients, there are at least three ethical principles to consider: integrity, competence, and promoting client well-being.

The first consideration is the ethical principle of integrity. This principle is based on the assumption that therapists do not impose their own prayer practices and beliefs on clients; therapists can legitimately consider utilizing prayer with clients for whom prayer is an important part of their life (West, 2000). A related assumption is that therapists are aware of their own biases and will disclose these to clients.

The ethical principle of competence requires that therapists only ethically utilize prayer as an intervention if they are sufficiently qualified by education, training, or experience. This ethical principle can easily be overlooked or rationalized by therapists eager to be responsive to client expectations. It has been observed that therapists too often rely on their personal beliefs and experience of prayer as their primary guideline when using prayer in psychotherapy (Magaletta & Brawer, 1998). In other words, just because a therapist engages in personal prayer does not qualify them as competent in using prayer as a therapeutic intervention.

With regard to the ethical principle of promoting the well-being of clients, therapists need to be mindful of the matter of power shifts that can result from using prayer. These include therapists using prayer to gain power over clients, clients using prayer to gain power over their therapists, or both therapists and clients losing power to the God being prayed to (Magaletta & Brawer, 1998). Furthermore, therapists also need to be cognizant of the power they have when they suggest an intervention that includes prayer. They must ensure that prayer is implemented at the will and in the interest of the client, and not to appease the therapist. Therapists must fully assess the levels of spirituality of clients and identify their expectations regarding the implementation of prayer in psychotherapy. Finally, therapists should be aware of the benefits and risks of using prayer as an intervention, as well as sensitivity to possible cultural factors that might be operative (Weld & Erikson, 2007).

There are also ethical considerations involved in praying *for* clients. The question arises: does a therapist need a client's permission to pray (outside of the session) for the client's healing and well-being? In other words, is it ethical to pray for a client without the client's awareness of such practice? It has been argued that this form of prayer is not unethical if the therapists intends such prayer as a means of grounding or as a method of preparation for sessions. "Using prayer as a support mechanism in this way engenders a sense of the client being upheld and brings with it a lightening of the load" (Gubi, 2001, p. 429). In fact, a case can be made that therapists have an ethical imperative to do whatever is appropriate and reasonable to increase the efficacy of the treatment process. If the therapist "believes in the effectiveness of praying for clients away from their presence, then it could be argued that it is unethical for her to withhold it" (p. 429).

A related ethical consideration is the discussion of prayer with supervisors. A qualitative study was reported regarding therapists' use of supervision in the implementation of prayer in psychotherapy. Results indicated that many therapists were afraid to discuss the practice of prayer with their supervisors (Gubi, 2007). The fear of discussing prayer with a supervisor led some therapists to disguise the labels and language that they used to describe prayer. Among therapists with more than one supervisor, some would discuss prayer with a supervisor who was perceived as receptive to the practice, but chose not to with a supervisor from whom they feared ridicule. Arguably, supervisors need "to create a culture of openness and a collaborative working alliance where all aspects of the counseling process can be explored" (Gubi, 2007, p. 119). Beyond concerns associated with therapists not being comfortable to discuss prayer in supervision, there are no clear guidelines for supervision when implementing spirituality in psychotherapy (West, 2000). Accordingly, additional training and guidelines are needed for therapists and supervisors alike who desire to integrate spirituality into psychotherapy.

Legal Considerations

There are a number of legal considerations in the practice of psychotherapy. They include duty to warn, privileged communication, practicing without proper credentials, and scope of practice. Of these scope of practice may be the most salient legal consideration in the practice of spiritually integrated psychotherapy. Interestingly, it is both a legal and ethical consideration. Accordingly, it is the main focus of this section.

Scope of Practice

A major ethical consideration in the Code of Ethics of all the mental health professions involves practicing within one's "scope of practice" (American Counseling Association, 2014; American Psychological Association, 2017). Scope of practice requires that a psychotherapist must have sufficient formal training, supervision, and experience in a specialized area to practice ethically, legally, and competently.

Ethical and legal concerns involving the practice of spiritually integrated psychotherapy can be quite complex and challenging. As Pargament (2009) has observed: "ethical complexity is to be expected when working in this area because people are by nature complex, multidimensional, bio-psycho-socio-spiritual beings" (p. 392). Amid this complexity is the issue of demarcating the boundaries of psychotherapeutic practice, where the goal is primarily psychological change or transformation, and spiritual practice, as in spiritual direction, where the goal is primarily spiritual transformation.

This means that psychotherapists can only ethically integrate spiritual and religious interventions in their psychotherapy practice when they have sufficient training and clinical competence to recognize and deal with related ethical issues (Association for Spiritual, Ethical and Religious Values in Counseling, 2009; Vieten & Lukoff, 2022). Even among highly competent psychotherapists, spiritual and religious issues can arise in their clinical practice that require consultation, additional training, collaboration, or referral.

Scope of practice raises a number of ethical considerations when spiritual and religious issues are involved. For instance, can a psychotherapist offer spiritual direction in the course of psychotherapy when spiritual direction is not typically within the legally defined scope of practice for psychology in a given state? Unfortunately, there is no single, definitive answer to the first question. Two factors need to be considered.

The first is that psychotherapists are licensed by the state in which they practice, while spiritual directors are not, and although pastoral counselors may not need to be licensed, they practice under the authority of a religious institution. If a psychotherapist begins offering spiritual direction or pastoral counseling services, they risk practicing outside of the scope intended by the psychology licensing board.

The second factor is that spiritually integrative psychotherapy can foster spiritual transformation, and some psychotherapists specify spiritual transformation as a therapeutic goal or target. Since spiritual transformation is not a standard psychotherapeutic goal, it may well be that this goal is outside the psychotherapist's scope of practice. Accordingly, it is recommended that they carefully consider the issue of professional accountability and communicate with their licensing board regarding scope of practice (McMinn, 2009).

Informed Consent

It can be relatively easy and natural to discuss the place of spiritual and religious issues in providing "informed consent" to a client who has expressed such an interest or concern.

Assuming that a licensed psychotherapist is not also ordained, certified, or otherwise authorized to provide pastoral care, pastoral counseling, or spiritual direction, the following suggestion is offered that provides both information and clarification of scope of practice.

One way this can be accomplished is to have a brief description of spiritually integrated psychotherapy printed in a brochure, on the therapist's website, or within an informed consent document to be signed by the client. Here is such a description:

> Spiritually integrated psychotherapy is a broad designation that refers to approaches provided by therapists that integrate the essential psychotherapy competencies as well as spiritual resources in addressing spiritual issues and struggles to resolve psychological and relational problems. Although it can also foster spiritual change and growth, spiritually integrated psychotherapy accomplishes this as a by-product that accompanies psychological change.

Psychotherapists would do well to briefly emphasize the last statement that any spiritual change that may result is a "by-product that accompanies psychological change" as it addresses the scope of practice consideration. An additional statement of how spiritual and religious issues are processed might also be added.

Ethical Guidelines for Culturally and Spiritually Sensitive Practice

To summarize and highlight much of the discussion of this chapter, the following eight practice guidelines are offered—clinicians should:

- become familiar with the various spiritual traditions present in their client population
- become self-aware of their own background and worldview, and how these might bias their response to clients with different backgrounds and worldviews
- refrain from proselytizing or imposing their worldview on clients
- remain mindful of factors that influence the appropriateness of their disclosure to clients, including disclosures that are congruent with the treatment approach used, facilitative of treatment, and necessary to address potential value conflicts that could impede treatment
- make ethically sensitive clinical decisions about utilizing specific interventions based on whether they are safe, effective, and appropriate for a given client
- make appropriate clinical referrals when clients express a strong preference for a therapist with a different spiritual background and this preference persists after reasonable attempts to engage the client, or when the nature of the presenting problem exceeds the therapist's competence despite relevant supervision or consultation
- respect spirituality as an important cultural domain and be mindful of the multiple ways this domain relates to other cultural factors, i.e., ethnicity, race, age, gender, and sexual orientation
- gain competence in working with clients of diverse spiritual backgrounds through consultation, continuing education, and supervised experience and practice within the scope of that training.

Continuation of the Case of Maria

Here is a summary of the cultural and spiritual dynamics of Maria as noted in Chapter 6. Maria is a third generation Cuban American who identifies herself as an upper middle class American. She is highly acculturated as are her parents. She is married to a fourth generation Irish American who also is highly acculturated. They have no children. Maria is a college graduate and a special education teacher.

Spiritually, she images God as demanding, critical, and withholding, and she reacts to others with anger and suspicion when distressed. Her discomfort with and limited contact with community support, particularly her church, seems related to feelings of unworthiness and perceived non-acceptance by others. The spiritual practices she described—limited to formula prayer and church attendance—were consistent with her religious tradition and limited to being both fear- and duty-based. It is noteworthy that her religious beliefs about "earning" salvation appear to reinforce her own perfectionistic beliefs and behaviors. She had been quite involved in a parish community in a leadership capacity, although for the past three years she has not been involved in that community.

The place of culture, particularly cultural identity and acculturation level, cannot be ignored or underestimated in a client's presentation, case conceptualization, and intervention plan. In the case of Maria, it was concluded that cultural dynamics were not prominent. The reason for this conclusion is that high levels of acculturation were identified in Maria, her husband, and her parents. In addition, there was no indication that other cultural dynamics such as prejudice or microaggressions were operative, and that personality dynamics were dominant in accounting for her presentation. As a result, culturally sensitive treatment was not indicated.

Suppose that the cultural dynamics differed, and Maria's cultural identity was Cuban, with a low level of acculturation, living in a primarily Cuban community in the southeastern US. As a result, it is more likely that she would be a homemaker and mother rather than a college graduate and professional teacher, and her presenting problems would not likely include job-related distress. Or suppose that her level of acculturation was high while her parents' acculturation level was low, and that she also reported considerable conflict and distress attributed to these acculturation differences, in addition to the stress associated with work and marriage. It is also possible that cultural dynamics would be more operative than personality dynamics (perfectionism might be less dominant), and that some types of culturally sensitive treatment might be indicated.

Given the interactive relationship between culture and spirituality, it is likely that Maria's spiritual dynamics would also differ. While her God image may be the same or similar, her spiritual beliefs reflecting perfectionism might be less prominent. The spiritual practices she engaged in might have been more culturally based, and it is unlikely that she would have engaged in centering prayer or other forms of meditation which are more common among those with higher levels of acculturation. Furthermore, it is more likely that she would have taken a more supportive rather than leadership role in her church community. In short, not only her presentation but also her case conceptualization and type and course of treatment might have differed to reflect other cultural and spiritual dynamics.

Concluding Note

The basic message of this chapter is that therapists who engage in spiritually integrated psychotherapy must recognize and practice in a manner that is consistent with several cultural, ethical, and legal considerations. Among these are ethically sensitive and effective clinical decisions that require the evaluation of potential interventions to determine whether they are safe, effective, and appropriate for a given client. Following the seven practice guidelines can facilitate a healthy therapeutic alliance, productive therapeutic process, and positive clinical outcomes.

References

American Counseling Association. (2014). *ACA code of ethics*. Author.

American Psychological Association. (2017). *Ethical principles of psychologists and code of conduct*. American Psychological Association.

Association for Spiritual, Ethical and Religious Values in Counseling (ASERVIC). (2009). Competencies for addressing spiritual and religious issues in counseling. *Interaction*, *10*(10), 3.

Bullis, R. (1996). *Spirituality in social work practice*. Taylor & Francis.

Corkery, J. (2005). Spirituality and culture. In P. Sheldrake (Ed.), *The new Westminster dictionary of Christian spirituality* (pp. 25–31). John Knox Press.

Costantino, G., Malgady, R. G., & Rogler, L. H. (1986). Cuento therapy: A culturally sensitive modality for Puerto Rican children. *Journal of Consulting and Clinical Psychology*, *54*, 639–645.

Gellerman, D., & Lu, F. (2011). Religious and spiritual issues in the outline for cultural formulation. In J. Peteet, W. Narrow, & F. Lu (Eds.), *Religious and spiritual considerations in psychiatric diagnosis: A research agenda for DSM V* (pp. 207–224). American Psychiatric Press.

Gubi, P. M. (2001). An exploration of the use of Christian prayer in mainstream counseling. *British Journal of Guidance & Counselling*, *29*, 425–434.

Gubi, P. M. (2007). Exploring the supervision experience of some mainstream counsellors who integrate prayer in counseling. *Counselling and Psychotherapy Research*, *7*, 114–121.

Hathaway, W. L., & Ripley, J. (2009). Spirituality and ethics. In J. Aten & M. Leach (Eds.), *Spirituality and the therapeutic process* (pp. 25–52). American Psychological Association.

Hays, P. (2016). *Addressing cultural complexities in practice: Assessment, diagnosis, and therapy* (3rd ed.). American Psychological Association. https://doi.org/10.1037/14801-000

Hays, P., & Iwanasa, G. (Eds.). (2006). *Culturally responsive cognitive-behavioral therapy: Assessment, practice, and supervision*. American Psychological Association.

La Roche, M., & Christopher, M. (2008). Culture and empirically supported treatments: On the road to a collision? *Culture and Psychology*, *14*, 333–356.

Li, C., & He, Y. (2008). Morita therapy for schizophrenia. *Schizophrenia Bulletin*, *34*(6), 1021–1023.

Magaletta, P. R., & Brawer, P. A. (1998). Prayer in psychotherapy: A model for its use, ethical considerations, and guidelines for practice. *Journal of Psychology and Theology*, *26*, 322–330.

Martsolf, D. (1997). Cultural aspects of spirituality in cancer care. *Seminars in Oncology Nursing*, *13*, 231–236.

McMinn, M. (2009). Ethical considerations with spiritually oriented interventions. *Professional Psychology: Research, and Practice*, *40*, 393–395.

Paniagua, E. (2005). *Assessing and treating culturally diverse clients: A practical guide* (3rd ed.). Sage.

Pargament, K. (2009). The psychospiritual character of psychotherapy and the ethical complexities that follow. *Psychology: Research and Practice*, *40*, 391–393.

Segal, Z. V., Williams, M., & Teasdale, J. D. (2013). *Mindfulness-based cognitive therapy for depression* (2nd ed.). Guilford Press.

Sperry, L. (2007). *The ethical and professional practice of counseling and psychotherapy*. Allyn & Bacon.

Sperry, L. (2018). Mindfulness, soulfulness, and spiritual development in spiritually oriented psychotherapy. *Spirituality in Clinical Practice*, *5*(4), 291–295.

Sperry, L. (2022). *Highly effective therapy: Developing essential clinical competencies in counseling and psychotherapy* (2nd ed.). Routledge.

Sperry, L., & Sperry, J. (2020). *Core competencies in counseling and psychotherapy: Becoming a highly competent and effective therapist* (2nd ed.). Routledge.

Vieten, C., & Lukoff, D. (2022). Spiritual and religious competencies in psychology. *American Psychologist*, *77*(1), 26–38. https://doi.org/10.1037/amp0000821

Weld, C., & Erikson, K. (2007). Issues and insights: The ethics of prayer in counseling. *Counseling and Values*, *51*, 125–137.

West, W. (2000). *Psychotherapy and spirituality: Crossing the line between therapy and religion*. Sage.

Chapter 11

Spiritually Integrated Psychotherapy

The Present to the Future

From Era I to the Present

For perspective it is helpful to recall that the word psychology is derived from the Greek word psyche which means soul or spirit. It provides a useful context for understanding how and why spiritually integrated psychotherapy developed as it did. In one form or another, psychotherapy with a religious and spiritual focus existed for centuries. However, the early twentieth century witnessed external attacks on religion, as the field of psychology sought to dissociate itself from its roots in moral philosophy and become a value-free scientific discipline (Era I). Religion in psychology was only formally recognized as a Division of APA in 1976 at a time when research, clinical practice, and training were still quite limited (Era II). As APA recognized diversity in 2017, religion and spirituality gained additional recognition as research, clinical practice, and training increased slowly (Era III). Research, clinical practice, and training expanded considerably in the next era as spiritually integrated psychotherapy became increasingly recognized (Era IV). Throughout these eras there remained a small but committed group who endeavored to keep psychology, religion, and spirituality connected.

An objective observer might conclude that in this current era, psychology has largely regained its "soul" and "spirit." Still research, clinical practice, and training in this specialty lags nearly a decade behind conventional psychotherapy research and practice. As noted in the commentary on the four eras in Chapter l, to "close the gap" will require increased attention in research, training, and clinical practice on routine outcome monitoring, the other essential psychotherapy competencies, particularly therapist effects and expertise, and the mechanism of change in spiritually integrated psychotherapy. Furthermore, research on specific spiritual interventions and practices must be a priority. Finally, because of the increasing number of researchers, clinicians, students, and other resources like training and research grants, Era V will build on these achievements and resources and further close the gap.

DOI: 10.4324/9781003425991-12

Recent Therapeutic Applications

There is a sense of excitement that this psychotherapy specialty is continuing to grow, particularly with the number of spiritually integrated psychotherapies that have and continue to emerge. At the same time the incidence of moral injury (MI) has increased while therapists seek treatment strategies to deal with it. Recently two spiritually integrated psychotherapies that address MI and sacred moral injury (SMI) stand out and this section describes both.

Spiritually Integrated Cognitive Processing Therapy

When MI is conceptualized in psychological terms only, conventional psychotherapy and even cognitive processing therapy (CPT) were found to be insufficient. When co-occurring with PTSD, standard psychological treatments, including CPT, were also found insufficient. In contrast, when conceptualized in moral, psychological, and spiritual terms, treatments such as spiritually integrated cognitive processing therapy (SICPT) have been shown to be effective. Preparing therapists to deal with this new condition and its sequelae is and will continue to be a major challenge for the field during this current era when the numbers of those in need of spiritually integrated therapies have increased dramatically.

SICPT was developed to treat the religious, spiritual, and moral symptoms of MI that psychological approaches like CPT were not addressing. Accordingly, SICPT extended CPT to address religious symptoms such as religious struggles and loss of religious faith, and spiritual and moral symptoms like loss of meaning and purpose, difficulty forgiving, feeling abandoned by God, and general moral concerns. SICPT also addresses psychological symptoms such as guilt, shame, feelings of betrayal, loss of meaning, trusting others, and self-condemnation (Koenig et al., 2019, 2023).

Treatment Protocol

SICPT is a 12-session manual-based approach that utilizes cognitive restructuring as well as a client's own spiritual resources including spiritual beliefs and practices, values, and motivations. These resources are supplemented with religious and spiritual practices such as confession, forgiveness, scripture memorization, and involvement in a spiritual community for ongoing support. SICPT is a group or individual intervention conducted in 50-minute weekly sessions. Religion-specific modules are also available for addressing MI among those from Christian, Jewish, Muslim, Buddhist, and Hindu faith traditions (Pearce, 2023).

Five of the sessions appear to be more focused on spiritual symptoms and concerns. These include Session 2: Meaning of the Event and Spirituality; Session 3: Spiritual Resources and Moral Injury; Session 5: Challenging Questions and Spiritual Distress; Session 10: Power, Control, and Spiritual Discrepancies; and Session 11: Intimacy and Spiritual Partnerships. Five other sessions appear more focused on moral and religious symptoms and concerns: Session 4: Kind Attention and Compassion; Session 6: Confession Ritual and Problematic Thinking; Session 7: Forgiveness I and Challenging Beliefs; Session 8: Trust and Forgiveness II; and Session 9: Esteem and Making Amends (Pearce, 2023).

Researchers conclude that "this is the first report on the efficacy of SICPT for MI among individuals with PTSD. Significant reductions in both MI and PTSD were observed in the first three patients enrolled in this single-group experimental study, providing initial support for the broader use of SICPT in the treatment of MI among those with severe trauma who find religious beliefs to be at least somewhat important in their lives" (O'Garo & Koenig, 2023, p. 661). Other clinical trials of this manualized treatment approach are also underway (O'Garo & Koenig, 2023).

Spiritually Integrated Psychotherapy for Sacred Moral Injury

Basically, SMI involves both an individual moral failure and a systemic moral failure. The individual moral failure is that of the abuser—betrayer. The systemic moral failure is that of the religious organization which is complicit with the abuser. Distinguishing SMI from PTSD, MI, and betrayal trauma is essential for effective recovery (Sperry, 2021a; 2021b; 2023).

SMI has been further defined as: a trauma syndrome with lasting biological, psychological, social, organizational, and spiritual effects which emerges from the experience of betrayal of a sacred trust by a perpetrator of a religious organization whom the victim perceives as representing God. Typically, the religious organization supports the perpetrator by covering up the event and invalidating the victim. Because it is both an individual moral failure and a systems or organizational failure, recovery from it requires that both failures be addressed (Sperry, 2021a; 2021b; 2023).

It is necessary to acknowledge that the abuser's immoral behavior may be denied, condoned, or covered up by the religious organization. While MI and betrayal trauma may involve an organizational or institutional moral failure, SMI moral injury always involves it.

Treatment Protocol

Unfortunately, as SICPT does not focus on loss of the sense of the sacred (McGraw et al., 2019) nor betrayal of sacred trust, it is unlikely to be effective with SMI. That is because recovery from the trauma of SMI involves restoring the sense of the sacred. Because the abused person has experienced betrayal of sacred trust by a priest or minister whom the abused perceives as God's representative, a loss of trust in God occurs. Accordingly, recovery requires overcoming sacred betrayal and regaining trust in God and God's representative. It also requires reducing the short- and long-term biopsychosociospiritual effects of the betrayal.

Because SMI is more than a medical or psychological condition, psychotherapy, apologies, and compensation are seldom sufficient. For abused persons, this process is an extended journey requiring the telling of their story and its acceptance by others, along with necessary and sufficient accountability. Since full recovery requires that both moral and organizational failures are addressed, the offending religious organizations must do more than listen, apologize, and provide therapy and compensation. Systemic changes in the organization's structure, leadership, and culture must also be involved (Sperry, 2021a).

A five step treatment strategy is usually necessary for recovery from this type of trauma. It involves: (1) listen, acknowledge, and validate; (2) offer apology and facilitate; (3) facilitate atonement and compensation; (4) provide effective spiritually integrated psychotherapy that has a trauma focus like SICPT; and (5) encourage systemic or organizational change (Sperry, 2021a). While there is a logical progression of the guidelines, the recovery process does not necessarily follow this order. That means that the person who has been abused may begin with psychotherapy before encountering the offending organization. To the extent that this five step strategy is operative, a full recovery can possibly be achieved.

Increasingly, religious organizations employ victim assistance coordinators whose role is to be the initial point of contact for persons who have been abused and are seeking healing with the religious organization. Therapists who can provide spiritually integrated psychotherapy are central to the process. Other religious personnel such as chaplains, spiritual directors, and pastoral counselors with training or experience in the healing of SMI may also be involved as the healing process unfolds.

Spiritually Integrated Psychotherapy Research

Research on spiritually integrated psychotherapy has increased in Era III and is likely to increase even more throughout Era IV. Two areas of this research are unique to Era IV. The first are clinical trials, both evidence-based and practice-based studies, of specific factors such as therapists' behaviors and spiritual practice, rather than treatment modalities as a whole. The second is the emergence of the practice-based network. These developments are described in this section.

Research on Specific Factors and Spiritual Practices

Spiritually integrated psychotherapy appears to be catching up with contemporary psychotherapy research with regard to specific factors such as therapist effects that influence retention compared to premature termination. Another important development in spiritually integrated psychotherapy involves clinical trials on specific spiritual practices. Both are briefly discussed here.

Specific Factors

It is now recognized that therapists who discuss the spiritual aspects of their clients' presenting concerns in the first session are more likely to retain their clients in therapy when compared with therapists who did not discuss such concerns. A recent study reported that specific spiritual interventions used in the first session were differentially predictive of treatment retention and engagement. Researchers collected data on 154 therapists who practiced spiritually integrated psychotherapy from 33 settings that were part of a practice-research network. They reported that some 80% of therapists utilized at least one spiritual intervention in the first session. The most commonly used spiritual interventions included (1) listening and discussion of spiritual concerns and solutions; (2) affirming clients' divine worth; (3) discussing compassion and hope; and (4) efforts to trust God. Overall, about 20% of clients did not return for a second session.

Listening and discussion of the client's spiritual concerns and solutions was empirically linked with clients' engagement in a second session, with a 118% greater probability that those clients stayed in therapy. In contrast, discussion of compassion and hope was linked with a 40% decrease in treatment engagement. This study highlights the potential opportunities and risks for using spiritual interventions when attending to clients' spiritual and religious concerns at the start of spiritually integrated psychotherapy (Currier, McDermott et al., 2024a). So, therapists' sensitivity and responsiveness to clients' spiritual concerns, instead of prematurely offering hope, affirming their divine worth, or suggesting that they trust God, is critically important. This important study confirms that therapist effects and expertise does matter.

Spiritual Practices

Some spiritual practices that are clinically useful in working with the spiritual concerns of clients were described in Chapter 8. Among the spiritual practices are meditation, mindfulness, centering prayer, Examen, discernment, as well as forgiveness, kindness, gratitude, and compassion. These and others are discussed and illustrated with case material in Thomas

Plante's (2024a) book, *Spiritually Informed Therapy*. There is also a clinically useful accompanying client workbook (Plante, 2024b).

While there is research on utilizing mindfulness, forgiveness, and gratitude with various psychological conditions, there is relatively little about its application with spiritual concerns. Until recently there has been little or no clinical trials on spiritual practices like centering prayer and the Examen. Besides writing about these spiritual practices, Plante has undertaken clinical trials on some of them.

A published study implemented the Examen as a cognitive-behavioral tool in a clinical trial with an addiction treatment population. Use of the Examen was compared to a treatment-as-usual mindfulness intervention. The study found that both the Examen and mindfulness were equivalent in clinical outcomes with measures of depression, anxiety, stress, and substance craving (Buenrostro & Plante, 2024).

A second study investigated the effects of centering prayer on mental health and well-being. The research involved students enrolled in a college religious studies course that incorporated centering prayer. Using a comparison group from another religious studies course, the study examined whether practicing this form of prayer for seven weeks can lead to changes in anxiety, stress, depression, mindfulness, satisfaction with life, hope, and compassion. Multivariate analyses of covariance indicated trends suggesting that centering prayer may contribute to decreased anxiety and increased hope and compassion. While no significant changes in these outcomes were observed ($p > .05$), the study highlighted the potential therapeutic benefits of this spiritual practice.

Practice-Based Research Networks

As mentioned in Chapter 5, practice-based evidence (PBE) focuses on whether treatment as usual provides benefits to the kinds of clients seen at a specific treatment site by a given psychotherapist. PBE is in line with the American Psychological Association's official stance on evidence-based practice, which encourages practice-based studies and evaluation of outcomes in everyday practice (APA Presidential Task Force on Evidence-Based Practice, 2006).

A practice-based research network (PBRN) is a group of psychotherapy practices that focus on the care of their clients and evaluate the processes and outcomes that occur within these practices. These networks can study the effectiveness of spiritually integrated psychotherapies without the use of manualized treatments. Instead, the therapeutic efforts of specific therapists are studied rather than a treatment modality as a whole. Such networks foster an atmosphere wherein a therapist can be both a clinician and a researcher at the same time, something that was often held up as the epitome of clinical practice in graduate training. The therapists that I know who are affiliated with a network feel more professionally enriched than they were before becoming involved in the network.

The largest PBRN studying spiritually integrated psychotherapy is the Bridges Research-Practice Network. Bridges has funded and undertaken a number of PBE research studies that include the routine monitoring of treatment processes and outcomes of spiritually integrated treatment approaches as they naturally occur in actual mental health treatment sites. It is noteworthy that they have not funded RCTs of spiritually oriented treatment approaches (Richards et al., 2015).

One of their studies involved 19 research teams who collected data from 400+ therapists and 40,000+ therapy sessions with routine monitoring of outcomes. The main finding was that when clinicians conducted a spiritual assessment, listened to their clients' spiritual issues, and discussed the spiritual dimensions of problems and solutions, both clients' psychological and spiritual distress were significantly reduced (Richards, Allen et al., 2023a).

A more recent Bridges PBRN study involved 164 therapists practicing spiritually integrated psychotherapy in 37 clinical settings. Routine outcome monitoring instruments were collected at each session from 1227 clients over a 12-week period. Three major findings were reported. First, clients who were engaging in spiritually integrated psychotherapy across sites displayed reductions in psychological distress with improvement occurring most strongly in the first four weeks of the study. Second, clients who struggled with religious and spiritual concerns and were more psychologically distressed displayed less clinical improvement. Third, therapists who closely attended to their clients' religious and spiritual concerns with specific spiritual interventions increased the rate and duration of clients' symptom reduction. Furthermore, this is the most comprehensive PBE study on spiritually integrated psychotherapy conducted to date (Currier, Swift et al., 2024b). Since 2022 the Bridges Institute for Spiritually Integrated Psychotherapies has continued the spiritually integrated psychotherapy research of the Bridges Research-Practice Network.

Spiritual Neuroscience

William James was the early pioneer in psychology who studied and wrote on the varieties of religious experience (James, 1902). Now more than a century later, researchers are again exploring religious and spiritual experiences. This new field is called spiritual neuroscience which is the study of the relationship between the brain and religious experiences. It utilizes neuroscience, neuroimaging, and other methods to identify the biological aspects of spirituality and correlate them with an individual's spiritual and religious beliefs, spiritual practices, and spiritual experiences. When it incorporates the theological dimension, the term neurotheology is used to describe this field of inquiry (Newberg, 2018).

Magnetic resonance imaging and positron emission tomography are commonly used neuroimaging techniques to examine brain activity associated with spiritual practices such as prayer, meditation, and yoga. This research has identified increased activity in the frontal lobe, decreased activity in the parietal lobe, and other changes in brain activity (Yaden et al., 2016).

The purpose of this research is to understand the neurobiological mechanisms underlying spiritual experiences and spiritual practices and correlate them with subjective measures of spiritual experiences. Presumably, this research will further increase our understanding and appreciation of the relationship between spirituality and the brain (Yaden & Newberg, 2022).

Neurotheology

Neurotheology is the interdisciplinary field that combines neuroscience and theology. It explores the relationship between the brain and religious and spiritual experiences. Recent research has focused on the therapeutic effects of meditation and the influence of psychedelic experiences on mental health. It has also begun addressing theological and philosophical questions about the nature of sin, revelation, and free will (Newberg, 2018).

Neurobiological Correlates of Spirituality and Religion with Mental Health Conditions

While considerable research on neuroscience and spirituality and religion has been reported, "the majority of neurobiological research on S/R has neglected mental health" (Rosmarin et al., 2022, p. 100). In their systematic review of the neurobiological benefits of spirituality and religion for depression, anxiety, alcohol use, and psychosis, these researchers found that spirituality may confer benefits on depression and alcohol use.

In their review of studies on depression they concluded that spirituality and religion appear to protect individuals against depression by either increasing cortical thickness or preventing cortical thinning. Specifically, spirituality was associated with thicker cortex and higher pial surfaces among individuals at high risk for depression. Also, increased white matter was noted in the superior and middle frontal gyrus, bilateral insula, and postcentral gyrus among those who reported a high level of importance of spirituality and religion in their lives, particularly for those with high familial risk of depression (Rosmarin et al., 2022). Miller (2021) reported similar findings.

These researchers also reported that the neurological correlates of alcohol use can respond to the spiritual intervention of prayer. Individuals in an experimental prayer group experienced fewer alcohol cravings when exposed to an alcohol-related image as well as increased activation in several brain regions such as the left-anterior middle frontal gyrus, left superior parietal lobule, and bilateral posterior middle temporal gyrus. They suggested that prayer may have reduced alcohol cravings and increased attention and control processes in the brain (Rosmarin et al., 2022).

Psychological symptoms that are associated with a number of medical conditions may well respond to spiritual interventions such as mindfulness or yoga. For example, anxiety and depression are common in individuals living with Parkinson's disease. A recent clinical trial reported that yoga reduced anxiety and depressive symptoms and increased spiritual well-being.

What are the clinical applications of these early research findings? Confirmatory research as well as clinical experience as therapists mull the implications of these findings will provide answers. Given that neuroscience research has already improved our health and well-being there is every reason to hope that additional spiritual neuroscience research will improve our spiritual health and overall well-being.

Training of Spiritually Integrated Psychotherapists

At the outset of Era IV there were more training opportunities in spiritually integrated psychotherapies than in the previous era. Nevertheless, it was not coordinated or consistent across programs, nor was it likely to be empirically informed. That is beginning to change.

First, efforts have been made to collect and disseminate information on available training programs. Second, there has been a large and ambitious project to train all mental health professionals in the basic competencies for attending to their clients' religion and spirituality. These are major initiatives that will increase the likelihood that this psychotherapy specialty will continue to develop.

Richards and colleagues (Richards, Currier et al., 2023b) acknowledge that while there are several dozen mental health graduate programs with faculty who can provide mentoring and research opportunities in spirituality to students, there is minimal graduate coursework available. Accordingly, they review four continuing education programs that offer training and other resources about spiritually integrated psychotherapy (SIP) that are available for practicing mental health professionals. These include the SCT-MH online course; the ACPE (Association for Clinical Pastoral Education) SIP program; the Solhiten Institute training program in SIP; and the Bridges Institute for Spiritually Integrated Psychotherapies.

They note that there are other training programs but they consider these four to be of high quality (Richards, Currier et al., 2023b).

The Spiritual and Religious Competencies Project was launched in 2022 and was funded by a $5.1 million Templeton grant. Its aim is to improve mental health care and promote human flourishing by ensuring every mental health professional possesses the basic competencies to attend to their clients' religious faith or spirituality in clinical practice through training and research (Currier et al., 2023). Basic competencies will presumably include the empirically based spiritual and religious competencies in psychology (Vieten & Lukoff, 2022) that were described in Chapter 5.

The stated long-term goal of this project is that every mental health professional will possess the basic competencies needed to sufficiently address the spiritual and religious dimensions of their clients. Accordingly, the project is taking a strategic and focused approach to facilitate research on competency training, establish consensus about the relevance and composition of these competencies, and disseminate resources for assessment and training to counseling, marriage and family therapy, psychology, and social work programs.

Concluding Note

In the midst of Era IV, research, training, and the practice of spiritually integrated psychotherapy are continuing to evolve. Because of the exciting developments sketched in this chapter, the future for this psychotherapy specialty looks quite hopeful. What and how the rest of this era and Era V will look is not yet known. What is clear, however, is that psychology has largely recovered its spirit and soul because of the vision and dedication of the cadre of faculty, mentors, practitioners, researchers, students, trainers, and trainees who have made a difference, and will continue to pursue the vision of responding to the spiritual and religious concerns of clients.

References

APA Presidential Task Force on Evidence-Based Practice. (2006). Evidence-based practice in psychology. *American Psychologist*, *61*(4), 271–285.

Buenrostro, C. M., & Plante, T. G. (2024). A clinical trial of the Examen and mindfulness within a secular substance use disorder treatment program. *Journal of Addictions & Offender Counseling*, *45*(1), 36–54.

Currier, J. M., Fox, J., Vieten, C., Pearce, M., & Oxhandler, H. K. (2023). Enhancing competencies for the ethical integration of religion and spirituality in psychological services. *Psychological Services*, *20*(1), 40–50. https://doi.org/10.1037/ser0000678

Currier, J. M., McDermott, R. C., Sanders, P., Barkham, M., Owen, J., Saxon, D., & Richards, P. S. (2024a). Practice-based evidence for spiritually integrated psychotherapies: Examining trajectories of psychological and spiritual distress. *Journal of Counseling Psychology*. https://doi.org/10.1037/cou0000727

Currier, J. M., Swift, J., Sanders, P., & Richards, P. S. (2024b). Preventing dropout in spiritually integrated psychotherapies: What are the effective methods of attending to clients' spirituality? *Psychotherapy*. https://doi.org/10.1037/pst0000530

James, W. (1902). *The varieties of religious experience: A study in human nature; being the Gifford lectures on natural religion delivered at Edinburgh in 1901–1902*. Longmans, Green.

Koenig, H., Ames, D., & Pearce, M. (2019). *Religion and recovery from PTSD*. Jessica Kingsley Publishers.

Koenig, H. G., Carey, L. B., & Wortham, J. (2023). *Moral injury: A handbook for military chaplains*. Kindle/Amazon.

Kwok, J. Y., Kwan, J. C., Auyeung, M., Mok, V. C., Lau, C. K., Choi, K. C., & Chan, H. Y. (2019). Effects of mindfulness yoga vs stretching and resistance training exercises on anxiety and depression for people with Parkinson disease: A randomized clinical trial. *JAMA Neurology*, *76*(7), 755–763.

McGraw, D. M., Ebadi, M., Dalenberg, C., Wu, V., Naish, B., & Nunez, L. (2019). Consequences of abuse by religious authorities: A review. *Traumatology*, *25*(4), 242–255. https://doi.org/10.1037/trm0000183

Miller, L. (2021). *The awakened brain: The new science of spirituality and our quest for an inspired life*. Random House.

Newberg, A. (2018). *Neurotheology: How science can enlighten us about spirituality*. Columbia University Press.

O'Garo, K. G. N., & Koenig, H. G. (2023). Spiritually integrated cognitive processing therapy for moral injury in the setting of PTSD: Initial evidence of therapeutic efficacy. *The Journal of Nervous and Mental Disease*, *211*(9), 656–663. https://doi.org/10.1097/NMD.0000000000001686

Pearce, M. J. (2023). *Treatment manuals for spiritually integrated cognitive processing therapy for moral injury in the setting of PTSD*. Available on request from Michelle.Pearce@umaryland.edu.

Plante, T. G. (2024a). *Spiritually informed therapy: Wisdom and evidence based strategies that work*. Cognella.

Plante, T. G. (2024b). *Living better with spiritually based strategies that work: Workbook for Spiritually informed therapy*. Cognella.

Richards, P. S., Allen, G. E., & Judd, D. K. (2023a). *Handbook of spiritually integrated psychotherapies*. American Psychological Association.

Richards, P. S., Currier, J. M., Jones, R. S., Pearce, M., & Stephens, D. (2023b). Training opportunities and resources for spiritually integrated psychotherapists and researchers. In P. Richards, G. Allen & D. Judd (Eds.), *Handbook of spiritually integrated psychotherapies* (pp. 423–447). American Psychological Association.

Richards, P. S., Sanders, P. W., Lea, T., McBride, J. A., & Allen, G. E. (2015). Bringing spiritually oriented psychotherapies into the health care mainstream: A call for worldwide collaboration. *Spirituality in Clinical Practice*, *2*(3), 169–179.

Rosmarin, D. H., Kaufman, C. C., Ford, S. F., Keshava, P., Drury, M., Minns, S., … & Sacchet, M. D. (2022). The neuroscience of spirituality, religion, and mental health: A systematic review and synthesis. *Journal of Psychiatric Research*, *156*, 100–113.

Sperry, L. (2021a). Moral injury in Christian settings: Sacred moral injury. In J. Peteet, S. Moffic, A. Hankir, & H. Koenig (Eds.), *Christianity and psychiatry* (pp. 113–127). Springer Nature. https://doi.org/10.1007/978-3-030-80854-9_8

Sperry, L. (2021b). Collaborative healing of clergy sexual abuse and sacred moral injury. *Journal of Christian Healing*, *37*(2), 5–13.

Sperry, L. (2023). Psychotherapy alone is insufficient: Treating clergy sexual abuse and sacred moral injury. *Spirituality in Clinical Practice*, *10*(4), 350–357.

Vieten, C., & Lukoff, D. (2022). Spiritual and religious competencies in psychology. *American Psychologist*, *77*(1), 26–38. https://doi.org/10.1037/amp0000821

Yaden, D. B., Iwry, J., & Newberg, A. B. (2016). Neuroscience and religion: Surveying the field. In N. K. Clements (Ed.), *Religion: Mental Religion* (pp. 277–299). Macmillan.

Yaden, D. B., & Newberg, A. B. (2022). *The varieties of spiritual experience: 21st century research and perspectives*. Oxford University Press. https://doi.org/10.1093/oso/9780190665678.001.0001

Glossary

Brain, Mind, and Mind-Brain Problem Brain refers to the enlarged, anterior part of the central nervous system within the skull. Its outer layer, the cerebral cortex, contains more than 10 billion nerve cells. **Mind** refers to consciousness and cognitive activities and functions which are presumed to be brain mediated. The **mind-brain problem** refers to the problem of how to address the relation between mental phenomena and neural or physical phenomena. It remains one of the fundamental philosophical and scientific questions that psychology faces. *See* Mind; Psychological Domain; Neurotheology.

Character Character is a central construct of the moral domain. It refers to an individual's moral and ethical qualities. It consists of the beliefs and moral principles that guide their actions. While character is often used synonymously with personality the two constructs are quite distinct. Personality is the sum of an individual's physical, psychological, emotional, and relational qualities that are reflected in their behavior. *See* Moral Domain.

Clinical Outcomes and Routine Outcomes Monitoring Clinical outcomes refers to measurable change in symptoms, ability to function, overall health, quality of life. Common outcomes in psychotherapy include symptom relief and improved life functioning. These and other outcomes are more likely to occur when client progress is regularly measured and monitored with standardized self-report measures. Routine outcome monitoring (ROM) occurs when the results of the standardized measures are fed back in real time to the clinician and client so that any needed change to the treatment plan can be made. Since 2006 APA has recommended that ROM be incorporated into the treatment process. *See* Spiritually Integrated Psychotherapy; Competence and Competencies.

Competence and Competencies Competence in the practice of psychotherapy refers to the basic attitudes, knowledge, and skills necessary to provide effective treatment that all therapists should possess, rather than advanced expertise. Essential psychotherapy competencies include the therapeutic alliance, clinical assessment, case conceptualization, treatment selection and intervention, and routine outcomes monitoring. *See* Spiritual and Religious Competence and Competencies; Spiritually Integrated Case Conceptualization; Clinical Outcomes and Routine Outcomes Monitoring.

Conscience Conscience is a central construct of the moral domain. It involves judgment of reason by which individuals recognize the moral quality of their actions. *See* Moral Domain.

Conversion Conversion is a reorientation of one's life involving both turning away from a past life of sin and turning toward God, resulting in an interior transformation of the person. It may result from a single event but is often an ongoing process. *See* Moral Domain; Spiritual Domain.

Ethical Practice of Psychotherapy Confidentiality, conflict of interest, informed consent, and therapist competence are the core ethical considerations in psychotherapy practice, particularly spiritually integrated psychotherapy practice. Of these, therapist competence is the critical ethical consideration as it involves ongoing clinical decision making throughout the therapeutic process. Three questions need to be answered in the positive for psychotherapy, particularly spiritually integrated psychotherapy, to be ethically practiced: (1) Is the intervention and/or process effective?; (2) Is it safe?; and (3) Is it appropriate for that client? *See* Spiritually Integrated Psychotherapy.

Forgiveness Forgiveness is a response to being harmed that requires a willful release of feelings of resentment toward the one who has done harm. It requires the voluntary transformation from resentful feelings to an expression of compassion toward the offender. When appropriate, forgiveness can be a useful intervention in psychotherapy. *See* Spiritual Interventions.

God Representations God representations (God images) refer to the way in which individuals view or represent God. A child's God representation appears to be linked to their perception of their parents or that the child projects their father onto their image of God. Positive God representations are correlated to well-being and negative God representations tend to be correlated with psychological distress. Research suggests that an adult's God image changes as a result of successful psychotherapy, i.e., harsh, negative images before therapy shift to loving, caring images at the completion of therapy. *See* Spiritually Integrated Psychotherapy.

Mind Mind in its broad sense refers to all intellectual and psychological phenomena of an organism, encompassing motivational, affective, behavioral, perceptual, consciousness, and cognitive systems. More narrowly it refers to only cognitive activities and functions, such as perceiving, attending, thinking, problem solving, language, learning, and memory. The nature of the relationship between the mind and the body, including the brain and its mechanisms or activities, has been, and continues to be, the subject of much debate. *See* Brain.

Mindfulness Mindfulness is the form of awareness that results from paying attention, intentionally, in the present moment, without judgment. It involves breathing methods, guided imagery, and other practices to relax the mind and body and reduce stress. *See* Spiritual Interventions; Psychospiritual.

Moral Domain The moral domain refers to moral thinking, decision making, and actions involving all relationships in one's life. It includes conscience formation and the development of character and virtue, as well as moral codes and professional codes of ethical practice. It is reflected in a person's response to moral distress and moral injury. *See* Character, Conscience; Virtue; Moral Distress; Moral Injury; Spiritual Struggles.

Moral Distress Moral distress is the feeling of unease stemming from situations where organizationally required behavior does not align with moral principles. This can be as a result of a lack of power or agency or structural limitations such as insufficient resources, staffing, training, or time. The individual experiencing moral distress need not be the one who has acted or failed to act; it can also be caused by witnessing the moral transgressions of others. *See* Moral Injury.

Moral Injury Moral injury is a form of trauma following a violation of one's conscience or moral values which leads to extended feelings of guilt, shame, and the inability to trust others and organizations to uphold a moral code of conduct. It can arise when sustained moral distress leads to impaired functioning or longer-term psychological harm. *See* Moral Distress; Sacred Moral Injury.

Neurotheology Neurotheology is the interdisciplinary field that combines neuroscience and theology. It explores the relationship between the brain and religious and spiritual experiences. Recent research has focused on the therapeutic effects of meditation and the influence of psychedelic experiences on mental health. It has also begun addressing theological and philosophical questions about the nature of sin, revelation, and free will. See Spiritual Domain; Brain, Mind, and Mind-Brain Problem.

Pastoral Counseling Pastoral Counseling is a type of counseling in which insights and principles derived from theology and psychology are used to help individuals, couples, families, and groups achieve healing and growth. Pastoral counselors typically have advanced training in psychology, theology, and pastoral care. Also called pastoral psychotherapy. *See* Spiritual Direction; Spiritually Integrated Psychotherapy.

Prayer Prayer is a vital and personal relationship with the living and true God, and the raising of one's mind and heart to God. Different forms of prayer include praise, petition, thanksgiving, and intercession. *See* Spiritual Practices.

Psychological Domain Psychological domain refers to the mind, behavior, and psychological well-being. It includes cognition, emotion, perception, motivation, memory, consciousness, personality, and mental health. It interconnects with the spiritual domain with the designation psychospiritual, and the moral domain in the subspecialty of moral psychology. See Psychospiritual; Moral Domain; Spiritual Domain.

Psychospiritual Psychospiritual refers to the relationship between the psychological and the spiritual domains. While there is currently no consensus definition of it, therapeutic systems which utilize both psychological and spiritual methods such as meditation, mindfulness, yoga, and breathwork in an integrated manner have been designated as "psychospiritual." *See* Psychological Domain; Spiritual Domain; Mindfulness.

Religion and Spirituality Religion refers to a social institution that involves a set of doctrinal beliefs and practices that are shared by a community. Spirituality refers to an individual's search for or sense of connection with the sacred, supernatural, or ultimate reality. For some individuals religion is separate from spirituality while others integrate both in their lives. Religiosity refers to religiousness which is reflected in the range of religious beliefs, activities, and practices in which individuals participate. The designation "R/S" is commonly used by writers and researchers to reflect these terms.

Religious and Spiritual Problems (V-Code) DSM-5-TR provides a V-Code (Z65.8) for specifying a Religious or Spiritual Problem. It is used when the focus of clinical attention includes distressing experiences such as lost or questioned faith, psychoemotional issues surrounding conversion to a new faith, or questions involving spiritual values as well as spiritual struggles, moral distress, and moral injury. Clinicians are encouraged to use this code to provide a fuller understanding of clients beyond their symptom disorder and/or personality disorder diagnoses. *See* Spiritual Distress; Spiritual Struggles; Moral Distress.

Sacred Moral Injury Sacred moral injury is a form of trauma with lasting psychological and spiritual effects which emerges from the experience of betrayal of a sacred trust by a perpetrator of a religious organization whom the victim perceives as representing God. Typically, the religious organization supports the perpetrator by covering up the event and invalidating the victim. Because it is both an individual moral failure and an organizational failure, recovery from it requires that both failures be addressed. *See* Sacred Moral Injury.

Scope of Practice Scope of practice refers to the services a state or territory allows a licensed or certified professional to perform. Typically, this includes the presenting issues and diagnoses that psychotherapists are experienced in treating, the age range with which they work, and the modalities and interventions designated by their training and licensure. Psychotherapists can expand their scope of practice through additional training, supervision, certification, and experience. *See* Spiritually Integrated Psychotherapy.

Self Self refers to the totality of the individual, consisting of all characteristic attributes, conscious and unconscious, mental and physical. Apart from its basic reference to personal identity, being, and experience, the term's use in psychology is wide-ranging. *See* Psychological Domain; Self-Capacities.

Self-Capacities Self-capacities refer to the extent to which an individual is able to accomplish three tasks: (1) maintain a sense of personal identity and self-awareness across various experiences; (2) tolerate and control strong impulses, i.e., impulse control, strong emotions without resorting to avoidance, i.e., affect regulation, and distressing or ruminative thoughts, i.e., thought stopping; and (3) develop and maintain meaningful relationships with others that are not disturbed by dysfunctional behavior or excessive preoccupation with interpersonal danger, rejection, or abandonment. *See* Self; Spiritual Interventions.

Soul Soul is the non-physical aspect of a human being, considered responsible for the functions of mind and individual personality and often thought to live on after the death of the physical body. Because the existence of the soul has resisted empirical verification, science has generally ignored the concept, and those who adhere to materialism, positivism, or reductionism reject it absolutely. Despite this, the term survives in the general language to mean the deepest center of a person's identity and the seat of their most important moral, emotional, and aesthetic experiences. *See* Spiritual Domain; Spirit.

Spiritual and Religious Competence and Competencies Spiritual and religious competence is a form of multicultural competence involving the basic attitudes, knowledge, and skills needed to provide effective treatment that all therapists should possess. Examples of spiritual and religious competencies include: becoming aware of one's own religious, spiritual, or non-religious/non-spiritual views and how they might influence or bias one's work as a therapist; inquiring about religious and spiritual concerns in clinical settings; being able to effectively assess a client's spiritual and religious background, beliefs, and practices; and incorporating background, beliefs, and practices into the assessment, case conceptualization, and treatment intervention when indicated, or being willing to refer and collaborate with clergy if needed. *See* Competence and Competencies.

Spirit Spirit is vital force seen as animating the bodies of living creatures, sometimes identified with the soul and seen as surviving death. *See* Spiritual Domain; Soul.

Spiritual Abuse Spiritual abuse is the use of religious texts or beliefs to coerce, control, manipulate, or abuse someone, and if severe and continued may result in the trauma associated with sacred moral injury. *See* Sacred Moral Injury.

Spiritual Assessment Spiritual assessment is a tool to evaluate a client's spiritual beliefs, needs, and expectations in a clinical context. It is part of the assessment and case conceptualization process. It usually includes specific questions and/or a spiritual assessment inventory to determine whether they should be addressed in treatment and used as healing and coping resources. *See* Spiritually Integrated Case Conceptualization

Spiritual Direction Spiritual direction is a method and process for spiritual growth in which a trained director guides and models this growth process through active listening, discernment, and instruction in prayer and other spiritual practices. While there is some overlap with pastoral counseling and spiritually integrated psychotherapy, spiritual direction differs considerably in focus, training, and practice. It can be provided to individuals or groups, but mostly practiced one-to-one on a monthly basis. *See* Pastoral Counseling; Spiritually Integrated Psychotherapy.

Spiritual Distress Spiritual distress occurs when one is unable to find meaning, peace, comfort, strength, hope, or connection in life. It can occur when experiencing change, challenges, physical and emotional pain, serious illness, or losses. *See* Sacred Moral Injury.

Spiritual Domain The spiritual domain refers to the need for meaning, purpose, and fulfillment in life. It includes one's belief, spiritual practices, and the will to live. It may or may not be informed by religious beliefs or affiliation but is reflected in one's attainment of an overall sense of health, well-being, and quality of life, as well as in the experience of spiritual distress. *See* Religion and Spirituality; Spiritual Distress.

Spiritual Interventions Spiritual Interventions are interventions that directly target spiritual concerns. These include forgiveness, mindfulness, spiritual journaling, praying silently for clients, as well as the use of spiritual practices.

Recent applications for interventions from Ignatian spirituality have been described and advocated. These include the Examen and Discernment which is a four-step process that clients can use for making life decisions. These and other spiritual interventions can be a useful adjunct or alternative to common psychological interventions like behavioral activation, cognitive restructuring, controlled breathing, roleplaying, relaxation training, and thought stopping. *See* Spiritual Practices; Spiritually Integrated Psychotherapy.

Spiritual Practices Spiritual practices are interventions that can be used in conjunction with spiritual interventions or employed by individuals outside of a therapeutic context who are seeking spiritual growth. These include prayer, meditation, mindfulness, fasting, almsgiving, confession, spiritual reading, and practicing gratitude. *See* Spiritual Interventions.

Spiritual Struggles Spiritual struggles are tensions, strains, and conflicts over what an individual holds as sacred. Three types are described: supernatural struggles involving perceptions of deities or evil forces; intrapsychic struggles that reflect strains and tensions about religious/spiritual beliefs, moral issues, and ultimate meaning; and interpersonal struggles involving conflicts with others about religious/spiritual issues. *See* Spiritual Domain.

Spirituality Spirituality refers to a sensitivity to concerns of the spirit or soul in contrast to materialistic concerns. Specifically, it is a concern for God and a sensitivity to religious experience, which may include the practice of a particular religion, or may not. *See* Spiritual Domain.

Spiritually Integrated Case Conceptualization Case conceptualization is a method and clinical strategy for obtaining and organizing information about a client, understanding and explaining the client's situation and maladaptive patterns, guiding and focusing treatment, anticipating treatment challenges, and preparing for successful termination. A clinically effective case conceptualization links assessment and treatment. A spiritually integrated case conceptualization is based on an accurate spiritual assessment and is essential in practice. *See* Spiritual Assessment; Spiritually Integrated Psychotherapy.

Spiritually Integrated Cognitive Processing Therapy Spiritually integrated cognitive processing therapy is a trauma-focused therapy approach that appears to be effective in treating moral injury likely because of its focus on forgiveness and reconciliation. Currently, it is a structured approach that is provided in a group setting. *See* Moral Injury.

Spiritually Integrated Psychotherapy Spiritually integrated psychotherapy is a broad designation that refers to approaches provided by therapists that integrate the essential psychotherapy competencies as well as spiritual resources in addressing spiritual issues and struggles to resolve psychological and relational problems. Although it can also foster spiritual change and growth, spiritually integrated psychotherapy accomplishes this as a by-product of psychological change. It is distinct from pastoral counseling and spiritual direction in its treatment focus and training. *See* Pastoral Counseling; Spiritual Direction.

Virtue Virtue is a central construct of the moral domain. It refers to the habitual and firm dispositions to do good. The virtuous individual pursues the good and chooses it in their concrete actions. *See* Moral Domain; Character.

Index

Page numbers in **bold** denote tables.

Kolibri 360 GmbH
Ferdinand-Jühlke-Straße 7
99095 Erfurt, Deutschland
produktsicherheit@kolibri360.de